THE PRACTICE
of Patient
Education

THE PRACTICE
of Patient Education

Barbara Klug Redman, RN, PhD, FAAN
Dean and Professor
Wayne State University College of Nursing
Detroit, Michigan

Ninth Edition

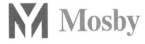 Mosby

A Harcourt Health Sciences Company

St. Louis   London   Philadelphia   Sydney   Toronto

7/02   Amazon / 38.00 / Nursing

ᴍ Mosby

A Harcourt Health Sciences Company

Vice President, Nursing Editorial Director: Sally Schrefer
Senior Editor: Susan R. Epstein
Developmental Editor: Maria Broeker
Project Manager: Deborah Vogel
Production Editor: Kelley Barbarick
Design Manager: Bill Drone

NINTH EDITION

Mosby, Inc.
A Harcourt Health Sciences Company
11830 Westline Industrial Drive
St. Louis, Missouri 63146

Printed in the United States of America

Library of Congress Cataloging in Publication Data

Redman, Barbara Klug.
   The practice of patient education / Barbara Klug Redman. — 9th ed.
         p.   cm.
   Includes bibliographical references and index.
   ISBN 0-323-01279-5
   1. Patient education.   2. Nurse and patient.   I. Title.

   RT90. R43   2000
   615.5′071—dc21   00-046297

00   01   02   03   04   GW/FF   9   8   7   6   5   4   3   2   1

To
Darlien Klug and to the memory of Harlan Klug
In grateful appreciation
for years of sustenance of various kinds

Preface

This book is written for all health care providers who want to know more about how to teach patients and families. Because the book began as a nursing text and because nursing has such a rich philosophic and conceptual heritage in patient education, much of the background is still drawn from that field. Students should be ready to use the book when they recognize in their patients the need for learning, when they have enough knowledge to be able to teach the subject matter, and when they are competent in their interactions with patients.

This book was inspired by students who were interested in and excited about teaching patients. It has been nourished over the years by extensive contact with providers who develop and manage programs of patient education.

This book is organized into two basic sections—the first describing the process of learning and teaching and the second reflecting the development of the major fields of patient education practice in place today.

Throughout, it reflects numerous new developments in the field. Examples given are not meant to be exhaustive; they are only illustrative of the teaching-learning process. It will be advantageous if the student already has a basic understanding of the psychology of learning because this complex subject must be abbreviated in a book of this size. Patient education is a dynamic field, absolutely essential to the innovations currently unfolding in the health system. Some of these innovations are described as are many of the fields of practice.

Barbara Klug Redman

Contents

Appendixes

THE PRACTICE
of Patient
Education

Part I

The Practice of Patient Education

The Practice of Patient Education: Overview

Patient education is a central part of the practice of all health professionals. While the modern movement of patient education into health care is now 35 years old, the field has evolved slowly because it faced a history of paternalism in not sharing information with patients. Standards of expected practice in this field are still developing. Movement of the health care system from procedure-based reimbursement to managed care and capitated methods of payment has improved incentives for incorporation of patient education into care. In this new system individuals are expected to do more self-care; however, teaching resources to assure that they and their families are competent and confident to do so have not been assured. Provider shortages and use of more assistive personnel rather than licensed professionals have stymied the move toward competent self-care.

Because learning is at the center of humans' ability to adapt, all social institutions, including health care, make provision for teaching and learning. Much learning (a persistent change in human performance or performance potential) is incidental to experience. Instruction is the deliberate arrangement of conditions to promote attainment of some intentional goal.

This chapter provides an introductory overview of patient education practice, which will be expanded and developed in subsequent chapters. Patient education practice is based on a set of theories, on research findings, and on skills that must be learned and practiced. In addition to general theories of learning and instruction, each area of practice (e.g., diabetes, cardiac care, or parenting) has evolved with a tradition and a set of goals particular to that area.

Patient education services are delivered during direct caregiving by health care practitioners and also in separate programs such as a diabetes self-management program. The legal base of patient education has been developed through case law and regulations governing professional practice and accreditation of health care institutions and most especially through the doctrine of informed consent. Its ethical base is still being defined. Ethical practice requires the competent practice of patient education by professionals, avoidance of the harms that this intervention can induce (such as debilitating confusion or loss of self-confidence), and serious examination of the reasons one is asking the patient or family members to change beliefs and practices, frequently at great cost to themselves. It must be devoid of gender, ethnic, and age bias and effective for persons of widely varied levels of formal education.

Perhaps the field to which patient education is

most closely related conceptually is health education. Table 1-1 describes my views of the differences between these two fields, although movement of patient care to the community is blurring what used to be sharper distinctions.

THE PROCESS OF PATIENT EDUCATION

Patient education is practiced using a process of diagnosis and intervention. The needs-assessment phase determines the nature of a need and motivation to learn, and goals are mutually set with the patient. The intervention is constructed to provide instructional stimulation for the exact learning needs that patients have. Evaluation occurs throughout instruction, summarized at periodic intervals to determine whether the outcome goals are being met. Reteaching is frequently necessary because it is not possible to accurately predict which instructional intervention will yield the desired learning by a

particular patient. In most instances, follow-up reinforcement and reteaching are needed over time, particularly for patients who are managing chronic health problems or learning how to prevent them.

The process of teaching can be summarized as follows.

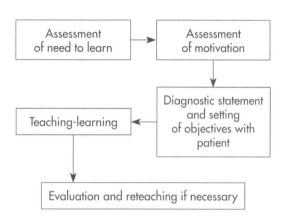

TABLE 1-1	Comparison of Patient Education and Health Education	
Focus	**Patient Education**	**Health Education**
Philosophy	Patient use of information and skills for whatever purpose is desired	Behavior change for health promotion and compliance with medical regimen
Unit of service	Individuals, families, and other groups	Specific populations
Delivery system	Part of clinical care by all direct-care providers in any setting	Campaigns that include mass media and work through community institutions
Content	Patient experiences, coping, helping patient develop self-management skills, decisional support	Risk factors, health behaviors
Theory base	Direction from field's theory of practice, learning, and instructional theory	Behavioral science, epidemiology
Ethical concerns	Scientific stability and cultural bias of what patients are asked to learn; subtle manipulation possible in provider-patient relationship; inadvertent side effects (e.g., loss of self-confidence)	Scientific stability and cultural bias of what patients are asked to learn; manipulation by government, under which many programs are carried out; inadvertent side effects such as "blaming the victim"
Literature	Integration of literature of disease entity or health problem	Public health literature and certain specialized health education journals
Challenges	Reliable delivery system, including outcome measurement	Accessing very powerful provider-patient relationship

Little is known about how this process is actually used by practitioners, but what seems clearest is that it does not flow in an orderly, sequential fashion, as shown in the preceding diagram. One starts at the beginning of the process but subsequently skips from step to step; however, the elements do serve as checkpoints to ensure that the relevant variables that affect the teaching–learning activity have been considered. Although teaching does not have a complete set of commonly used diagnostic categories, the objectives can serve such a purpose. In addition, as nursing diagnostic categories have been refined and expanded, they have become useful but incomplete in categorizing patient learning needs.

The teaching process can be seen as parallel to the nursing process in that each has an assessment, diagnosis, goals, intervention, and evaluation phase (Table 1-2). Because learning about health is pertinent to nursing practice, some general screening questions should be part of the general nursing assessment; for example, what do patients know and how do they perceive their present problems? If at any time during care the ongoing assessment indicates a patient learning problem that teaching can alleviate, a more refined assessment of need and readiness is made and that problem is dealt with through the teaching process.

Of course, the most cogent question concerns the quality of use of either the nursing process or the teaching process and whether (at least in the psychosocial realm) fine points used in the process make any difference in patient outcome. I believe that there are gross errors in the practice of patient education that make a difference. Errors in practice are probably made in this order: (1) omission of assessment of the patient's need to learn, so that no activity in patient education is initiated; and (2) omission of any given step, for example, omitting the assessment of readiness, the setting of goals, or the systematic evaluation, but not omitting the actual intervention. Of course, it is impossible not to have at least implicit goals when one teaches, but the goals may not be related to a particular patient's readiness and the instruction may not be constructed to meet those goals.

With adequate practice, providers can become proficient in thinking through the required steps of the teaching process. They can become sensitive to expressions of readiness that may be part of an ordinary conversation with the patient and can learn to organize care to elicit measurements of readiness. The teaching that many

TABLE 1-2	**Relationship of Teaching Process to Nursing Process**				
Assessment	**Diagnosis**	**Goals**	**Intervention**	**Evaluation**
Nursing Process				
General screening questions to detect patient's need to learn	One of problem statements may be a need to learn or a nursing diagnosis	Learning goals are a subset of goals	Teaching intervention may be delivered with other intervention	Evaluating whether nursing care outcome was met
Teaching Process				
Refined assessment of need and readiness to learn	Learning diagnosis	Setting of learning goals	Teaching	Evaluating learning

patients require can be accomplished in the same amount of time that the nursing process takes if it is done at the proper level of proficiency.

SUMMARY

Patient education is an expanding and evolving field, now seen as central to achieving adequate outcomes of care. It is integrated throughout care to individuals and groups in all settings. A diagnostic-intervention-evaluation process model is used to practice patient education.

 Study Questions/Activities

1. During a few days of clinical practice, keep a log of instances of paternalism on the part of staff members toward patients. Did these instances occur because the patients involved could not understand the decisions about their care, or did they occur for other reasons? Are these reasons justifiable?
2. T. Berry Brazelton[1] has written: "Demonstrating the behavior of a newborn baby to an inexperienced mother can be both exciting and revealing. The mother's comments as the baby performs are likely to be meaningful in terms of her past experience and present expectations. As her baby goes from sleep to crying in an all-too-short period, the examiner might describe the speed of the state change without labeling it with a value judgment. The mother may then feel it safe to say: 'I just get frantic when he cries and I don't know how to stop him.' The pediatrician or nurse practitioner can then join her, recognizing her anguish and offering to participate with her by saying, 'Well, I don't know how either yet but we can work on it together.' A tacit but powerful alliance between the two is struck, with the baby's behavior a common ground for open communication."

Label the parts of the teaching-learning process, as discussed in this chapter: assessment of need and readiness to learn, diagnoses and goal setting, intervention, and evaluation.

References

1. Brazelton TB: Demonstrating infants' behavior, *Children Today* 10(4):5, 1981.

Chapter 2

Motivation and Learning

MOTIVATION

Motivation is a term that describes forces acting on or within an organism that initiate, direct, and maintain behavior. Motivation also explains differences in the intensity and direction of behavior. In the teaching-learning situation, motivation addresses the willingness of the learner to embrace learning. The term *readiness* describes evidence of motivation at a particular time. This chapter discusses theories of motivation in general, with specific application to health. It also describes assessment of motivation as part of the teaching-learning process and presents teaching practices that stimulate and develop motivation.

Six general theories of motivation can be used to direct learning in a variety of situations.[39]

Reinforcers. In behavioral learning theory the concept of motivation is tied closely to reinforcement of repeated behaviors. For example, behaviors that have been reinforced in the past are more likely to be repeated than are behaviors that have not been reinforced or that have been punished. Reinforcement histories and schedules of reinforcement help explain why some individuals learn better than others.

Needs. Satisfaction of needs for food, shelter, love, and maintenance of positive self-esteem explains the concept of motivation for other theorists. Persons differ in the degree of importance they attach to each of these needs.

Cognitive dissonance. Cognitive dissonance theory holds that individuals experience tension or discomfort when a deeply held value or belief is challenged by a psychologically inconsistent belief or behavior. To resolve the discomfort, patients may change a behavior or a belief, or they may develop justifications or excuses that resolve the inconsistency.

Attribution. To make sense of the world, individuals will often try to identify causes to explain why something has happened to them. Persons are particularly motivated to conduct attributional searches in ambiguous, extraordinary, unpredictable, or uncontrollable situations. Attributions may occur after a diagnosis, an exacerbation of chronic illness, an accidental injury, or the relief or cure of a symptom or illness. We know that attributions can have powerful effects on psychological adjustment, behavior, and morbidity. In a study of patients with myocardial infarctions, attributions of patients and their spouses (Why did this happen to me?) significantly predicted whether the family considered itself rehabilitated. Individuals make attributions about disease severity and treatment efficacy. They use these ideas to regulate self-management of their diseases.[22] Thus it is always important to know patients' beliefs about the cause of their present situation because their actions are guided by these attributions.

A concept central to attribution theory is *locus*

of control. Those with an internal locus of control in a situation attribute success or failure to their own efforts or abilities. Those with an external locus of control believe that success or failure depends on luck, task difficulty, or other persons' actions.

Personality. Motivation in personality theory describes a general tendency to strive toward certain types of goals such as affiliation or achievement. An extreme motivation to avoid failure is learned helplessness, which causes persons to believe that they are doomed to failure no matter what. This behavior can arise from an inconsistent and unpredictable use of rewards and punishments by teachers. The problem can be avoided or alleviated by giving learners opportunities to realize success in small steps and by giving them immediate, positive feedback with consistent expectations and follow-through.

Coping styles may also be part of personality. Some individuals are vigilant and seek information from all available sources. If these persons find discrepancies in the information they receive, they feel anxious. Others use a coping style of avoidance. They want little information because it constitutes a source of stress. Monitors typically scan the environment for threat-relevant information and rehearse and amplify the threats cognitively, whereas blunters cope with aversive health events by distraction. Patients fare better psychologically, behaviorally, and physiologically when the information they receive is tailored to their coping style. Monitors do better when given more information that can be used constructively and more emotional support. Those with blunting styles do better with less information (Miller).[26]

Expectancy. Expectancy theories of motivation hold that a person's motivation to realize a goal depends on the perceived chance of success, as well as on how much value that person places on success. The theory of reasoned action posits that volitional behavior is predicted by the person's intention to perform the behavior. Intention is, in turn, a function of beliefs about the consequences of the behavior and norms about the behavior that are held by significant others.[29]

Summaries of research have shown a powerful relationship between perceived self-efficacy and adequate performance. How individuals judge their capabilities to produce and regulate events in their lives affects their motivation, their thought patterns, their behavior, and their emotions. Those who believe that they will not be able to cope well dwell on their personal deficiencies and imagine that potential difficulties will be more formidable than they really are. Self-efficacy increases notably when persons' experiences contradict their fears and when they gain new skills in managing threatening activities. Repeated failures lower self-efficacy, especially if failure occurs early in the course of events and does not reflect lack of effort or adverse external circumstances.[2]

Judgments about self-efficacy are based on the following sources of information: performance attainments (the most influential), vicarious experiences of observing performance of others, verbal persuasion and other social influences, and physiological states. Self-efficacy probes during a course of treatment can provide helpful guides for implementing a program of personal change. Adopting attainable subgoals that lead to more impressive future goals can provide the patient with clear markers of progress to verify a growing sense of self-efficacy.[2]

Finally, humanistic interpretations of motivation emphasize personal freedom, choice, self-determination, and a striving for personal growth. Although generally not expressed as a theory in the scientific sense, important assumptions made by humanists cause us to reflect on learners' resolutions to become motivated and to make their own decisions about whether to pursue a course of action.

Two theoretical models used to assess and stimulate motivation in patients follow. Seeking care and adapting to illness are examples of tasks that require motivation on the part of patients and may well be the focus of educational programs.

Health Belief Model

The health belief model[36] affirms that individuals are not likely to take a health action unless

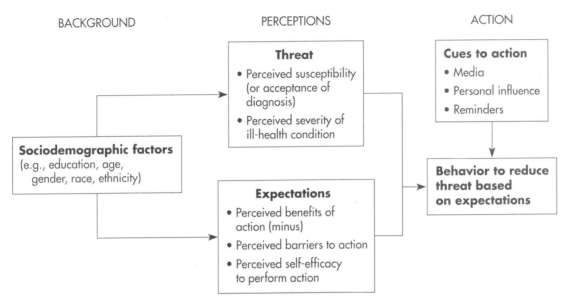

BACKGROUND   PERCEPTIONS   ACTION

Figure 2-1 Schematic diagram of components of health belief model. (From Rosenstock IM, Strecher VJ, Becker MH: The health belief model and HIV risk behavior change. In Di Clemente RJ, Peterson JL, editors: *Preventing AIDS: theories and methods of behavioral interventions*, New York, 1994, Plenum Press.)

(1) they believe that they are susceptible to the ill-health condition in question; (2) they believe that the condition would seriously affect their lives if they should contract it; (3) they believe that the benefits of action outweigh the barriers to action; and (4) they are confident that they can perform the action (self-efficacy). Cues, such as an interpersonal crisis or the nature and severity of symptoms, trigger action. This model, which is depicted in Figure 2-1, is an example of the value-expectancy approach, developed to explain an individual's health actions under conditions of uncertainty.

In patient education practice, the health belief model has been used to assess whether an individual holds these beliefs, and if not, to direct teaching at missing skills or information. Kloeblen and Batish[20] provide an example of the applicability of the health belief model to understand the intention among low-income pregnant women to permanently follow a high-folate diet for protection against neural tube defects. Items used to measure each construct in the model may be seen in Box 2-1. Among the group of women studied, perceived benefits were most predictive of folate intention.[20]

A summary of 16 studies found that use of the health belief model did not accurately predict an individual's actions in seeking screening, taking risk-reduction action, or adhering to a medical regimen. Difficulty with measurement of the constructs in the model and the lack of clarity about how they interact affected this outcome.[14]

Transtheoretical Model

A second model relevant to motivation is the transtheoretical model of change. It holds that intentional change requires movement through discrete motivational stages over time, the active use of different processes of change at different stages, and modifications of cognitions, affect, and behaviors. Although it has been most thoroughly studied with addictive behaviors such as smoking, it is also useful for prediction of, and intervention in, behaviors more open to the effects of patient education, such as exercise, diet change, and mammography screening. Progression through the stages is not usually linear; for

Box 2-1   Application of Health Belief Model for High Folate Diet

Perceived susceptibility statements

1. If I do not eat a diet high in folic acid prior to my pregnancy and very early in my pregnancy, I could have a baby with a neural tube defect (NTD), which is a type of birth defect.
2. I could get pregnant and my unborn baby could be sick without my even knowing it.
3. I could get pregnant sometime (besides now) and not know it right away.
4. I could have a baby with a birth defect someday.
5. I get colds and illnesses all of the time.

Perceived severity statements

1. Having a NTD, which is a type of birth defect, is a very serious condition.
2. Having a NTD would leave a child disabled for life.
3. Complications in an infant with a NTD are severe and could even result in death.
4. Having a baby with a birth defect would be very expensive.
5. Having a baby with a birth defect would negatively affect my social life, my family life and my ability to work.

Perceived benefits statements

1. Eating more foods high in folic acid all of the time, even when I am not pregnant, could prevent or reduce my risk of having a baby with a NTD (a type of birth defect).
2. My family and friends would be proud of me if I improved my diet to contain more foods high in folic acid.
3. Improving my diet to include more foods high in folic acid could make me feel better and be a healthier person overall.
4. Changing my diet to include more foods high in folic acid all the time in case I get pregnant would make me feel good about myself.
5. Eating a diet high in folic acid all the time could save me money and time by helping to keep me from having a baby with a NTD that would be expensive and would require a lot of time to care for.
6. Eating a diet high in folic acid all the time could help keep me healthy and help keep my baby healthy if I were to get pregnant again.

Perceived barriers statements

1. I think that eating a diet high in folic acid would be expensive.
2. I don't know enough about what foods are high in folic acid. I don't like most foods that are high in folic acid.
3. I think it would take too much time to change my diet to include more foods high in folic acid all of the time.
4. I think it would be too hard to change my diet to include more foods high in folic acid all of the time.
5. My friends and family would not like the changes in my diet if I tried to eat foods high in folic acid all of the time.

Self-efficacy statements

1. I am confident that I could eat a diet high in folic acid all of the time if I tried.
2. I feel that I would be able to follow a diet high in folic acid if I wanted to.

Cues to action statements

1. If a health professional reminded me to eat a diet high in folic acid when I came in for a doctor's visit, that would help me remember to eat more foods high in folic acid all of the time.
2. Seeing something on television about folic acid would help remind me to follow a diet high in folic acid all of the time.
3. If a friend or someone I know told me about folic acid, that would help me to be sure I get plenty of folic acid in my diet all of the time.
4. Reading pamphlets or seeing posters about folic acid would help me remember to eat more foods high in folic acid all of the time.
5. Have you ever talked about folic acid with someone else like a nutritionist, doctor, nurse, friend or family member? (in % yes)
6. Do you know someone who had a baby with a NTD or who has lost a baby with a NTD? (in % yes)
7. Have you ever had a baby with a NTD? (in % yes)

From Kloeblen AS, Batish SS: Understanding the intention to permanently follow a high folate diet among a sample of low-income pregnant women according to the Health Belief Model, *Health Educ Res* 14:327-338, 1999.

most health-behavior problems the majority of individuals relapse and return to earlier stages of the model before eventually succeeding in maintaining change.

The stages of change are as follows[33]:

1. *Precontemplation.* Individuals are not considering change within the next 6 months. They may be resistant, have lack of knowledge, or be overwhelmed by the problem.
2. *Contemplation.* Individuals are seriously thinking about changing within the next 6 months, but because of ambivalence, they may remain in this stage for years.
3. *Preparation.* Individuals are seriously planning to change within the next month and have already taken some steps toward action.
4. *Action.* This stage, which involves overt modification of the problem behavior, can last from 3 to 6 months.
5. *Maintenance.* This period begins after 6 months of continuous successful behavior change. Individuals can remain in maintenance from 3 to 5 years and yet still experience temptations to relapse.

In early stages the decisional balance is stronger for the cons—that is, against taking the action—than for the pros—that is, for taking it. Before action occurs, the balance must swing so that the pros outweigh the cons. For example, in the adoption of exercise behavior, the pros might include helping to relieve tension, liking the body better, having a more positive outlook on life, sleeping more soundly, and having more energy. The cons might include feeling too exhausted to exercise, exercise taking too much time, and feeling uncomfortable from getting out of breath.[24] Predictably, perceived self-efficacy (confidence that I can succeed in taking this action) is lowest during the early stages and rises as one progresses.

Typically, about 40% of populations at risk are in the precontemplation stage, another 40% are in the contemplation stage and stuck there for long periods of time by ambivalence, and only 10% to 20% are in the preparation stage. These ratios hold across a number of behaviors: smoking, alcohol and substance abuse, anxiety and panic disorders, eating disorders and obesity, high-fat diets, AIDS prevention, mammography screening, unplanned pregnancy prevention, and sedentary lifestyle. Relapse occurs from action or maintenance to an earlier stage, although usually not as far back as precontemplation.[37] It is essential that the instructional strategy be matched to the stage; many educational programs are implicitly designed for individuals who are ready to take action. Boxes 2-2 and 2-3 provide examples of questions asked to determine what stage an individual is in and intervention approaches appropriate for the various stages.

Seeking Care

Available evidence indicates that seeking health care is influenced by many factors and by the interplay among them. A single factor, such as ignorance, is often not solely responsible for delay or promptness in seeking health care. Denial may play a part. Economic need for care is bound up with health beliefs and with values about the priority of health, among other motivations. The individual's, the family's, and the culture's answers to the following questions help to determine whether care will be sought: What is the meaning attached to a symptom located at a particular body site? How are hospitals, health care personnel, surgery, and the body itself viewed? Does the family support the health action psychologically and financially? How do individuals view their responsibility for their own health? How important is the individual? What kinds of care facilities are acceptable for use? All these factors influence the way that persons select, perceive, and interpret information and services available to them.

Certainly the development of anxiety helps to determine action in seeking health care. Mild anxiety is useful because it causes the individual to act. However, greater degrees of anxiety interfere with adaptive action. Fear of negative reactions from high-status medical personnel may prevent some individuals from going to the

Box 2-2	*Staging Questions for Dietary Fat Reduction*

Note, the item in brackets was asked of Sample B but not of Sample A. This item was not included in the staging algorithms for either sample.

1. Have you ever changed your eating habits to decrease the amount of fat in your diet?
    Yes 1
    No 2 (Skip to #2)

1A. IF YES, Are you currently limiting the amount of fat in your diet?
    Yes 1
    No 2 (Skip to #2)

1B1. IF YES, How long have you been limiting the amount of fat in your diet?
    Less than 30 days 1
    1-6 months 2
    7-12 months 3
    Over 1 year 4

[1B2. IF YES, Would you say you are now eating a low-fat diet?]
    Yes 1
    No 2

2. In the past month, have you thought about changes you could make to decrease the amount of fat in your diet?
    Yes 1
    No 2

2A. How confident are you that you will make some of these changes during the next month?
    Very confident 1
    Somewhat confident 2
    Mildly confident 3
    Not at all confident 4

Staging algorithm

Stage	Question(s)	Answer(s)
Precontemplation	1 or 1A	No
	2	No
Contemplation	1 or 1A	No
	2	Yes
	2A	Mildly or not at all confident
Decision	1 or 1A	No
	2	Yes
	2A	Somewhat or very confident
Action	1 and 1A	Yes
	1B1	6 months or less
Maintenance	1 and 1A	Yes
	1B1	7 months or more

From Curry SJ, Kristal AR, Bowen DJ: An application of the stage model of behavior change to dietary fat reduction, *Health Educ Res* 7(1):97-105, 1992.

Box 2-3	*Stages of Change*				
	PRECONTEMPLATION (UNAWARE)	CONTEMPLATION (NOT QUITE READY YET)	PREPARATION (INTENTION SOON)	ACTION (MODIFYING TARGET BEHAVIOR)	MAINTENANCE (STABILIZING NEW BEHAVIOR)
Assess	Cognitive insights Attitudes Beliefs	Coping skills Risk status	Instrumental skills Social support	Self-management skills	Positive momentum Role of relapse
Advise	Messages that raise pros and lower cons	Personalize risk messages	Multiple cognitive and behavioral strategies	Criterion for altered behavior	Upward spiral may regress temporarily
Agree	Think seriously about target behavior	Build commitment Optimism	Small steps toward action	Alter target behavior	Anticipate relapse situations
Assist	Tailor information to educational needs Provide consistent message that health is important	Insight Clarification Cognitive restructuring	Therapeutic alliance Self-monitoring Goal setting	Stimulus control Positive reinforcement Life change counseling	Positive reinforcement Substitute behaviors
Arrange	Create awareness of need for change Provide patient education material Note in medical record that patient not ready (labeling) Reassess readiness to change at next appropriate opportunity	Environmental context Evaluation Risk assessment	Self-help materials Define role of medication Cue sheets	Follow-up Social support Skills training Group programs Linkage with community resources	Relapse prevention training

From Elford RW and others: A practical approach to lifestyle change counselling in primary care, *Patient Educ Couns* 24(2):175-183, 1994.

provider with an "insignificant" symptom. Often, persons have no clear understanding of their disorder and will wait for symptoms that they consider worthy of medical attention and treatment and that they are no longer willing to tolerate.

Especially for those with chronic illness, uncertainty is constant and results from unpredictable and inconsistent symptom onset or recurrence and inability to distinguish symptoms of the chronic illness from other bodily changes. Unresolved uncertainty is significantly associated with poorer mood states. Some patients are able to make it through periods of disorganization from an illness to a new reality of living with it.[27]

Providers have assumed that the physical symptoms of those patients seeking care accurately reflect the extent of tissue abnormality. However, recent evidence indicates that the symptoms of organic disease vary widely among patients with the same tissue abnormality. For example, myocardial ischemia may not generate a report of chest pain for the following reasons: (1) the patient is hyposensitive to visceral sensation; (2) the patient is coping with the threat of heart disease by denying pain; or (3) the patient misunderstands the cause and significance of a vague or ambiguous cardiac sensation. Also, many patients with symptoms have no demonstrable electrocardiographic findings, and numerous patients with arrhythmias do not report symptoms. Between 10% and 30% of patients with angina-like pain that is severe enough to warrant coronary angiography are without significant coronary stenosis. Similarly, the existence of a peptic ulcer is only weakly related to symptoms, arthritic pain cannot be predicted from x-ray studies of the spine, dyspnea reported by asthmatic patients corresponds poorly to objective measures of airway obstruction, and symptoms of diabetes correlate better with depression levels than with glycosylated hemoglobin levels. Do these patterns occur because patients acknowledge and selectively attend to only those symptoms that alert them to an aberration in health and body? Or is something additional occurring?[6]

One conceptual model of how individuals decide to seek health care, shown in Figure 2-2,

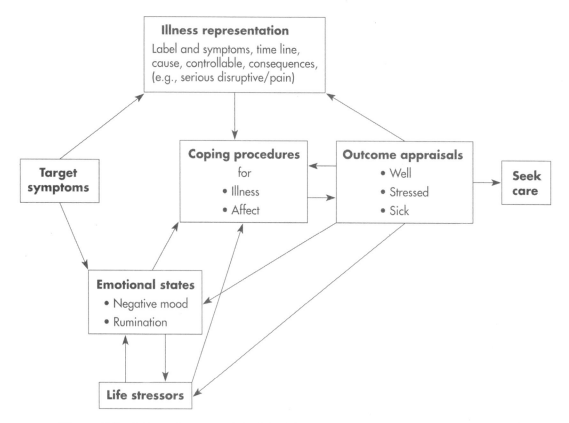

Figure 2-2 Self-regulatory model of health and illness behavior. (From Cameron L, Leventhal EA, Leventhal H: Symptom representations and affect as determinants of care seeking in a community-dwelling, adult sample population, *Health Psychol* 12:171-179, 1993.)

builds on the self-regulatory theory of health and illness behavior.[7] According to this model, symptoms are key factors in the cognitive representation of health threats. These somatic changes are compared with memories of prior episodes of symptoms, thus generating a notion of identity, duration, consequences, causes, and expectations of controllability. Failure to cope either with the symptom episode or with the distress induced by the episode can motivate health care use. A person's interpretation of a symptom and

the ways in which the individual is coping with it can, of course, be elicited in a patient assessment. This model acknowledges that other factors, such as inability to perform social roles, may also affect care seeking.

Adapting to Illness

The experience of illness carries with it certain adaptive tasks that occur in stages and that very much focus motivation. Table 2-1 describes one such model specific to adapting to living with

---

TABLE 2-1 Fredette Model for Improving Cancer Patient Education: Summary

Period	Adaptation Stage	Content	Strategies
1	Existential plight: impact distress, disbelief, shock	Talk about the cancer as it relates to: harms, threats, resources. Discuss disease: personal aspects, family, social concerns.	Be present whenever diagnosis and therapy are discussed by physician. Move out of denial/avoidance. Use one-on-one approach, pamphlets, discussion—short frequent sessions; provide what is asked for.
2	Existential plight proper, developing awareness	Correct misinformation. Expand knowledge base. Re-explain concepts formerly blocked. Explain treatment plan. Teach self-care. Teach about coping strategies, especially information seeking.	Continue one-on-one. Be accepting of anger and crying. Watch for a "teachable moment." Have short frequent sessions. Toward end of period, use simple audiovisuals always followed by discussion.
3	Mitigation, reorganization, restitution	Strengthen coping. Introduce new ideas and options about disease, treatment side effects, treatments for side effects. Reteach facts presented in earlier period. Teach anxiety reduction methods. Model expression of feelings. Use "I Can Cope" program.	Use pamphlets, videotapes, films, self-learning packages, longer sessions, group education. Continue to reserve time for questions/discussion. Include family.

From Fredette SL: A model for improving cancer patient education, *Cancer Nurs* 13(4):207-215, 1990.   *Continued*

TABLE 2-1		Fredette Model for Improving Cancer Patient Education: Summary—cont'd	

Period	Adaptation Stage	Content	Strategies
4	Accommodation, resolution and identity change	Discuss new identity, further therapy, treatment of side effects, second opinions, work, sexuality, interpersonal issues, fear of recurrences, coping with a chronic illness, living as a cancer survivor. Teach stress reduction. Use "Living With Cancer" program.	Use group teaching, support groups, all other methods. Encourage all free expression.
5	Decline and deterioration, stages of dying	Answer questions asked. Interpret what is happening in the illness. Explain/discuss options. Validate patient's right of choice. Stress hope for comfort rather than cure.	Use one-on-one. Take cues from patient for when and what to teach.
6	Preterminality and terminality, stages of dying	The dying process. The grieving process. Spiritual-existential concerns. Physical symptom management. Psychological symptom management. Interpersonal/communication problems. Need for open, honest communication.	Use one-on-one. Include family. Use short verbal explanations. Use periods of acceptance and physical comfort. Take cues from patient. Have patience with "middle knowledge phenomenon."

From Fredette SL: A model for improving cancer patient education, *Cancer Nurs* 13(4):207-215, 1990.

cancer, with suggestions for content and teaching strategies appropriate to the stage the patient is experiencing. Assessments and interventions are designed to assist the patient and family to move forward through the grieving and adaptation process, including decision-making and self-management.[11]

General Principles of Motivation

Basic principles of motivation exist that are applicable to learning in any situation.

The environment can be used to focus the patient's attention on what needs to be learned. It should provide an atmosphere in which learning is reinforced and the patient is encouraged to practice what is learned, with feedback for correction.

Internal motivation is longer lasting and more self-directive than is external motivation, which must be repeatedly reinforced by praise or concrete rewards. Individuals who want to learn are internally motivated, as are those who become absorbed in the task and achieve a sense of accomplishment from it. Some individuals have little capacity for internal motivation and must be guided and reinforced constantly.

Learning is most effective when individuals are ready to learn, that is, when they want to do something. Sometimes a patient's readiness to learn comes with time, and the caregiver's role is to encourage its development. If the need for behavior change is urgent, a teacher will need to stimulate motivation.

Motivation is enhanced by the way in which the instructional material is organized. In general, the best-organized material makes the information meaningful to the individual. One method of organization includes relating new tasks to those already known.

None of these techniques will produce sustained motivation unless the goals are realistic for the learner. The basic learning principle involved is this: success is more predictably motivating than is failure. Ordinarily, individuals will choose activities of intermediate uncertainty rather than those that are difficult (little likelihood of success) or easy (high probability of success). For goals of high value there is less tendency to choose more difficult conditions. Having learners assist in defining goals increases the probability that they will understand them and want to reach them.

Because learning requires change in beliefs and behavior, it normally produces a mild level of anxiety, which is useful in motivating the individual; however, severe anxiety is incapacitating. During an emergency, teaching-learning is at a minimum because other goals are more important and because anxiety is high. Individuals with less severe health crises may also react with intense anxiety because they feel threatened by what has occurred. If anxiety is severe, the individuals' perception of what is going on around them is limited. They are oriented more toward gaining relief than toward attending to learning, and they show physical signs and symptoms of anxiety. For this reason, mothers who are highly distressed because of their children's illness may be unable to learn the skills to care for them.

It is important to help each learner set goals and to provide informative feedback regarding progress toward those goals. Setting a goal demonstrates an intention to achieve and activates learning from one day to the next. It also directs the learner's activities toward the goal and offers an opportunity to experience success.

Both affiliation and approval are strong motivators. Individuals seek out others with whom to compare their abilities, opinions, and emotions; they also may seek acknowledgment that they are doing well.

Many behaviors result from a combination of motives.

Acquiring a new behavior is a process, not an event, and often entails learning by performing successive approximations of the behavior, with completion of each step developing readiness for the next step. This increasingly prevalent view of learning and motivation in health suggests that we think of interventions as a series, highly specific to each step to be mastered.[17]

These general principles of motivation are interrelated. A single teaching action can use many principles simultaneously. For example, having a display of teaching pamphlets available in the patient lounge of a maternity clinic can focus the patients' attention on things to be learned, taking advantage of their natural curiosity about subjects such as breastfeeding or postpartum exercises. The content of teaching pamphlets is aimed at helping patients set and attain realistic goals and often is organized to relate new material to that which most women know. Such a display can encourage patients to ask questions as well as convey the staff's interest in their learning.

Finally, it should be noted that an enormous gap exists between knowing that health behavior is motivated and identifying the specific motivational components of any particular act. Providers must focus on learning patterns of motivation for an individual or group, with the realization that errors will be common.

Assessment of Motivation

It is important to begin with a needs assessment, which can be used to establish what a patient needs to learn. For example, while conducting an admission assessment, a provider might ask these questions: What do you know about your

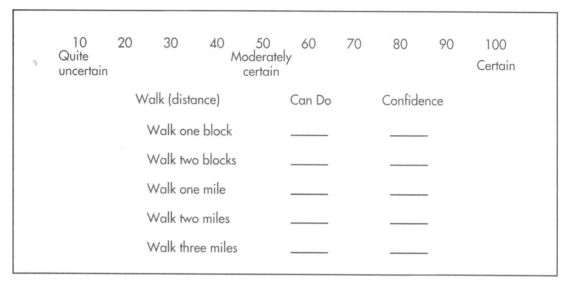

Figure 2-3   Self-efficacy scale. (From Houston-Miller N: Questions and answers, *J Card Rehabil* 4:104-106, 1984.)

disease and treatment? How do you cope with symptoms? How do you manage stressful situations? How do you prefer to learn new information? What concerns you the most right now?[42]

Assessments should also be conducted to tailor an educational program to the particular needs of the specific group of people who will receive it. For example, a "community needs" assessment structured by the health belief model was used to assess women who needed mammograms. The women in this particular community believed they were susceptible to breast cancer and were cognizant of the benefits of mammography. Fear of pain, radiation, and embarrassment proved to be significant barriers for some of the women. Also, women older than 65 rarely had physicians who recommended mammography; therefore the intervention included educating physicians and using senior citizen groups to encourage older women to be more assertive in asking for referrals. Because the assessment also found a need to reach Spanish-speaking Hispanics, a bilingual mammography facility guide was developed.[28] The intervention was validated by

an increase in the number of women obtaining mammograms.

Following are two examples of specialized measuring tools that may be used to assess patients' needs for education and their ability to learn. The self-efficacy scale (Figure 2-3) measures cardiac patients' perceived ability to perform various physical tasks. The value of the method results from the close relationship that exists between self-efficacy and the probability that a given activity will be attempted. These scores can also be used to evaluate interventions, such as exercise testing when it is followed by an explanation of test results by staff members. This scale measures perceived self-efficacy for walking. Results probably would not hold true for dissimilar tasks.[16] Also, a brief test to assess the baseline knowledge of pregnant women with overt diabetes is shown in Box 2-4; it could also be used to evaluate the outcomes of instruction.[40] This test should be used with other assessment devices. Although knowledge is necessary, it alone is not sufficient to achieve most positive health outcomes.

Box 2-4	*Diabetes in Pregnancy Knowledge Screen*

Below are questions about diabetes during pregnancy. Answering these questions will help us determine your current knowledge about diabetes during pregnancy and enable us to provide the best care possible during your pregnancy. Many questions have more than one answer; therefore circle "I don't know" rather than guessing. By answering to the best of your knowledge, we will be able to counsel you most effectively about diabetes during your pregnancy.

1. Which of the following feelings may result from a reaction? (Circle all that might happen, not just those that have happened to you)
   a. Difficulty thinking
   b. Blurred vision
   c. Nervousness or shaky
   d. Numbness
   e. Sweating
   f. I don't know
2. What should you do if you have a reaction? (Circle all that apply)
   a. Walk it off
   b. Sit down and rest
   c. Eat crackers or cheese
   d. Drink milk
   e. I don't know
3. Glycosylated hemoglobin levels are drawn about once per month during pregnancy. Why are these levels taken?
   a. They measure previous blood sugar control
   b. They measure the amount of iron in your blood
   c. They measure how helpful your diet is in controlling your blood sugar
   d. I don't know
4. When planning vigorous exercise (e.g., swimming, playing tennis), what changes should you make in your daily diabetes routine? (Circle all that apply)
   a. Decrease insulin
   b. Carefully time when to do your exercising
   c. Increase the amount of carbohydrates (e.g., bread, fruits) you eat
   d. Increase the amount of protein (e.g., meat, cheese) you eat
   e. I don't know
5. On days when you are sick, what steps should you take to control your diabetes?
   a. Increase the amount of water or other fluids
   b. Stop your insulin
   c. Call your doctor
   d. I don't know
6. The normal range for blood sugar during pregnancy is:
   a. 40-150 mg/dl
   b. 60-120 mg/dl
   c. 100-200 mg/dl
   d. I don't know
7. A specific meal plan has been devised for you by the dietitian. Which of the following statements about your meal plan are correct? (Circle all that apply)
   a. You should eat everything on your meal plan
   b. You can reduce the amount of food you eat if you're not hungry
   c. You should control the amount of food you eat all the time
   d. You can eat your meals any time during the day as long as you eat everything on your plan
   e. I don't know

Continued

Box 2-4	*Diabetes in Pregnancy Knowledge Screen—cont'd*

8. Bedtime snacks are an important part of your meal plan because they help you avoid having reactions overnight. (Circle one)
   True or false
9. Margarine is mainly:
   a. Protein
   b. Carbohydrate
   c. Fat
   d. Mineral and vitamin
   e. I don't know
10. Rice is mainly:
   a. Protein
   b. Carbohydrate
   c. Fat
   d. Mineral and vitamin
   e. I don't know
11. If you don't feel like having the egg on your diet for breakfast, you can: (Circle two)
   a. Have extra toast
   b. Substitute one small chop
   c. Have an ounce of cheese instead
   d. Skip the egg, and don't eat anything else
   e. I don't know
12. If you have problems controlling your blood sugar during pregnancy, what are some of the possible effects on your baby after birth? (Circle all that apply)
   a. Could be born with low blood sugar (hypoglycemia)
   b. Could be a large baby making delivery more difficult
   c. Could have breathing problems after birth
   d. I don't know
13. What does glucagon do?
   a. Helps liver release more sugar into blood
   b. Makes liver stop releasing sugar into blood
   c. Helps pancreas release more insulin
   d. Stops pancreas from releasing insulin
   e. I don't know
14. After using glucagon, it's most important to:
   a. Drink plenty of fluids
   b. Get plenty of rest
   c. Eat a meal so your blood sugar doesn't drop
   d. None of the above
   e. I don't know

From Spirito A and others: Screening measure to assess knowledge of diabetes in pregnancy, *Diabetes Care* 13:712-718, 1990.

Finally, tools for motivation assessment and readiness to learn exist within the context of the patient-provider relationship. Rapport within this relationship is necessary to obtain evidence about motivation, and data from tools must be synthesized with data from interactions with the patient. In addition, teachers frequently stimulate motivation by questioning, caring, and helping the patient reach a learning goal, as well as by encouraging the sense of commitment a patient develops toward a caregiver.

Teachers must consciously activate motivation before activating learning and help the patient maintain motivation during learning. The construction of goals is important, especially ones that are specific, moderately difficult, and attained quickly. Such goals enhance motivation and encourage persistence because they provide clear standards for judging performance. Teachers also must provide clear feedback on the quality of the learners' performances, help them feel pride and satisfaction in their achievements, and assist as the learners try to maintain manageable levels of anxiety.

LEARNING

Instructional practices are also based on the psychology of learning and on material that has produced results for practitioners in the past. Although bright and motivated individuals can learn a great deal without a teacher, their efforts to learn can be quite inefficient. Individuals who need to learn health information and skills, even if they are motivated, often do not have sufficient orientation to health matters to attain the goal alone. Learning is defined as change in an individual caused by experience and does not include changes caused by development.[39]

Theories of Learning

Learning involves changing to a new state—it is a state that persists. What can be learned? New thinking strategies, new motor skills, and new attitudes are learned in complex patterns that can promote a new performance. General conditions exist (such as reinforcement and transfer) that are applicable to all kinds of learning and learners. Particular conditions that facilitate particular kinds of learning are also present.

Twentieth century learning theories may be classified into two broad categories: behavioral and cognitive, with Bandura's social cognitive theory containing many key elements of both.[3] Recently, theories/philosophies of constructivism suggest that learners are helped to construct their own meaning in real environments—frequently in teams working together to solve problems. Conscious learning and conceptualization emerge from this activity instead of preceding it, transmitted by teacher to learner in artificial environments.[19]

Behavioral Learning Theory

The most important principle of behavioral learning theory is that behavior changes according to its immediate consequences. Pleasurable consequences strengthen behavior (reinforce it), whereas unpleasant consequences weaken it. Reinforcers may be food, water, warmth, praise, recognition, grades, or paychecks, varying from one individual to another. Extinction is a process used to decrease a previously reinforced behavior by ceasing reinforcement. Also, punishment delivered immediately in response to a particular behavior may decrease that behavior; however, the results of punishment are unpredictable. The Premack principle theorizes that a particular behavior performed by a person frequently can be used to reinforce a low-frequency behavior. Shaping involves applying reinforcements in accordance with gradually changing criteria. As the performer begins to roughly approximate the target behavior, closer approximations of the final response are needed before reinforcement can be delivered.[39]

In teaching, one must be sure that effective reinforcement is applied to a well-defined behavior so that learners will understand what they did to warrant the reward. As new behaviors are learned, reinforcement is frequent; however, after behaviors are established, reinforcement is given at random to encourage persistence of the behavior.

Staffs in nursing homes use these principles to teach shaving and dressing behavior to residents.

Cognitive Learning Theory

In cognitive theory, learning is the development of insights or understandings that provide a potential guide for behavior. New insights lead to a reorganization of the individual's cognitive structure, which is stored internally in visual images and in propositional networks and schemata. Within this framework, learning makes change in behavior possible, although not necessary. Motivation to take action results from a need to make sense of the world and solve problems.

Teachers using this theory determine the schemata of the learner and organize content so that it can be assimilated easily into the existing schema. Some learning can be described as an accumulation of new information in memory; however, the basic goal is to direct a longitudinal development of increasingly sophisticated mental models. Each level of learning addresses a larger set of problems. Novices can relate only superficially to the problem area or to the subject matter and must use pre-existing schemata to interpret these isolated pieces of data. Experts, on the other hand, quickly identify the problem and know how to approach it, consolidate information in meaningful ways, and monitor and accurately predict the outcome of their performance.[12] In contrast to general learning skills, expertise is increasingly viewed as specific to a particular domain of knowledge or thought.

Social Cognitive Theory

Social cognitive theory as developed by Bandura[3] is largely a cognitive theory but incorporates principles of behaviorism. According to this theory, humans respond primarily to cognitive representations of the environment rather than to the environment itself.

Individuals acquire information, values, attitudes, moral judgments, standards of behavior, and new behaviors through observing others. Infants who are several months old model behavior with competency and continue to do so throughout their lives. Individuals can learn and

formulate rules of behavior by observing persons, films or videotapes of models, symbolic models (written accounts of a performance), or sets of instructions (compressed accounts of a performance). This coded information serves as a guide for future action. The learner also gets information about the probable consequences of modeled action. Individuals visualize themselves executing the correct sequence of actions; therefore cognitive rehearsals and actual performances increase the proficiency of individuals, give them a sense of efficacy, and reduce the tendency to forget learned behaviors.

In social cognitive theory, behavior is regulated by expectations for similar outcomes on future occasions. Individuals will persist for some time in actions that go unrewarded on the expectation that their efforts will eventually produce rewarding results. Extrinsic incentives are especially necessary in early stages of developing competencies (such as playing the piano) until competency becomes self-rewarding. The natural social environment is often inconsistent, contradictory, and inattentive. To ensure that the individual's newly acquired skills generalize and endure under these less than favorable circumstances, transitional practices must gradually approximate those of the natural social environment.

Much behavior is motivated and regulated by internal standards and self-evaluative reactions to the individual's own actions, including self-incentives and self-concepts of efficacy. To function competently requires skills and perceived self-efficacy. Perceived self-efficacy is a belief in one's ability to realize a certain level of performance. It must be distinguished from outcome efficacy, which judges the likely consequence certain such behaviors will produce. Judgments of self-efficacy are based on four principal sources of information: (1) performance attainments, the strongest of the sources, which involve acting out the desired behavior, with repeated failures lowering self-efficacy; (2) vicarious experiences through observing the performances of others, especially if the model is similar to the learner in ability, age, sex, and experiences; (3) verbal persuasion; and (4) perceived physiological states from which individuals partly judge their capability, strength, and vulnerability. Self-efficacy also lessens unsettling emotions such as stress and depression.[4] For example, cardiac rehabilitation programs are structured to provide information from these four sources, and the patient's perceived self-efficacy to perform various tasks is closely related to whether he or she will attempt those activities.

Types of Learning

Transfer of Learning

Transfer of learning, the effect of prior learning on subsequent learning, is one of the most important products of education, inasmuch as no learner can practice for all situations that will arise. It is more efficient for an individual to learn general information, skills, and ways of thinking and apply them to a variety of situations than to learn specifically for each situation. Teaching for transfer is based on evidence that individuals forget nonsense material and isolated facts. However, individuals remember general ideas, attitudes, ways of thinking, and skills that are meaningful to them and that they have thoroughly learned and applied.

For the transfer of learning to occur, individuals must also recognize that the new situation is similar to previously learned situations and they must remember which specific thoughts or behaviors are appropriate. In behavioral learning theory, transfer has an increased probability for responses occurring in the future because of past performance or because of the appearance of identical stimuli. In cognitive learning theory, transfer is not automatic; when it occurs, it is in the form of generalizations, concepts, or insights that have been developed in one situation and are being used in other situations.

Many studies provide evidence that generally positive transfer increases when overall training and application conditions coincide. Practice in a variety of contexts enhances transfer (less like the original learning). Indeed, extensive, varied practice based on imitating a model and driven by reinforcers can lead to the automatic triggering of a well-learned behavior in a new context. Use of examples aids transfer, especially if one extracts the rule from the present example and uses it in new situations.[37] Instruction must be planned to ensure that transfer will occur.

Memory

Forgetting learned material is one of the banes of our existence. Not using learned material, interference of other learning, loss during reorganization of ideas, and motivated forgetting (which may be subconscious) constitute explanations for not remembering learned materials. Nevertheless, ideas are remembered for a long time, whereas facts are not.

The cognitive process involves the following: (1) selective perception of stimuli from the environment; (2) storage in short-term memory persisting for as long as 20 seconds; (3) encoding (leaves short-term memory and enters long-term memory); (4) storage in a meaningful mode as concepts, propositions, schema, and imagery in long-term memory; (5) retrieval; (6) response generation; (7) performance (patterns of activity that can be observed); and (8) feedback. Instruction can aid each of these steps by providing, for example, differentiation of features facilitating selective perception, verbal instruction or pictures that suggest encoding schemes, or cues that aid retrieval. Retrieval time is slow except for the short-term memory, which holds only six to nine items. Forgetting is characteristically a progressive loss of precise information about an event rather than the total loss of a stored item and usually occurs because of the ineffectiveness of search and retrieval processes.

Information is stored in long-term memory in networks of connected facts or concepts called schemata. Information that fits into an existing schema is more easily understood, learned, and retained than is information that does not.[39]

Ways to increase memory retention include fostering intent to learn and to remember, overlearning, finding meaning in material to be learned, applying newly learned material to practical situations (practicing), rehearsing remembering, chunking information (related ideas together) to decrease memory load, using organizing strategies and visual imagery, and learning over a period of time. Use of projects or plays gives learners vivid images they can remember.

Ley[23] completed a series of studies on patient memory of clinical advice, which is summarized in an excellent article. Neither age nor intelligence showed any consistent relationship with recall. Diagnostic statements were best recalled and those concerned with instructions and advice most poorly recalled. These findings seemed to result from perceived "importance" effects. Four methods were found to increase recall: use of shorter words and sentences, explicit categorization, repetition, and use of concrete-specific rather than general-abstract statements (general: "You must lose weight"; specific: "You must lose 7 pounds"). Using these tactics plus giving instructions and advice and stressing their importance resulted in significant differences in the amount of information recalled by patients.

Professionals have been shocked and dismayed at patient recall of informed consent conversations that generally include explanation of diagnosis, the nature of the illness, proposed surgery, risk of death or complications, benefits, and alternate methods of management, with the chances for failure or success. Patients frequently remember fewer than half the items covered, as verified against recordings of the initial conversation. Certainly use of the approaches just outlined would improve retention.

Problem Solving

Problem solving is frequently a desired goal in learning situations. Problem tasks are more complex if they have one or more of the following characteristics: (1) incompletely defined alternatives, (2) existence of a number of subproblems, (3) several ways to reach the goal, (4) need for a large number of information sources to solve the problem, or (5) a rapidly changing problem situation.[8] Problem solving can be broken into a series of steps: (1) identification of the problem, (2) determination of possible actions and their probable results, (3) selection of one action, (4) implementation of the chosen action, and (5) evaluation of problem-solving effectiveness. Frequently, breaking the problem into parts is helpful. Learners may need help at any of the stages of problem solving. Assessing this need can be accomplished by problem solving out loud or teaching a novice learner how to solve the problem.

The following is an example of a nurse helping a patient solve his problem: An elderly man who lives alone has had heart damage and is about to be discharged from the hospital with permanent limitation of activity. He will have a problem caring for himself as he did before his illness. Although he recognizes the situation as a problem, he needs help in defining its breadth—the extent to which this restriction will affect his daily pattern.

The nurse is a source of information to clarify the meaning of activity restriction. She also knows the amount of energy the patient will expend in different activities and can help him consider how he can economize in the use of his resources. The patient, with the help of the nurse, concludes that he can meet the restrictions and remain living alone by having his groceries delivered and by allowing a daughter to do his cleaning, washing, and ironing. It is agreed that these new living arrangements will be judged by the amount of energy he must expend, by how tired or how contented he is, and by his and the provider's opinion about his state of health.

The patient then goes home and tries out the hypothesized solutions, evaluating them as determined. At this stage he again needs the nurse's help, best given in his home, in assessing his subjective feelings of tiredness and the total amount of energy he expends. By visiting the home, the nurse is able to think of new possible solutions to try. Of course, the situation in this example may be altered slightly or considerably by such factors as the patient's ability to understand the situation, his emotional readiness to deal with it, a decrease in income, the daughter's moving away, or a change in his health status.

This example is not meant to imply that each patient has only a single problem—such difficulties are often interrelated.

Attitude Learning

Attitudes pervade all spheres of learning. They may be defined as learned, emotionally toned predispositions to react in particular ways toward an object, an idea, or a person. Values, which are similar but more permanent, are expressions of how individuals believe an object or relationship affects them. Over the years feelings are developed, become well established, and are reflected in behavior. Often we do not realize that we are acquiring attitudes. Membership in groups, particularly primary ones, seems to influence acquisition of attitudes.

Suggestions for teaching attitudes follow directly from knowledge about how they are learned and include employing someone to teach whose attitudes the learner can view and imitate. This model might not be a health care professional but possibly another patient with whom the learner can identify, which is the reason for establishing colostomy and ileostomy clubs and other such groups. Another way of influencing attitudes is to provide satisfying experiences, so that the person develops a positive response to ideas or feelings associated with the experiences. For example, personnel in a health care clinic should try to provide experiences of the sort that help patients have positive feelings about the clinic.

Psychomotor Learning

Anyone recalling the awkwardness of a puppy or a child, or the unsteadiness of an old man, and comparing it with the sure coordination of a skilled artist can observe a variation in motor skills. These skills can vary with strength, reaction time, speed, balance, precision, and flexibility of tissues. Motor skills are usually composed of an ordered sequence of movement that must be learned. Separate parts of a motor act can be learned and practiced separately as part-skills.

To execute a particular skill, a person must possess a neuromuscular system that is capable of performing the skill and must have an ability to form a mental image of the act. A mental image is created when the learner watches a demonstration that shows the skill and points out relevant cues for a successful performance. Relevant cues often involve muscular cues of balance and pull; cues may also be seen or heard. When learning to walk with crutches, a person must see the floor or objects that might get in the way, hear persons approach from behind, and feel whether he or she is balanced. The cues must be obvious to the beginner and often are not noticed much in advance of the action. The person experienced in using the motor skill can use many cues rather than just the obvious ones. He or she is not confused by irrelevant cues, attending to them with less conscious concentration. Also, the person experienced in certain motor skills reacts faster and can take advantage of cues far in advance of action. The goal is a smooth, coordinated sequence of action with a minimum expenditure of energy.

The learner practices to develop a proficient performance. The mental image is a guide. At first, however, the teacher may need to guide the person's body so that he or she experiences the physical sensations that accompany correct motions. For example, one might guide a child's hands as she learns to drink from a cup. It is best for the learner to practice in a situation that provides cues similar to those in the environment where the skill will be used. For example, the person with a colostomy is taught in a setting that simulates a bathroom at home. During the crucial early stages of practice, information about the patient's progress, or lack of it, is important. Learners often need help in judging their own performances, even though they can judge someone else's. Eventually, learners receive messages from their own physical sensations and can decide if their objectives have been accomplished.

It is generally recommended that practice periods be short and infrequent enough to avoid fatigue. If intervals between practices are too long, the learner may forget. Once a motor skill

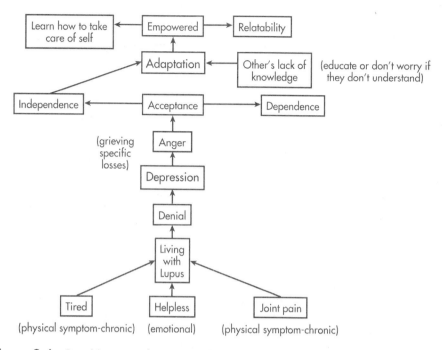

Figure 2-4   Cognitive map of a 33-year-old woman living with lupus. Note: Statements in parentheses are additional explanations by the participant. (From Wiginton KL: Illness representations: mapping the experience of lupus, *Health Educ Behav* 26:443-453, 1999.)

has been learned, it can be quickly recaptured even after an interval of many years.

Cognitive Learning

Cognitive learning theory holds that behavior is structured by the way people think about their experiences. Research on the structure of lay theories of health consistently finds five dimensions around which the experience of illness is organized: identity, cause, consequences, time line, and controllability. An individual's representation of a particular illness is made up of his or her answers to these questions. In Western society, having a causal theory about one's illness is related to better adjustment.[38] These schemas are important to know. For example, representations of medication show that patients interpret side effects as a sign that the drug is working and absence of them as distressing. Adherence issues may be explained by beliefs that if medicine is taken continuously it becomes less

effective and carries the risk of dependence or addiction and that it is important to give the body a rest. Research shows that medication representations correlate with adherence.[15]

Concept mapping provides an opportunity to understand an individual patient's cognitive representations in an area in which learning is important to tailoring the content of instruction. This technique involves identifying key concepts in a subject matter and their linkages, thus describing the individual mental model. The mental model or cognitive map of a woman living with lupus may be found in Figure 2-4.[43]

Developmental Phases

Adult Learning

The dominant current theory of adult learning builds on the cognitive tradition, and the kind of learning most characteristic of the adult phase is transformative learning. The challenges of adulthood involve a process of traveling through an uncertain number of changes that transform the individual. A disorienting dilemma or an integrative circumstance usually provides motivation to reflect about one's perspectives and assumptions and to conclude that previous approaches are no longer adequate. Although adult learners do not return to old perspectives once transformation occurs, passages involve difficult negotiation and compromise, stalling, and backsliding. Self-deception and failure are common. The crucial difference between this transformation lag and primary (child) socialization is that adults are capable of being critically reflective while children are not. Assistance with perspective change involves helping adults to see their problems and providing access to alternate-meaning perspectives to help individuals interpret the unreality. Adult learners then can examine their assumptions critically by using stories and pictures that pose hypothetical dilemmas, with conflicting rules and assumptions in the areas of critical concern. Little is known about why some dilemmas lead to perspective transformation and others do not.[41]

Indeed, support groups often involve adults who come together in response to the same life dilemma. These groups foster critical reflection. They help the participants gain and apply insights to their own lives. One can study the outcomes of this kind of education by interviewing group participants and by comparing movement in problem awareness, expectations, and goals.[25] Health-threatening situations frequently cause individuals to feel disoriented and precipitate self-reflection.

Adaptation to the usual auditory and memory changes that frequently accompany aging must be built into instruction. Learning through alternate modalities (e.g., use of audio tapes if one does not see well) is important. Decline in memory can be compensated for by providing short instructional sessions focused on a few skills. Frequent practice until the material is overlearned and use of memory aids such as pill boxes that organize doses of medication are helpful.

Learning in Children

Ability to learn depends on maturation, and a great deal of maturation occurs in childhood. Readiness to learn in childhood changes considerably, beginning with visual, auditory, and motion stimulation of infants. The primary dimension of children's development is the degree of differentiation they make between the self and others. Children move toward a clearer distinction between the internal and the external self. The general principles and comments about learning outlined in previous sections of this chapter are applicable to children within their readiness level.

Intellectual development moves from concrete to abstract. During the preschool years, children can use language to represent objects or experiences and can solve problems by direct manipulation of physical objects. Young children are egocentric and interested in only what affects them. They want explanations for everything but are not concerned with supplying reasons for their questions. If children have a background of direct nonverbal experience during the elementary school years, they can verbally manipulate relationships between ideas without having the objects present. As they grow toward adolescence and then adulthood, they gradually come to understand and manipulate relationships between abstractions without any reference to the concrete. Eventually, they can formulate and test hypotheses based on the possible combinations of several ideas.

Children must develop motor skills and feelings, as well as grow intellectually. Developing trust in the first 2 years is crucial. At that point children become more autonomous—learning to walk, run, jump, and feed themselves. Between the ages of 3½ and 7, children develop imagination and learn to take initiative. During the early school years they become industrious, turning their attention to the outside world. As adolescents they develop their identities.

Knowledge of growth and development suggests that teachers should determine realistic objectives and explain them in a way that children can understand. Allowing children to handle equipment, such as a breathing mask, seems to encourage acceptance of treatment. This is especially true during the years when direct nonverbal experience is important. Because children younger than 5 years experience egocentricity and fear of injury, they need to know how procedures will affect them. For example, it can be explained to children that during a chest x-ray examination they will just have to stand still, hold their breath for a few seconds, and not worry because they will not feel anything.

Research has consistently reported limited periods of behavioral upset followed by rapid recovery after discharge from the hospital. (Children between 6 months and 4 years are the most vulnerable.) Young children, in particular, consider illness to be self-caused and punitive. It has been suggested that if a child is younger than 4 years, explanation of anatomy and physiology is not useful because the child does not have the necessary understanding and is prone to develop undesirable fantasies. There is confusion between cause and effect and lack of differentiation between illnesses. Separation anxiety in this age group is a primary problem. Therefore, teaching should stress that the same provider needs to care for the child, and the parents should be encouraged to help.

For children older than 7 years, more sophisticated language and drawings can be used. Children of school age also benefit from tours of hospital playrooms and wards and from discussion in which they can learn about their illness, its origins, and proposed plans of treatment. Because school-age children have a maturer concept of causality than younger children possess, they have the capacity to understand that neither illness nor treatment is imposed on them because of their own misdeeds. These children are able to cooperate with treatment because they can think before they act. Inasmuch as they can express their feelings in words and have a greater grasp of time sequences, they can better tolerate a separation from their parents.

Children's health attitudes and behaviors show a critical period of change around the time they enter the third grade. Third graders are able to decide whether to report illness or injury. They have developed cognitive abilities, and they have learned the social rules that govern illness and when to seek care. By the sixth grade these abilities are refined.

Adolescents must master the ability to think in abstractions and to imagine the possibilities that are inherent in a variety of situations. Many adolescents need help in thinking through behavioral alternatives. They may need guidance through steps of problem solving and planning. Role playing in peer groups can help illustrate appropriate norms of behavior. It can also translate abstract information into stories that are easier to remember.

Chronically ill children become increasingly able to understand their illnesses as they develop intellectually. Cognitive development brings with it the ability to grasp the meaning of a poor prognosis or of functional limitations.

Adolescents frequently display particular thought patterns involving an imaginary audience or a personal fable, consistent with a stage of intense preoccupation with themselves. They believe that if everyone is watching them and thinking about them, thanks to the imaginary audience, they must be something special, unique, or different. Teenagers with chronic illness may stop taking medications because they believe they are special and different and can manage without the medications. Believing that they are immune to the natural laws that other persons must obey can also cause them not to use contraceptives. Unprotected intercourse may not be viewed as a risk by the adolescent.[10] Pestrak and Martin[31] believe that many adolescents are functioning at a cognitive level that renders them unable to practice most forms of birth control effectively. The authors conclude that the effective practice of birth control requires that individuals accept their sexuality and acknowledge that they are sexually active, anticipate the present, and view potential future sexual encounters realistically.

Pridham, Adelson, and Hansen[32] have developed a useful tool (Table 2-2) describing how features of development are pertinent in helping children deal with procedures.

Application of Learning Theories

All of the theories described in the early part of this chapter are frequently used in health situations. Although they do show overlap, often more than one theory is needed. In this section clinical examples of learning theory application are provided.

Behavioral learning theory suggests use of a patient-provider contingency contract. Desired behaviors, rewards, punishments, and time frames are discussed, written, and signed by the patient. An example of such a contract may be seen in Figure 2-5. Research shows that the patient-provider contingency contracts yield at least short-term, positive effects across a variety of medication conditions and health-related behaviors. However, long-term results show considerable recidivism.[18]

Parents have been taught to use behavior modification with their children and can learn how to modify any class of overt child behaviors. Behavioral management skills that parents frequently need to learn include (1) obtaining the child's attention before issuing a request, (2) issuing one request at a time, (3) waiting after each request for 8 to 15 seconds without talking, (4) helping the child, (5) assuming a threatening or cajoling expression until the requested action is completed, (6) issuing discipline when the child is noncompliant after the first repetition of the request, (7) praising the child's compliance, and (8) requiring time-out when appropriate.[35]

Cognitive learning theory suggests a focus on attributions (a form of cognitive interpretation about why something happened) and schemata. A persuasive theory suggests that individuals tend to attribute the cause of serious illness to their emotional state, their health behaviors, confidence in their ability to control the outcome of the problem, or the ability to contend with uncertainty regarding their condition. This may explain why attributions predict morbidity in some serious illnesses.[1]

Some examples may be helpful. Bar-On and Cristal[5] report a study of male patients younger than 60 years who had experienced their first myocardial infarction. Their attributions about the cause and outcome of the infarction formed five clusters: (1) some of the patients attributed the myocardial infarction to fate, luck, or the pressures of life; (2) some denied the problem and said that the infarction was a matter of chance and that they would continue to do what they had been doing; (3) some wanted to control the future by building their bodies and following their physicians' advice; (4) some believed that their anger had caused the attack and that with the help of physician and family, they would be able to cope; and (5) some believed that their bodies were vulnerable because of inherited tendencies, smoking, or bad habits; however, they believed that medication would help. Those with the fourth pattern of attribution were more likely to recover and return to work.

Likewise, a study of parents who cared for their adult children with schizophrenia discovered four patterns of attribution for the cause of the illness and for appropriate caretaking: (1) schizophrenia was caused by chemical imbalance, and care should be oriented to monitoring and limiting the ill family member's intake of chemicals; (2) the adult children could be persuaded to respond to reason; (3) symptoms were largely out of the individual's control but could be reduced if he or she avoided certain environments that exacerbated symptoms; and (4) because the symptoms were the patient's way of coping with the confusion, the appropriate model of care was gentle support.[9]

Finally, Gray[13] studied parents' explanatory models of autism, a condition in which both etiology and prognosis are poorly understood, effectiveness of treatment is limited, and the disabling nature of the disorder presents serious difficulties for parenting. There is no confirming biological test, and families reported that diagnosis frequently took up to a year. This uncertainty

Text continued on p. 34

TABLE 2-2   Features of Development that are Pertinent to Helping Children Deal with Procedures

	Birth-2 Years	2-7 Years	7-12 Years	Adolescence
How the child thinks and problem solves	Sensory-motor experience develops schema (well-defined and repeated sequences of actions and perceptions). Memory is obvious by 3-4 months and is demonstrated in second year by child's imitations of parents' activities. Between about 18 and 24 months, use of symbols for thought-reasoning communication appears.	Preoperational stage (thinking is dominated by the child's perceptions rather than logic). Verbally communicated information is increasingly important in learning; exploratory manipulation of objects also helps the child to learn. Child watches, listens, asks questions (why? how?). Child can (a) label (classify) familiar things; perception is often limited to a single, salient feature, making it difficult for child to see things in a context or differentiate unessential from essential properties of an experience; (b) use memory to reconstruct past events; (c) use imagination to deal with events, people, objects; (d) about age 4, begin to infer outcomes; (e) define objects/events in terms of their use/function. Thinking relies on the	Concrete operational phase. Child learns from observing/interacting with peers as well as from own experiences. Can use symbols to organize thoughts and represent experience. Features of thinking include increasing capacity to (a) understand viewpoints of others; (b) see the relative nature of things (e.g., that this hurts a little; that hurts a lot); (c) use deductive logic in respect to tangible (concrete) experiences (if this, then that); (d) classify things in terms of several characteristics, implying that the child can view things in context, for example, "The shot hurt, but it will make me feel better"; (e) evaluate painful intrusive actions in terms of logical function rather than in terms of	Stage of formal operations. At this point, there is use of reason and logical thinking and interest in theoretically possible problems and questions. The adolescent can engage in self-reflection and think about own thinking and can learn from verbally presented ideas and arguments.

		child's own point of view (egocentricity), since children do not have the capacity to identify a point of view other than their own. As the child gets older, he or she begins to be able to think in terms of quantities (e.g., to recognize variation in quantity; to use numbers to count). Attention is increasingly selective as the child's schema or perceptual sets become more refined.	punishment; and (f) understand unseen body mechanics/functions. Child can make use of sensory as well as procedural information.	
Major fears and worries	After about 6 months: separation from parents; unfamiliar people/experiences/places, especially when not accompanied by parent.	Separation from parents; harm to body, including fears of castration after about age 3; punishment for wrongdoing	Body injury; disability (loss of body functions); loss of control; loss of status.	Uncertainty about selves as persons (especially early and middle adolescence); concern about whether or not body, thoughts, and feelings are "normal."
Understanding cause and effect	By about 3 months, may associate an action with a result. In second year: magical thinking: belief that what is wished for happens.	Beliefs: (a) everything happens by intention; (b) imminent justice—misbehavior is followed by punishment; (c) belief that events that in fact are associated only by happenstance are connected.	Child 6-8: conclusions are based on perceptions. Child 9-12: applies logical operations (deductive thinking) to concrete (immediately experienced) circumstances. Prior to about 9 years, children are likely to view their illness as a consequence of transgressions of rules. (Rules	Can use formal rules of logic and evidence to assess cause and effect.

From Pridham KF, Adelson F, Hansen MF: Helping children deal with procedures in a clinic setting: a developmental approach. *J Pediatr Nurs* 2:13-22, 1987.

Continued

TABLE 2-2   Features of Development that are Pertinent to Helping Children Deal with Procedures—cont'd

	Birth-2 Years	2-7 Years	7-12 Years	Adolescence
			exist in their own right and misdeeds have their own inherent punishment.) Prior to 9 years, children are likely to believe that illness is caused by germs whose presence is sufficient for illness. At about 9 years, children begin to understand that (a) an illness may have multiple causes; (b) the body's response to an agent or a combination of agents may vary; and (c) host factors interact with agent(s) to cause illness.	Can synthesize the past, present, and future in thinking.
Concept of time	By about 3 months, shows anticipation for feedings. Can wait as a consequence of perceiving clues of a familiar and desired activity.	Organized around familiar/routine activities of daily living. By about age 4, has concept of time and day and knows days of week.	Has a concept of the past and future as well as of the present. Can understand time intervals between events and can tell time by a clock. Sense of time is thus more independent of perceptual data, e.g., activities of daily living.	

Intentions, goals, and plans	By about 4 months, may show signs of intention/a sense of making an effort to get a result. In second year, child can make a choice of two options.	About age 4, begins to plan and anticipate actions in the near future; has objectives for activities.	Plans more elaborate projects that involve others to a greater extent.	By mid adolescence (about age 15), makes future plans for self. Can think in terms of tasks as well as responsibilities in relation to them.
Handling emotion	By about 7 months, the child cries for attention, help, or when distressed. By about 9 months, begins to express fears (e.g., separation) in play.	Expresses emotion motorically and through play. Learns to label feelings. Needs trusted adult to reassure, set limits, prevent loss of self-control.	Has a greater capacity to express emotion in verbal terms; can describe fears. Can use projective methods to describe fears (e.g., explain how another child might feel or respond in a specific situation).	May use a range of modalities, from relatively sophisticated verbal or written expression to motoric activity and, perhaps, regressed ways of behaving. Thoughts, feelings, and fears may be shared with friends, especially peers.
Relationship with parent/clinicians	Developing a sense of self/others. In latter half of first year, beginning to sustain the memory of parent in parent's absence, at least for a short time. Depends on adult to know child's wants/needs.	Child is likely to have had experience in relating needs and worries to day-care or church school teachers or clinicians. Children may not expect clinicians to perceive/understand how they feel about things until about the age of 10 years.	May test limits set by caretaker/clinician.	By mid adolescence, has begun to learn how to negotiate a relationship with a clinician.
Self-evaluation	Feelings about self are derived from feeling tones communicated by others and perceived by the child.	Develops expectations of self; learns to inhibit own actions. Begins to use other children as models.	Evaluates self in terms of performance relative to that of peers and in relation to the set of norms that children believe to be predetermined for them.	May use a set of criteria consciously adopted to evaluate self.

From Pridham KF, Adelson F, Hansen MF: Helping children deal with procedures in a clinic setting: a developmental approach. *J Pediatr Nurs* 2:13-22, 1987.

Date _____

Heath-care contract

Contract goal: (Specific outcome to be attained)

I, (client's name), agree to (detailed description of required behaviors, time and frequency limitations)

in return for (positive reinforcements contingent upon completion of required behaviors; timing and mode of delivery of reinforcements)

I, (provider's name), agree to (detailed description of required behaviors, time and frequency limitations)

(Optional) I, (significant other's name), agree to (detailed description of required behaviors, time and frequency limitations)

(Optional) Aversive consequences: (Negative reinforcements for failure to meet minimum behavioral requirements)

(Optional) Bonuses: (Additional positive reinforcements for exceeding minimum contract requirements)

We will review the terms of this agreement and will make any desired modifications, on (date). We hereby agree to abide by the terms of the contract described above.

Signed: (Client) _____
Signed: (Significant other, if relevant)

_____

Signed: (Provider) _____
Contract effective from (Date) _____
to (Date) _____

Figure 2-5   Patient-provider contingency contract. (From Janz NK, Becker MH, Hartman PE: Contingency contracting to enhance patient compliance: a review, *Patient Educ Couns* 5:164-178, 1984.)

means that lay conceptions of the situation are essential to coping because they make sense of the illness, its cause, and course. The most common explanation offered by parents was trauma related to a difficult birth.

SUMMARY

Motivation and learning theory provide the base that is needed to plan and be successful in teaching. Learners are motivated by helping them set their own goals, expressing clear feedback about what they did right, providing effective praise and removing barriers to action. Individual differences in self-directedness, failure tolerance, attributional style, past experience with the task, and expectation of success influence choices to engage and persist in learning. Learning theory, research about kinds of learning, and develop-

mental phases describe conditions understood to be necessary in changing to a new state of understanding or behavior that persists.

Study Questions

1. It has been said that patients seek help when they are no longer able to cope with their problems at their current level of understanding. If this statement is at least partly true, what are the implications for health care services?
2. List the questions that you would ask to assess need and motivation to learn in each of the following nursing situations.
   a. You are to teach breast self-examination to groups of women in the waiting room of a gynecology clinic.

b. You are to teach a 10-year-old boy who is mentally disabled, blind, and suffering from cerebral palsy how to feed himself.

3. Because an increasing number of high-risk infants are discharged to home with complex medical needs, parents are receiving instruction in cardiopulmonary resuscitation (CPR). One study[21] showed that parents lost information over time and that those who were regularly reinforced with hands-on demonstration during clinic visits retained the most skills. Are you surprised by the findings? What learning principles were used?

4. Pelco and others[30] describe an approach to teaching a 4-year-old girl how to take a capsule, using behavioral learning principles. Label the behavioral approaches being used.

Teaching Action	Behavioral Approach
a. Child refused to accept any capsules.	
b. Therapist showed child how to swallow by putting capsule between his fingers, placing it on back of his tongue, taking a sip of juice, tilting his head, and swallowing.	
c. Explained to child that by doing what therapist asked, she could earn pennies to buy toys displayed in the room.	
d. When child refused to swallow, therapist placed his hand over child's and guided it through the steps, until she successfully swallowed capsule.	
e. Pennies and praise were given even if physical guidance was used and child swallowed smaller capsule. These steps were followed until child could consistently swallow prescription-sized capsules. Parent was trained how to maintain routine capsule acceptance postintervention.	

References

1. Affleck G and others: Attributional processes in rheumatoid arthritis patients, *Arthritis Rheum* 30: 927-931, 1987.
2. Bandura A: Self-efficacy mechanism in human agency, *Am Psychol* 37:122-147, 1982.
3. Bandura A: *Foundations of thought and action: a social cognitive theory*, Englewood Cliffs, NJ, 1986, Prentice-Hall.
4. Bandura A: *Self efficacy; the exercise of control*, New York, 1997, Freeman.
5. Bar-On D, Cristal N: Causal attributions of patients, their spouses and physicians, and the rehabilitation of the patients after their first myocardial infarction, *J Cardiopulm Rehabil* 7:285-298, 1987.
6. Barsky AJ and others: Silent myocardial ischemia, *JAMA* 264:1132-1135, 1990.
7. Cameron L, Leventhal EA, Leventhal H: Symptom representations and affect as determinants of care seeking in a community-dwelling, adult sample population, *Health Psychol* 12:171-179, 1993.
8. Campbell DJ: Task complexity: a review and analysis, *Acad Manage Rev* 13:40-52, 1988.
9. Chesla CA: Parents' illness models of schizophrenia, *Arch Psychiatr Nurs* 3:218-225, 1989.
10. Elkind D: Teenage thinking: implications for health care, *Pediatr Nurs* 10:383-385, 1984.
11. Fredette SL: A model for improving cancer patient education, *Cancer Nurs* 13:207-215, 1990.

12. Glaser R, Bassok M: Learning theory and the study of instruction, *Annu Rev Psychol* 40:631-666, 1989.

13. Gray DE: Lay conceptions of autism: parents' explanatory models, *Med Anthropol* 16:99-118, 1995.

14. Harrison JA, Mullen PD, Green LW: A meta-analysis of studies of the health belief model with adults, *Health Educ Res* 7:107-116, 1992.

15. Horne R: Representations of medications and treatment. In Petrie KJ, Weinman JA, editors: *Perceptions of health and illness*, Amsterdam, 1997, Harwood Academic Press.

16. Houston-Miller N: Questions and answers, *J Card Rehabil* 4:104-106, 1984.

17. Jackson C: Behavioral science theory and principles for practice in health education, *Health Educ Res* 12:143-150, 1997.

18. Janz NK, Becker MH, Hartman PE: Contingency contracting to enhance patient compliance: a review, *Patient Educ Couns* 5:164-178, 1984.

19. Jonassen DH, Peck KL, Wilson BG: *Learning with technology; a constructivist perspective*, Columbus, Ohio, 1999, Merrill Press.

20. Kloeblen AS, Batish SS: Understanding the intention to permanently follow a high folate diet among a sample of low-income pregnant women according to the Health Belief Model, *Health Educ Res* 14:327-338, 1999.

21. Komelasky AL, Bond BS: The effect of two forms of learning reinforcement upon parental retention of CPR skills, *Pediatr Nurs* 19:96-98, 1993.

22. Lewis FM, Daltroy LH: How causal explanations influence health behavior: attribution theory. In Glanz K, Lewis FM, Rimer BK, editors: *Health behavior and health education*, San Francisco, 1990, Jossey-Bass.

23. Ley P: Memory for medical information, *Br J Soc Clin Psychol* 18:245-255, 1979.

24. Marcus BH, Rakowski W, Rossi JS: Assessing motivational readiness and decision making for exercise, *Health Psychol* 11:257-261, 1992.

25. Mezirow J: *Transformative learning*, San Francisco, 1991, Jossey-Bass.

26. Miller SM: Monitoring versus blunting styles of coping with cancer influence the information patients want and need about their disease, *Cancer* 76:167-177, 1995.

27. Mishel MH: Uncertainty in chronic illness. In Fitzpatrick JJ, editor: *Annual Review of Nursing Research*, New York, 1999, Springer.

28. Morisky DE and others: The role of needs assessment in designing a community-based mammography education program for urban women, *Health Educ Res* 4:469-478, 1989.

29. Mullen PD, Hersey JC, Iverson DC: Health behavior models compared, *Soc Sci Med* 24:973-981, 1987.

30. Pelco LE and others: Behavioral management of oral medication administration difficulties among children: a review of literature with case illustrations, *J Dev Behav Pediatr* 8:90-96, 1987.

31. Pestrak VA, Martin D: Cognitive development and aspects of adolescent sexuality, *Adolescence* 20:981-987, 1985.

32. Pridham KF, Adelson F, Hansen MF: Helping children deal with procedures in a clinic setting: a developmental approach, *J Pediatr Nurs* 2:13-22, 1987.

33. Prochaska JO and others: The transtheoretical model of change and HIV prevention: a review, *Health Educ Q* 21:471-486, 1994.

34. Prochaska JO, Velicer WF: The transtheoretical model of behavior change, *Am J Health Promotion* 12:38-48, 1997.

35. Rickert VI and others: Training parents to become better behavior managers, *Behav Modif* 12:475-496, 1988.

36. Rosenstock IM, Strecher VJ, Becker MH: The health belief model and HIV risk behavior change. In Di Clemente RJ, Peterson JL, editors: *Preventing AIDS: theories and methods of behavioral interventions*, New York, 1994, Plenum Press.

37. Salomon G, Perkins DN: Rocky roads to transfer: rethinking mechanisms of a neglected phenomenon, *Educ Psychol* 24:113-142, 1989.

38. Schorloo M, Kaptein A: Measurement of illness perceptions in patients with chronic somatic illnesses: a review. In Petrie KJ, Weinman JA, editors: *Perceptions of health and illness*, Amsterdam, 1997, Harwood Academic Press.

39. Slavin RE: *Educational psychology: theory into practice*, Englewood Cliffs, NJ, 1994, Prentice-Hall.

40. Spirito A and others: Screening measures to assess knowledge of diabetes in pregnancy, *Diabetes Care* 13:712-718, 1990.

41. Taylor EW: Building upon the theoretical debate: a critical review of the empirical studies of Mezirow's transformative learning theory, *Adult Educ Quart* 48:34-59, 1997.

42. Volker DL: Needs assessment and resource identification, *Oncol Nurs Forum* 18:119-123, 1991.

43. Wiginton KL: Illness representations: mapping the experience of lupus, *Health Educ Behav* 26:443-453, 1999.

Educational Objectives and Instruction

Statements of goals and objectives provide direction for instructional activities that create conditions of learning. Together they constitute a plan for instruction, with use of interpersonal relationships and instructional materials and experiences to stimulate specific learning activities. Thus making knowledgeable decisions about objectives and stating them precisely is a crucial first step toward effective teaching.

EDUCATIONAL OBJECTIVES

The kinds of learning goals to be reached are frequently well developed by consensus and based on a body of research within various areas of patient education practice. Part II of this book describes a number of such areas of practice, some well established and others just becoming established. Against this set of common expectations, a needs assessment is completed for a particular patient or group, with whom learning objectives are negotiated.

Constructivist philosophies of learning suggest that patients should set their own goals and priorities and learn in "real" settings. Such an approach aims to avoid production of inert knowledge that is difficult to apply or transfer to meaningful contexts. Under this philosophy, specific learning objectives should be set, at least in part, by the learner. A study of patients with diabetes shows that they need a certain level of education before they are able to do this without leaving serious knowledge gaps that could affect self-management.[10]

A statement of objectives requires the use of terms with precise meanings, a statement of both a behavior and a content, and the classification of objectives in established taxonomies (classification systems), which helps one know what kind of instructional strategies are necessary to meet the objective. The objectives flowing from the situation described in Box 3-1 demonstrate these characteristics.

Examples of general nonspecific verbs and the much more useful specific verbs follow.[25]

Nonspecific	Specific
Knows	Defines, describes, identifies, lists, names, selects
Understands	Distinguishes, estimates, explains, gives examples
Applies	Predicts, prepares, solves, uses

Box 3-1 *Statement of Objectives*

Situation

A home health nurse is teaching a wife and a daughter how to care for a bedfast elderly husband and father. The patient moves little but has not been incontinent. He has had no skin breakdown to the present but, according to the wife, has been allowed to lie in one position for 4 hours. The main objective is part of the more encompassing objective, to avoid the harmful consequences of bedrest.

Main Objective

To avoid pressure ulcer formation (psychomotor, cognitive, affective)

Subobjectives

A. To recognize any evidence of tissue breakdown by inspecting at least once a day (cognitive, comprehension; psychomotor, perception)
B. To reposition the patient at least every 2 hours, so that the body is resting on the same surface only every fourth time (psychomotor, mechanism; cognitive, comprehension)
C. To keep all linen wrinkle free (psychomotor, mechanism; cognitive, knowledge)
D. To cleanse skin at the time of soiling and at routine intervals (psychomotor, mechanism; cognitive, comprehension)
E. To report to the nurse evidence of incontinence or skin breakdown, within 4 hours after it is observed (cognitive, knowledge)
F. To maintain adequate nutritional intake (cognitive, knowledge)

TAXONOMIES (CLASSIFICATION SYSTEMS) OF EDUCATIONAL OBJECTIVES

Behaviors are divided into three domains: (1) cognitive, dealing with intellectual abilities; (2) affective, including expression of feelings in the areas of interests, attitudes, values, and appreciations; and (3) psychomotor, dealing with skills commonly known as motor skills. Each domain is ordered in taxonomic form of hierarchy; that is, complex behaviors at the upper end

of the taxonomy (number 5.00 or 6.00) diminish to simple behaviors at the lower end (numbered 1.00). (The taxonomies appear on pp. 39-42.) The cognitive and psychomotor domains are ordered on the concept of complexity of behavior, whereas the affective domain represents increasing internalization or commitment to a feeling, thus also requiring more complex behavior at higher levels.

Besides establishing definitions that facilitate communication, the taxonomy of educational objectives also clarifies certain teaching decisions. In the cognitive domain, learning at the lowest level—acquiring information—can be achieved by a great variety of learning experiences, including lectures, printed material, and pictures or illustrations. Attainment of the higher levels of the domain requires much more investment of time and energy on the part of the teacher and the learner, with the learner actively working through problems and the teacher helping the learner attain insight into the processes to be learned.

Boxes 3-2, 3-3, 3-4, and 3-5 have been prepared to give the reader an opportunity to relate the taxonomy to behaviors that are being taught.

INSTRUCTIONAL FORMS

Instruction is designed to ensure conditions that support learning. The following summary highlights the guidelines from motivation and learning introduced in the first two chapters[34]:

- Begin with objectives, including patients' objectives, and keep them in focus from planning through evaluation.
- Design instruction according to patients' abilities, knowledge structures, and expectations.
- Provide realistic tasks that patients can become competent at performing and believe that they can perform competently.
- Provide advance organizers to constitute "ideational scaffolding" in learning. These statements summarize the essence of the lesson and integrate it with previously learned material.

Text continued on p. 44

Box 3-2	*Taxonomy of Cognitive Domain*

1.00 Knowledge

Knowledge, as defined here, involves recall or remembering of information.

1.10 Knowledge of Specifics

Terminology, specific facts

1.20 Knowledge of Ways and Means of Dealing With Specifics

Corrections, trends and sequences
Classification, categories
Criteria, methodology

1.30 Knowledge of the Universals and Abstractions in a Field

Principles and generalizations, theories and structures

2.00 Comprehension

This represents the lowest level of understanding. It refers to a type of understanding. The individual knows what is being communicated and can make use of the material or idea being communicated without necessarily relating it to other material or seeing its fullest implications.

2.10 Translation

Comprehension is evidenced by the care and accuracy with which the communication is paraphrased or rendered from one language or form of communication to another. Translation is judged on the basis of faithfulness and accuracy, that is, on the extent to which the material in the original communication is preserved although the form of the communication has been altered.

2.20 Interpretation

The explanation or summarization of a communication. Whereas translation involves an objective part-for-part rendering of a communication, interpretation involves a reordering, rearrangement, or new view of the material.

2.30 Extrapolation

The extension of trends or tendencies beyond the given data to determine implications, consequences, corollaries, effects, and so forth which are in accordance with the conditions described in the original communication.

3.00 Application

The use of abstractions in particular and concrete situations. The abstractions may be in the form of general ideas, rules of procedures, or generalized methods. The abstractions may also be technical principles, ideas, and theories, which must be remembered and applied.

4.00 Analysis

The breakdown of a communication into its constituent elements or parts, that the relative hierarchy of ideas is made clear or the relations between the ideas expressed are made explicit, or both. Such analyses are intended to clarify the communication, to indicate how the communication is organized and the way in which it manages to convey its effects, as well as to indicate its basis and arrangement.

4.10 Analysis of Elements

Identification of the elements included in a communication.

From Bloom BS and others: *Taxonomy of educational objectives. Handbook I: Cognitive domain,* New York, 1984, Longman.

Continued

Box 3-2	*Taxonomy of Cognitive Domain—cont'd*

4.20 Analysis of Relationships

Identification of the connections and interactions between elements and parts of a communication.

4.30 Analysis of Organizational Principles

Identification of the organization, systematic arrangement, and structure that hold the communication together. This includes the "explicit" as well as "implicit" structure. It includes the bases, necessary arrangement, and mechanics that make the communication a unit.

5.00 Synthesis

The putting together of elements and parts to form a whole. This involves the process of working with pieces, parts, elements, and so forth, and arranging and combining them in such a way as to constitute a pattern or structure not clearly present before.

5.10 Production of a Unique Communication

The development of a communication in which the writer or speaker attempts to convey ideas, feelings, or experiences or all three to others.

5.20 Production of a Plan or Proposed Set of Operations

The development of a plan of work or the proposal of a plan of operations. The plan should satisfy the requirements of a task that may be given to the student or that he may develop for himself.

5.30 Derivation of a Set of Abstract Relations

The development of a set of abstract relations either to classify or explain particular data or phenomena, or the deduction of propositions and relations from a set of basic propositions or symbolic representations.

6.00 Evaluation

Judgments about the value of material and methods for given purposes: quantitative and qualitative judgments about the extent to which material and methods satisfy criteria; use of standard of appraisal. The criteria may be determined by the student or given to him.

6.10 Judgments in Terms of Internal Evidence

Evaluation of the accuracy of a communication from such evidence as logical accuracy, consistency, and other internal criteria.

6.20 Judgments in Terms of External Criteria

Evaluation of material with reference to selected or remembered criteria.

| Box 3-3 | *Psychomotor Domain: A Tentative Taxonomic System* |

1.00 Perception

Process of becoming aware of objects, qualities, or relations by way of the sense organs.

1.10 Sensory Stimulation

Impingement of a stimulus(i) on one or more of the sense organs.
- 1.11 Auditory
- 1.12 Visual
- 1.13 Tactile
- 1.14 Taste
- 1.15 Smell
- 1.16 Kinesthetic

1.20 Cue Selection

Identification of the cue or cues, associating them with the task to be performed, and grouping them in terms of past experience and knowledge. Cues relevant to the situation are selected as a guide to action; irrelevant cues are ignored or discarded.

1.30 Translation

The mental process of determining the meaning of the cues received for action; it involves symbolic translation, that is, having an image or being reminded of something, "having an idea," as a result of cues received, insight, sensory translation, and "feedback."

2.00 Set

A preparatory adjustment or readiness for a particular kind of action or experience.

2.10 Mental Set

Readiness, in the mental sense, to perform a certain motor act. This involves, as prerequisite, the level of perception already identified. Discrimination, using judgments in making distinctions, is an aspect.

2.20 Physical Set

Readiness in the sense of having made the anatomic adjustments necessary for a motor act to be performed, including sensory attending and posturing of the body.

2.30 Emotional Set

Readiness in terms of attitudes favorable to the motor act's taking place.

3.00 Guided Response

The overt behavioral act of an individual under the guidance of the instructor. Prerequisite to performance of the act is readiness to respond and selection of the appropriate response.

3.10 Imitation

The execution of an act as a direct response to the perception of another person performing the act.

3.20 Trial and Error

Trying various responses, usually with some rationale for each response, until an appropriate response is achieved.

4.00 Mechanism

Learned response has become habitual. The learner has achieved a certain confidence and degree of skill. The act is a part of his or her repertoire of possible responses to stimuli and to the demands of situations where the response is an appropriate one. The response may be more complex than at the preceding level; it may involve some patterning of response in carrying out the task.

5.00 Complex Overt Response

Performance of a motor act that is considered complex because of the movement pattern required. A high degree of skill has been attained, and the act can be carried out with minimum expenditure of time and energy.

5.10 Resolution of Uncertainty

Performance of a complex act without hesitation.

5.20 Automatic Performance

Performance of finely coordinated motor skill with a great deal of ease and muscle control.

6.00 Adaptation

Altering motor activities to meet the demands of new problematic situations requiring a physical response.

7.00 Origination

Creating new motor acts or ways of manipulating materials out of understandings, abilities, and skills developed in the psychomotor area.

Modified from Simpson EJ: In *Contributions of behavioral science to instructional technology: the psychomotor domain,* Mt Rainier, Md, 1972, Gryphon Press.

Box 3-4	*Taxonomy of Affective Domain*

1.00 Receiving (Attending)

1.10 Awareness

Awareness is almost a cognitive behavior. But unlike knowledge, the lowest level of the cognitive domain, awareness is not so much concerned with a memory of or ability to recall an item or fact as with the phenomenon that, given an appropriate opportunity, the learner will merely be conscious of something—that he or she will take into account a situation, face or event, object, or stage of affairs.

1.20 Willingness to Receive

At a minimum level we are describing here the behavior of being willing to tolerate a given stimulus, not to avoid it.

1.30 Controlled or Selected Attention

There is an element of the learner's controlling the attention here, so that the favored stimulus is selected and attended to despite competing and distracting stimuli.

2.00 Responding

2.10 Acquiescence in Responding

The student makes the response but he or she has not fully accepted the necessity for doing so.

2.20 Willingness to Respond

There is the implication that the learner is sufficiently committed to exhibiting a behavior so that he or she does so not just because of a fear of punishment, but "on his own" or voluntarily.

2.30 Satisfaction in Response

Behavior is accompanied by a feeling of satisfaction, an emotional response, generally of pleasure, zest, or enjoyment.

3.00 Valuing

3.10 Acceptance of a Value

The learner is sufficiently consistent that others can identify the value and sufficiently committed that he or she is willing to be so identified, but there is more of a readiness here to re-evaluate his or her position than would be present at higher levels of valuing.

3.20 Preference for a Value

Behavior at this level implies not just the acceptance of a value to the point of being willing to be identified with it, but more, a seeking it out and wanting it.

3.30 Commitment

Belief at this level involves a high degree of certainty. There is a real motivation to act out the behavior.

4.00 Organization

4.10 Conceptualization of a Value

At this level the quality of abstraction or conceptualization is added. It permits patients to understand how the value relates to those that they already hold or to new ones that they are learning to hold.

4.20 Organization of a Value System

Objectives properly classified here as those that require the learner to bring together a complex of values, possibly disparate values, and to relate them in an ordered fashion with one another. Ideally, the ordered relationship will be one which is harmonious and internally consistent.

5.00 Characterization by a Value or Value Complex

5.10 Generalized Set

A generalized set is a basic orientation that enables individuals to reduce and order the complex world about them and to act consistently and effectively in it. The generalized set may be thought of as closely related to the idea of an attitude cluster.

5.20 Characterization

Here are found those objectives that concern the individual's view of the universe, his or her philosophy of life . . . a value system having as its object the whole of what is known or knowable.

From Krathwohl DR, Bloom BS, Masia BB: *Taxonomy of educational objectives. Handbook II: Affective domain*, New York, 1984, Longman.

Box 3-5	*Examples of Health Teaching Objectives According to Taxonomies of Educational Objectives*

Cognitive Domain

Knowledge	To describe three main purposes of the cough, turn, deep-breathe regimen after surgery
	To state why the mother's diet may affect breastfeeding
Comprehension	To recognize, in changing a surgical dressing, when something has been contaminated
	To translate instructions on a medicine bottle into appropriate action
Application	To apply principles of asepsis to washing a wound with pHisoHex
	Given a general knowledge of safety, to plan how to rid a house of safety hazards
Analysis	To identify factors that cause bowel upsets
	To distinguish how an uninformed argument differs from scientific reasoning
Synthesis	To design an ileostomy bag that suits the patient's needs better than do available commercial ones
	To interpret to others the feelings experienced during illness
Evaluation	To assess the health care the patient is receiving in terms of its completeness, the patient's satisfaction with it, and the results obtained

Affective Domain

Receiving	To be aware that others are available to help
	To tolerate having a retention catheter
Responding	To cooperate with the insertion of a nasogastric tube
	To feel some satisfaction in caring for a baby
Valuing	To accept many of the limitations in life imposed by heart disease
	To desire good health rather than mere absence of disease
Organization	To relate to others in a manner consistent with rehabilitation goals
	To regularly choose those alternatives of action that are consistent with good parenting
Characterization by a value	To develop a code of behavior consistent with respect for the health of or value complex of the patient and others

Psychomotor Domain

Perception	To recognize the "feel" of holding a baby with good balance
	To recognize the difference between systolic and diastolic blood pressure sounds
Set	To demonstrate a well-balanced stance with crutches
	To demonstrate correct placement of sphygmomanometer and stethoscope
Guided response	To discover the most efficient method of diapering a baby through trial of various procedures
	To imitate the blood pressure measurement procedure after demonstration
Mechanism	To control the fall of mercury in the sphygmomanometer at 2 to 3 mm Hg per heartbeat
Complex overt response	To pass a tube through the nose into the stomach skillfully with a minimum of discomfort or danger to the patient
	To measure blood pressure in 1 minute, accurate to ± 5 mm Hg (mercury), in comparison with an expert
Adaptation	To perform one's own design for turning, moving, and transferring a hemiplegic person, weighing 100 pounds more than oneself, in a home environment
Origination	To design new materials to self-catheterize

- Provide models with whom patients identify and from whom they can learn.
- Match instruction to patients' stages of readiness.
- Divide complex tasks into smaller, achievable sequential learning units so that patients can experience satisfaction and a feeling of self-efficacy.
- Organize complex information in easy-to-remember structures such as graphics or schematics.
- Practice instruction in a variety of ways to match different learning styles. Ample learning time should be used for practice that is participatory, experiential, and uses different senses.
- Provide immediate feedback so that patients can improve their responses.
- Conclude instruction by having patients review what they have learned and feel confident they can do.

Most instructional forms are familiar to readers of this book. They have three basic components: (1) a delivery system, which is the physical form of the materials and hardware used to present stimuli to the learners, such as handouts, slides, computer-assisted instruction, or a person; (2) a content or message; and (3) a form or condition of abstractness. Figure 3-1 shows an example of the abstract-concrete continuum. Methods are also instructor-centered, interactive,

individualized, or experiential (see Box 3-6) and can be matched with domains and levels of learning (Table 3-1).

Patient education also fits within taxonomies of interventions describing the practice of particular professions. One of the several taxonomies for nursing is the Nursing Intervention Classification Project, which describes patient education as one class of intervention within the behavioral domain. The Project describes more than 400 nursing interventions categorized into classes and domains.[27] This work creates a standardized language for nursing treatments. More specific "Intervention Labels" related to patient education include participatory guidance, decision-making support, learning facilitation, childbirth preparation, learning-readiness enhancement, parent education, preparatory sensory information, teaching: disease process, teaching: group, teaching: individual, teaching: infant care, teaching: preoperative, teaching: prescribed activity/exercise, teaching: prescribed diet, teaching: prescribed medication, teaching: procedure/treatment, teaching: psychomotor skill, and teaching: safe sex. Box 3-7 shows one of the teaching interventions with its definition and activities. This class of teaching interventions is among those with the highest use among practicing nurses.[7]

Yet another taxonomy describes pediatric primary care nursing interventions. A major focus here is on self-care and patient education, which Kilmon[29] describes as:

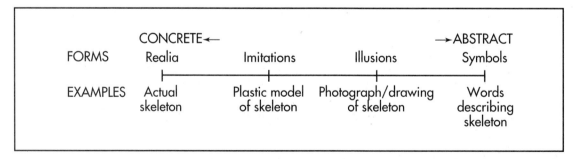

Figure 3-1 Form of instructional materials: the abstract-concrete continuum. (Modified from Weston C, Cranton PA: Selecting instructional strategies. *J Higher Educ* 57(3):259-288, 1986.)

Box 3-6   *Summary of Instructional Methods*

INSTRUCTOR-CENTERED	INTERACTIVE	INDIVIDUALIZED	EXPERIENTIAL
Lecture Passive students Efficient for lower learning levels and large classes	**Class Discussion** Must have small class size May be time-consuming Encourages student involvement	**Programmed Instruction** Most effective at lower learning levels Very structured Allows students to work at own pace Extensive feedback for students	**Field or Clinical** Occurs in natural setting during performance Active student involvement May be difficult for management and evaluation
Questioning Monitors student learning Encourages student involvement May cause anxiety for some	**Discussion Groups** Small class size Student participation Effective for high cognitive and affective learning levels	**Modularized Instruction** May be time-consuming Very flexible formats Allows students to work at own pace	**Laboratory** Requires careful planning and evaluation Active student involvement in realistic setting
Demonstration Illustrates an application of a skill or concept Students are passive	**Peer Teaching** Requires careful planning and monitoring Utilizes differences in student expertise Encourages student involvement	**Independent Projects** Most appropriate at higher learning levels May be time-consuming Active student involvement in learning	**Role-Playing** Effective in affective and psycho-motor domains Provides "safe" experiences Active student participation
	Group Projects Requires careful planning and monitoring Utilizes differences in student expertise Encourages student involvement	**Computerized Instruction** May involve considerable instructor time or expense May be very flexible Allows students to work at own pace Student involvement in varying activities	**Simulations and Games** Provide practice of specific skills Produce anxiety for some Active student participation
			Drill Most appropriate at lower learning levels Provides active practice May not be motivating for some students

Modified from Weston C, Cranton PA: Selecting instructional strategies, *J Higher Educ* 57(3):259–288, 1986.

TABLE 3-1 Matching Domain and Level of Learning to Appropriate Methods

Domain and Level	Method
Cognitive Domain	
Knowledge	Lecture, programmed instruction, drill and practice
Comprehension	Lecture, modularized instruction, programmed instruction
Application	Discussion, simulations and games, computer-assisted instruction, modularized instruction, field experience, laboratory
Analysis	Discussion, independent/group projects, simulations, field experience, role-playing, laboratory
Synthesis	Independent/group projects, field experience, role-playing, laboratory
Evaluation	Independent/group projects, field experience, laboratory
Affective Domain	
Receiving	Lecture, discussion, modularized instruction, field experience
Responding	Discussion, simulations, modularized instruction, role-playing, field experience
Valuing	Discussion, independent/group projects, simulations, role-playing, field experience
Organization	Discussion, independent/group projects, field experience
Characterization by a value	Independent projects, field experience
Psychomotor Domain	
Perception	Demonstration (lecture), drill and practice
Set	Demonstration (lecture), drill and practice
Guided response	Peer teaching, games, role-playing, field experience, drill and practice
Mechanism	Games, role-playing, field experience, drill and practice
Complex overt response	Games, field experience
Adaptation	Independent projects, games, field experience
Origination	Independent projects, games, field experience

From Weston C, Cranton PA: Selecting instructional strategies. *J Higher Educ* 57(3):259-288, 1986.

Box 3-7 *Teaching: Prescribed Diet*

Definition: Preparing a patient to correctly follow a prescribed diet

Activities

Appraise the patient's current level of knowledge about prescribed diet.

Determine the patient's/significant other's feelings/ attitude toward prescribed diet and expected degree of dietary compliance.

Inform the patient of the proper name of prescribed diet.

Explain the purpose of the diet.

Inform the patient how long the diet should be followed.

Instruct the patient how to keep a food diary as appropriate.

Instruct the patient on allowed and prohibited foods.

Inform the patient of possible drug/food interactions as appropriate.

Assist the patient to accommodate food preferences into prescribed diet.

Assist the patient in substituting ingredients to conform favorite recipes to prescribed diet.

Instruct the patient how to read labels and select appropriate foods.

Observe the patient's selection of foods appropriate to prescribed diet.

Instruct the patient how to plan appropriate meals.

Provide written meal plans as appropriate.

Recommend a cookbook that includes recipes consistent with prescribed diet as appropriate.

Reinforce information provided by other health care team members as appropriate.

Refer patient to dietitian/nutritionist as appropriate.

Include the family/significant others as appropriate.

From McCloskey JC, Bulechek GM, editors: *Nursing interventions classifications (NIC)*, ed 3, St Louis, 2000, Mosby.

an effort to assist parents with self-management of identified health problems. Anticipatory guidance entails education for healthy families with the goal of promoting healthy child and family development while avoiding injuries and other preventable health problems. The category of health problem supportive services includes teaching parents of a child with a significant health problem how to effectively utilize health care resources.

The seven major elements of Kilmon's taxonomy are anticipatory guidance, health problem supportive services, counseling, dietary modifications, immunizations, procedures, and medications. A number of other taxonomies also describe practice, all of which include patient education as a major intervention.

Interpersonal Teaching Forms

Probably the most potent learning occurs experientially in real situations, by patients making the judgments and doing the tasks they will need to do for themselves, directed by their sense of need to become competent. Learning from peers who have successfully completed the transition on which patients are embarking often provides models and an emotional identification that is motivating. Such conditions integrate cognitive, affective, and psychomotor learning in a single performance. These conditions must be reconstructed as a patient enters a new phase of readjustment and faces new challenges and goals. Because education has traditionally been delivered in settings in which highly technical health care is provided, learning conditions realistic to everyday life have been considerably underutilized. When patient education is taken seriously, realistic, experiential learning environments are created and tested. Considerable evidence shows that with a patient's mastering of a basic knowledge base, these realistic, motivating, learning environments will be the most effective of the methods known, even for patients with little formal education.

Groups provide an economical way to teach. The experience of having the support of a group, gaining motivation to learn from other members, decreasing feelings of isolation, and modeling the behavior of other individuals may be the best way for patients to meet their objectives.

For example, caregivers of persons with Alzheimer's disease and related disorders need groups that focus on education and support. Such help is necessary because of progressive deterioration of the patient's condition over a 7- to 10-year period. Experiences include role reversals, little support from peers or other family members, absent or misinterpreted feedback from the patient, and withdrawal from social networks. These unpleasant changes can result in progressive deterioration of the family system and depression for caregivers. Caregivers can learn specific skills, such as how to respond to the patient's behavior and cognitive impairments, how to modify his or her environment, and how to deal with legal and financial problems, sadness, frustration, and anger. It is less expensive for the family to be involved in effective educational and support groups than it is to institutionalize the patient if the caregiver fails to cope. One study of caregivers for frail elderly persons in the community finds that the institutionalization rate decreases from 17% to 5% when the caregivers are involved in educational or support groups. The educational program focused on assisting caregivers in dealing constructively with negative feelings, as well as on how to lift, move, and bathe the patient and how to administer medication. Social skills for dealing with the patient and other family members and relaxation techniques were also taught. The availability of a secondary caregiver was important.[24]

Annually, 6.4 million people participate in member-governed, problem-specific, low-fee self-help groups. Health professionals are involved with these groups in various ways but usually are not central to them. Some groups are small and local; others are nationally networked assemblies. Members are psychologically bonded by the compelling similarity of their concerns. They rely primarily on the collective experiential knowledge possessed by the membership. Acceptance by the group seems to be a vital step toward making the cognitive, emotional, and behavioral changes necessary for more effective functioning and an improved quality of life. One database in California found 188 distinct problem categories around which groups were formed. Support groups address problems such as alcoholism, anorexia, arthritis, parental bereavement, coping with various cancers, care taking of persons with Alzheimer's disease, diabetes, burns, drug abuse, impact of incest, and parental coping with handicapped children, as well as many others.[28]

Some groups form spontaneously. In one case, informal support groups were evolving as patients with ventricular tachycardia, who were in a hospital for electrophysiological studies and treatment, socialized in their rooms and in the lounge. The disadvantage of this development was that misinformation was easily passed on. Because the disease was life threatening and the treatment invasive, the disruption caused by misinformation could have been serious. A formal program was therefore developed with a teaching component that included information on normal electrical conduction in the heart and the pathology of ventricular tachycardia, electrophysiological studies, telemetry monitoring, medications, and preparation for discharge. Certification in cardiopulmonary resuscitation for family members and friends was also offered. Patients exhibiting severe anxiety, frank denial, or overt hostility were screened out of the group and taught individually.[14]

In another example, Kulik and Mahler[31] describe groups that formed even when not intended. Patients who had a roommate who had already had surgery before their own operations were less anxious preoperatively, they were more ambulatory postoperatively, and they were released 1.4 days more quickly than were patients whose roommates preoperatively also had not had surgery yet. Social comparison theory predicts that evaluative needs of individuals in unusual and stressful situations are best served by comparison with others who are in similar situations. Roommates' experiences may also provide patients with information preoperatively that will enable them to interpret postoperative sensations and events in a more accurate and less personally threatening manner. With today's

brief preoperative stays, such opportunities may no longer exist.

Sometimes it is important to form separate groups for patients and for families. It is also useful to prescreen individuals entering a group to assess whether their learning needs are generally the same or whether one individual would be disruptive to the group. Group appointments, in which patients and others with the same diagnosis are seen by a multidisciplinary team for extended visits, are gaining popularity in managed care settings.

Role-Playing

Role-playing is an excellent technique for diagnosis of motivation and readiness to learn, as well as for teaching ideas and attitudes. People are assigned to play themselves or someone else. A related technique is for the teacher to enact a role that the learner can model. For example, the teacher could enact a positive or desirable parental role in relation to a child's specific behavior and then discuss and label the behavior that has been portrayed.

Through role-playing, a desired behavior is rehearsed. Thus a person is taught the skills required and gains the confidence needed to carry them out. Reversal of the roles is a technique useful for sensitizing one person to the other's situation. Role-playing provides a kind of behavioral and mental rehearsal that is a form of practice. It is also a means of increasing retention in learning.

Role-playing techniques have been cited as useful in teaching persons from disadvantaged backgrounds. These techniques are effective in situations that have been described as physical, action-oriented, concrete, and problem-directed rather than those that are introspective. They are most effective when instruction is easy and informally paced. Role-playing may also reduce the role distance between patient and professional. The technique has considerable potential for reducing overintellectualization and for uniting understanding and feeling.

For all these reasons, school-aged children are often taught how to deal with their asthma by using puppets to role-play. At this stage of child development, the chief learning mode is visual and psychomotor (puppets), and teachers focus on helping the children develop an "I can do" attitude (role-playing). Box 3-8 contains suggested role-playing situations using puppets. The role-play is designed to help children manage an asthma attack, take their medications correctly, and cope with teasing from peers.

Role-playing is often incorporated as one technique in a program. For example, one educationally oriented support group for teenagers with diabetes began with a weekend camping experience to bond the group. The group wore identical T-shirts with a logo to aid in group identity. The members quickly discovered that the group was a place to meet with friends. Role-playing on how to relate to parents and other family members was a critical element of the program. Snacks were cooked, and awards were given for each teenager's special trait. Blood glucose was tested before and after exercise. The teenagers gained experience in solving actual problems, and they signed contracts agreeing to certain future behaviors.[11]

Verbal Teaching

Inasmuch as teaching is communicating, which is accomplished in large part by language, the teacher must be skilled in the use of language. Clinicians need special knowledge of language because of two conditions inherent in health teaching: medical terminology is foreign to much of the public, and individuals with considerable health needs often have poorly developed language skills that result in low levels of understanding.

The use of written information improves patients' retention of information. The use of another device, called "advanced organizers," produced significant increases in recall in a study by Ley and others.[33] The advanced organizers were

---

Box 3-8	*Suggested Role-Play Situations*

Lesson 1

Wheezing Willie is very allergic to grass. If he is near it, he will wheeze and may even have an asthma attack. He is at his friend's house for a birthday party and the children decide to do somersaults and cartwheels on the freshly cut grass. What should Wheezing Willie do?

Lesson 2

Healthy Heather has been given the assignment to tell the class what happens to the human body when it has an asthma attack.

Lesson 3

Wheezing Wendy and her family have just moved to a new neighborhood and she is going to a new school. In the morning of her first day, she begins to wheeze. The person sitting next to her hears her wheezing and starts to call her names. What should Wheezing Wendy do?

Lesson 4

Wheezing Willie has to take a breathing treatment and other medication every day at school during the lunch period. Because he has to take a treatment, he misses half of recess. Lately, Willie has been feeling well and has stopped going to the office to take his breathing treatment and medication. Do you think Wheezing Willie is doing the right thing? What should he do?

Lesson 5

Wheezing Wendy is at her friend Healthy Heather's house. She is having fun playing with Barbie dolls when she begins to have a headache and her throat starts to feel scratchy. These are two of Wheezing Wendy's early warning signs. Wheezing Wendy's mother is at work and won't be home for 2 more hours. What should she do?

From Ramsey AM, Siroky AS: The use of puppets to teach school-age children with asthma, *Pediatr Nurs* 14:187-190, 1988.

category names to organize the material, which consisted of the following statements:

1. You have a chest infection.
2. And your larynx is slightly inflamed.
3. But I think your heart is all right.
4. We will do some heart tests to make sure.
5. We will need to take a blood sample.
6. And you will have to have an x-ray examination of your chest.
7. Your cough will disappear in the next 2 days.
8. You will feel better in a week or so.
9. And you will recover completely.
10. We will give you an injection of penicillin.
11. And some tablets to take.
12. I'll give you an inhaler to use.
13. You must avoid cold drafts.
14. You must stay indoors in fog.
15. And you must take 2 hours' rest each afternoon.

The advanced organizers were used as follows[23]:

I am going to tell you:

what is wrong with you;
what tests we are going to carry out;
what I think will happen to you;
what treatment you will need; and
what you must do to help yourself.
First, what is wrong with you . . . (statements 1-3)
Second, what tests we are going to carry out . . . (statements 4-6)
Third, what I think will happen to you . . . (statements 7-9)
Fourth, what the treatments will be . . . (statements 10-12)
Finally, what you must do to help yourself . . . (statements 13-15)

Notice that the category names are not medical terms; rather, they are categories meaningful to patients.

Because of their backgrounds, health professionals may tend to overuse verbal instruction. They often value independence and symbolic learning. They may therefore choose a verbal means of instruction to motivate a person, when joining the patient in the health action would be more effective. Expressing the idea in words can serve to maintain a professional distance from patients and at the same time create a student-teacher role hierarchy and a status gap between helper and patient. It may fail as a teaching technique, especially if used exclusively.

Demonstration and Practice

Demonstration is a performance of procedures or psychomotor skills, which, combined with practice, is the method most suited to attaining skills. The purpose of the demonstration is to give the learner a clear mental image of how the procedure is performed. Presentations of a prime view by television or motion picture may be necessary if the groups are large. In some instances an over-the-shoulder view of the demonstrator provides learners with a clear idea of the way they must perform the action. When the demonstrator is removing fluids from a vial and giving an injection, the mirror image that viewers receive by facing the demonstrator is not entirely realistic.

Learners need practice to develop motor skills; therefore the teaching plan must incorporate a time for patients to practice. When equipment is sufficient and the group is small enough, practice may begin with the learner demonstrating the skill immediately after the teacher finishes. Additional practice should take place in a setting similar to that in which the skill will be used. The teacher must supervise enough to provide feedback for correct performance and to stimulate motivation if necessary.

Teaching Tools

Much teaching is accomplished by means of tools, both written and audiovisual, used within the context of an instructional plan. If these tools are well designed and have been shown to be effective in creating learning, and if they are well matched to the goals of instruction and to the learner's capabilities, they can be almost self-instructional.

Written materials are by far the most frequently used in patient education, despite persistent evidence that they are mismatched to the needs of many patients, particularly in their reading level. Printed teaching material can be described as a frozen language that is selective in its description of reality (which is both a strength and a weakness). It encourages limited feedback but is constantly available. Print partially relaxes time requirements and is more efficient than oral language (except for those who have not learned to read efficiently) because readers can control the speed at which they read and comprehend. Certain kinds of thinking seem to demand written expression. For example, a complex sequence of thoughts that incorporates definitions, qualifications, and logical constraints is expressed best in writing. Most people who have learned to read well generally prefer to acquire information by reading. Reading is ideal for understanding complex concepts and relationships. If the learning objective primarily requires skill in dealing with persons or things, then demonstrations, concrete experience with the activity, and oral coaching and guidance would be more effective than print media.

The various media that can be used for learning possess cognitively relevant characteristics in their technologies, symbol systems, and processing capabilities. Computers are distinguished by their extensive processing capabilities rather than by their access to a particularly unique set of symbol systems (they use words and pictures). In television the symbols can depict action; however, the symbols are transient.[22]

Although some students can learn a particular task regardless of the medium, others need the advantage of a particular medium's characteristics. For example, experts who learn from text can skim rapidly, using trigger words to read selectively and nonsequentially. When memory limits are reached, they stop and summarize the material they have learned. Such processing strategies cannot be used with audio tapes or lectures. Novices take advantage of the text's stability to slow the rate of information processing; as a result they are able to review the material. Pictures that illustrate information central to the text help the reader. If, however, the material is too difficult for the reader, he or she must expend a great deal of effort trying to decode the text, possibly increasing the risk of learning failure.[30]

Print Materials

Because different media have different strengths, use of a variety of media is likely to be more successful than is use of a single medium. Learning from print materials is an economical use of time, if they are well designed to promote learning and if they match a patient's reading and literacy levels. Approximately half the population in the United States struggles with basic reading skills. For many others the materials available are written at a higher level than they can comprehend. The reading levels of many individuals may be up to five grades below the grade they report to have completed.

Graphic design techniques that can increase readership, comprehension, and memory are summarized in Box 3-9.[9] For low-literacy readers, increase the amount of white space and use question and answer or bullet (not paragraph) format.[35] Photos and illustrations decrease the density of the text. In addition, authors of print materials should do the following:

- Make key messages easy to find.
- Use the first paragraph to communicate the benefits the audience desires most and the actions to obtain them.
- Provide true or fictional stories about people taking concrete actions and experiencing consequences that are interesting to them.
- Describe step-by-step the action requested.
- Provide pictures and words that evoke vivid imagery, which will be better remembered than abstract words.
- Write text in second person to convey information personally relevant to readers.
- Increase rehearsal of information by repeating it, highlighting it, or boxing it, and ask readers to perform specific activities.
- Provide materials sensitive to the culture of those with whom they will be used, addressing their lifestyles and using cultural language and symbols.

Box 3-9	*Graphic Design Guidelines for Easy-to-Read and Effective Written Materials*

To Direct Readers to the Message

Do

- Use arrows, underlines, bold type, boxes, white space, and bullets to direct readers' eyes to the key messages.

Don't

- Use italics, all capital letters, script, or screens of color over text.
- Require reader to look in many directions on the page to read copy and find the message.

To Select an Easy-to-Read Typeface

Do

- Use 10- to 14-point type size.

- Use a typeface with serifs in the body copy (e.g., Times Roman).

Don't

- Go below 10-point type size for good readers and 12-point for poor readers.
- Mix typefaces or use more than three sizes of print on one page.
- Use white letters on black background.

To Create Easy-to-Read Copy

Do

- Use 40 to 50 character-wide columns, left justified.
- Use lots of white space.
- Use highly contrasting colors for text and background such as black on white or cream.
- Use the same dark color for headings and body copy or colors with similar intensity.

Don't

- Break margins with illustrations or other graphics. If required, break only the right margin.

- Use light or unusual ink colors such as red, green, or orange.

To Create Clear Visuals

Do

- Convey one key message per visual. Print the message in a caption.
- Make the message easy to grasp at a glance.
- Show only the "desired" way to act in visuals.

- Use realistic drawings, photos, or human-like figures.
- Use visuals with which the audience can identify.

Don't

- Add any visuals simply to decorate the material.

- Include any details or background in the visual that are not required to communicate the message.
- Use highly stylized or abstract graphics.
- Portray blood cells and other body parts as cartoon characters.

From Buxton T: Effective ways to improve health education materials, *J Health Educ* 30(1):47-50, 61, 1999.

Of the plethora of studies on readability, most come to the conclusion that many persons who must use written patient education materials have limited ability to understand those that are available.

- The reading difficulty levels of one U.S. government publication, *Dietary Guide-*

lines, vary from sixth grade to college level; 75% of individuals in the Special Supplemental Food Program for Women, Infants and Children (WIC) who were studied were frustrated or needed instructional assistance to understand this publication.[8]

- Analysis of 63 patient package inserts accompanying drugs revealed a tenth-grade reading level on average, with only 11% written at the fifth- to seventh-grade level recommended for documents used by the general public. Half had small type or poor-quality printing.[3]

- In another study, the reading ability of parents of pediatric outpatients in one large public teaching hospital was at the seventh- to eighth-grade level, although the average last grade reported was 11.5. Eighty percent of 129 materials from the American Academy of Pediatrics, the Centers for Disease Control and Prevention (CDC), the March of Dimes, pharmaceutical companies, and commercial publishers on baby care required at least a tenth-grade reading level, with only 2% written at less than a seventh-grade level. The reading levels of these publications are cited in an article by Davis and others.[12] A federal act mandating that vaccine information pamphlets be given to parents also mandates that the materials be understandable; yet all three of the CDC vaccine pamphlets analyzed were written at a level well above the reading ability of two thirds of the parents tested in the study.

- Readability of consent forms is especially problematic because they have consistently been estimated to be written at a scientific or college level. Analysis of reading levels of consent forms for studies at the National Cancer Institute found them to range from grades 12 to 17.5, with a mean grade level of 14.3.[37]

- Analysis of readability of 209 low-cost brief nutrition education pamphlets found 68% at ninth-grade level or higher, 11% at sixth-grade level or below, and 2 publications written at the third-grade level.[16]

- Mean readability of 100 patient pamphlets developed by the American College of Obstetrics and Gynecology was seventh- to ninth-grade. Because the average reading level of U.S. citizens is eighth grade and one in five adults reads at the fifth-grade level or below, these materials are also mismatched with many of their intended users.[18]

- On average, patient material on the World Wide Web is written at tenth-grade reading level.[23]

The term "readability" refers to the understandabilitiy of written text. It is important to note that readability formulas indicate reading ease, not comprehension, although when the reading level is beyond the skill of the learner, comprehension is known to be decreased and recall is sketchy and inaccurate. Although not commonly used in everyday practice, several brief tests are available to estimate a patient's reading level.[40] In contrast to the amount of attention devoted to measuring readability of materials, little attention has been paid to measuring patient comprehension of, or learning from, educational literature. Other characteristics not captured in readability formulas are also important in written and other instructional materials. These include organization, including use of headings and outlines, appropriate sequencing of material, and clarity. Examples of materials written at high levels and revised to be read at much lower levels can be found in Boxes 3-10, 3-11, and 3-12.

Various readability formulas may be useful for different kinds of text. For example, the Fry readability formula, shown in Box 3-13 and in Figure 3-2, determines the level of materials from grades 1 through college; however, this formula is not useful with passages of fewer than 300 words. The FOG INDEX[SM] formula, shown in Box 3-14, uses the number of sentences and the number of polysyllabic words and is useful for grades 4 through college. The Flesch formula, shown in Box 3-15, uses average sentence length and word length and is useful for grades 5 through college. The SMOG formula, shown in Box 3-16 (see rules for testing in Box 3-17), counts the number of sentences and the number of words with three or more syllables and is useful for grades 5 through college. Meade and Smith[38] compared readability formulas based on the same health education materials and have found that the Flesch, FOG

Box 3-10 | *Examples of Reading Materials for Patients: Original and Revised Versions*

Example 1: Consent to Operation

Original (Twenty-fifth Grade Level)

I consent to the performance of operations and procedures in addition to or different from those now contemplated, whether or not arising from presently unforeseen conditions, which the above-named doctor or his associates or assistants may consider necessary or advisable in the course of the operation.

Revised (Sixth-Grade Level)

I agree to other operations or treatments. My doctors may learn more in surgery. They may think I need other treatments. My doctors will decide in surgery. I agree to let them do the things they think are needed.

Example 2: Patient Education Material

Original (Sixteenth-Grade Level)

Angina pectoris is a symptom and not actually a disease. The term refers to a pain in the chest, usually under the sternum (breastbone), which is brought on chiefly by exercise or emotional upsets in a person who has a heart problem. The pain is usually relieved by rest alone, but goes away more quickly with the use of a medicine which helps to bring more blood to the heart muscle.

Revised (Seventh-Grade Level)

Angina is a feeling. It is not really a disease. The word means a pain in the chest. The pain is felt under the breastbone. A person who has heart trouble may feel this. Exercise or getting upset can cause the pain. The pain usually goes away with rest. It goes away faster if you take medicine. The medicine helps to bring more blood to the heart.

From Davis TC and others: The gap between patient reading comprehension and the readability of patient education materials, *J Fam Pract* 31:533-538, 1990.

INDEX[SM], and Fry formulas correlate highly with each other.

Of the more than 30 formulas assessing readability,[20] Fry[21] developed one that can assess passages of 40 to 300 words. Fry's formulas use a dictionary that gives grade levels for 43,000 words. Also, several software packages can calculate readability formulas. The user selects several random samples (representative of the text) of 100 words, types the text into the computer, and receives the calculated readability score.[39]

A sample of a pamphlet for use by the lay public is shown in Figure 3-3. Consider the objectives that this pamphlet meets. Its statements seem to be correct. Some pictures are used to create interest or explain content. The organization of the pamphlet is clearly outlined and reinforced with visual cues throughout the body of the pamphlet. The final messages left with the reader are important ones about prevention and

taking action if one has symptoms of pneumonia. Check the readability level.

Many health agencies prepare some teaching aids of their own, often incorporating schedules or procedures specific to that agency. These written materials must also be considered in light of the objectives they must meet, the validity of the material, and the likelihood of patient comprehension.

The "Planning Home Care" guide for caregivers of persons with Alzheimer's disease is presented in Box 3-18. Its implicit objective is to develop self-efficacy for caregiver coping skills. It is organized around simple suggestions and accompanied with pictures to serve as visual cues to jog memory.

Literacy

While readability formulas are used to analyze text, tests of reading ability are administered to

Box 3-11 · *Sample Patient Information Handouts*

Sample A

The sample below is a typical patient information handout, written at the reading level of a high school graduate or higher, that would be given to patients whose reading ability appears to be at that level. Sample B is the same handout, rewritten at a fifth-grade level of reading ability, and more appropriate for those patients with less developed reading skills.

Strep Throat

The physician will treat your strep throat by first ordering a throat culture to make sure you have the streptococcus organism and, if you do, then prescribing medicine. You could receive either a penicillin injection or have to take oral antibiotic medicine for a prescribed length of time. It is essential that you take all the medicine your physician has ordered because if you don't, the infection could continue. When you have finished the oral antibiotic, you may have to come back and see the doctor and have another throat culture. Ask your doctor if you need to return and then call a week in advance for an appointment.

Here are some things you can do. It is important to rest and get sufficient sleep; naps are recommended. Try to drink plenty of water and juice. For example, drink at least five glasses of water and two glasses of juice every day; more if possible. If your throat is painful or you develop a fever, take one or two Tylenol not any more frequently than every four hours. A simple solution of salt water may help the soreness in your throat. Put ¼ teaspoon of salt in one cup of warm water and gargle gently with this as often as needed.

Do not return to work or school until your fever is gone and you have improved. In any case, you must wait at least 24 hours after you have had your shot to return to work or school and, if you are taking oral medication, you must wait at least 48 hours after beginning your pills to go back. This is so you will no longer be contagious when you return.

Follow these instructions and you should be feeling better soon. If you don't improve in a couple of days, however, call the office and ask to speak to the nurse.

Sample B

The sample patient handout below contains the same information as Sample A above but is written at a fifth-grade level of reading ability for those patients with weaker reading skills. Note the simpler vocabulary and sentence structure, the use of questions to focus reader attention on specific points, and the use of bold type to highlight important information.

Sore Throat Caused by Streptococcus

HOW WILL THE DOCTOR TAKE CARE OF MY STREP THROAT?

1. The doctor will order medicine for me. I may have to get a shot (penicillin). I may have to take __ pills (antibiotic) every day, for __ days.
2. It is very important that I take all my pills. Even when my sore throat goes away, I must finish taking my pills. If I do not take all my pills, I could get sick again.
3. I may have to come back to see the doctor again. When all my pills are gone, I might need a test (throat culture). If so, I will come back on ____.

HOW CAN I HELP MYSELF GET BETTER?

1. I need to sleep more. Naps are important to get more sleep.
2. I need to drink lots of water and juice. Try to drink 5 glasses of water and 2 glasses of juice a day.
3. TYLENOL medicine can be taken, if I feel hot or have a sore throat. Only take one or two pills of TYLENOL at one time. Do not take TYLENOL any more often than every four hours.
4. I can gargle with warm salt water to help my sore throat. Put a small amount of salt in a spoon and add to a cup of warm water. Gargle gently with the warm salt water as often as it helps.
5. I will not go back to work or school until ____. If I feel hot or sick, I will stay home and rest. If my sore throat does not go away in __ days, I will call the nurse at __ (telephone number).

When I have a bad sore throat, if I see a doctor and take all my pills and rest and drink lots of water, then I will soon feel better.

From Dixon E, Park R: Do patients understand written health information? *Nurs Outlook* 38:278-281, 1990.

Box 3-12   *Sample Material*

Written at the Thirteenth-Grade Level

The heart usually receives electrical signals from the sinoatrial node, an area in the top right chamber. In ventricular tachycardia the signals that orchestrate the rhythm originate in the ventricle, located below the atrium. This area of origin results in an erratic beat or rhythm. The erratic beat disables the ventricles from contracting; thus blood is unable to be pumped out adequately. Inadequate blood supply affects all body parts since oxygen and nutrients are located in the blood. When the brain does not receive adequate blood supply, symptoms that include fainting, dizziness, and unconsciousness can occur. Stroke and death are also potential results.

With the knowledge that ventricular tachycardia is an erratic and potentially fatal rhythm that can occur at unpredictable times, physicians usually prescribe medications to control or prevent that rhythm. When medications are unable to keep the erratic beat dormant, the heart may require defibrillation. Defibrillation resets the electrical circuit, allowing the sinoatrial node to once again dominate.

Rewritten at the Sixth-Grade Level

Electrical signals from the heart's pacemaker keep the heart beating in a normal way. The pacemaker is called the S-A node and is found in the top part of the heart. Signals can also come from the bottom part of the heart. If they come from the bottom part, an irregular or rapid beat results. Several rapid and irregular beats are called V Tach. V Tach means the heart is not able to pump blood. When this happens, the body is not able to get the blood it needs. Blood carries oxygen and food to the body. One of the body parts that needs blood most is the brain. When the brain does not get blood, it can make a person feel faint or dizzy. It can also cause a stroke or death.

Doctors order medicines to try to control or stop this irregular or rapid beat. The medicines usually control this type of beat. Sometimes they do not work. The heart may then need to be shocked. The shock is given by a machine called a defibrillator. The shock usually helps the heart to reset its signals. It then beats in a regular way. All parts of the body can then get the supply of blood they need.

From Evanoski CAM: Health education for patients with ventricular tachycardia: assessment of readability, *J Cardiovasc Nurs* 4(2):1-6, 1990.

Box 3-13   *Directions for Using the Readability Graph*

1. Select three one-hundred-word passages from near the beginning, middle, and end of the book. Skip all proper nouns.
2. Count the total number of sentences in each hundred-word passage (estimating to nearest tenth of a sentence). Average these three numbers.
3. Count the total number of syllables in each hundred-word sample. There is a syllable for each vowel sound; for example: cat (1), blackbird (2), continental (4). Don't be fooled by word size; for example: polio (3), through (1).

Endings such as -y, -ed, -el, or -le usually make a syllable, for example: ready (2), bottle (2). I find it convenient to count every syllable over one in each word and add 100. Average the total number of syllables for the three samples.

4. Plot on the graph the average number of sentences per hundred words and the average number of syllables per hundred words. Most plot points fall near the heavy curved line. Perpendicular lines mark off approximate grade level areas.

Example

	Sentences Per 100 Words	Syllables Per 100 Words
100-word sample page 5	9.1	122
100-word sample page 89	8.5	140
100-word sample page 160	7.0	129
	3)24.6	3)391
Average	8.2	130

Plotting these averages on the graph, we find they fall in the 5th grade area; hence the book is about 5th grade difficulty level. If great variability is encountered either in sentence length or in the syllable count for the three selections, then randomly select several more passages and average them in before plotting.

From Fry E: A readability formula that saves time, *J Reading* 11:513-516, 1968.

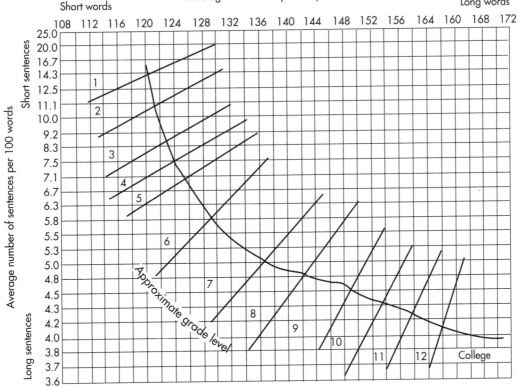

Figure 3-2 Graph for estimating readability. *Directions:* Randomly select three 100-word passages from a book or article. Plot average number of syllables and average number of words per sentence on graph to determine area of readability level. Choose more passages per book if great variability is observed. (From Fry E: A readability formula that saves time, *J Reading* 11:513-516, 1968.)

Box 3-14   *Gunning FOG INDEX^{SM} Scale*

1. Select a sample of writing 100 to 125 words long. If the piece is long, take several samples and average the results.
2. Calculate the average number of words per sentence. Treat independent clauses as separate sentences. "In school we studied; we learned; we improved" counts as three sentences.
3. Count the number of words of three syllables or more. In your count, omit capitalized words; combinations of short words like *bookkeeper* or *manpower*; or verbs made into three syllables by adding "-es" or "-ed." Divide the count of long words by the passage length to get the percentage.
4. Add the results of 2 (average sentence length) and 3 (percentage of long words). Multiply the sum by the factor 0.4, and ignore the digits following the decimal point.

The result is the years of schooling needed to read the passage with ease. Few readers have over 17 years of schooling, so any passage over 17 gets a FOG INDEX^{SM} of "17-plus."

From Gunning R, Kallan R: *How to take the fog out of business writing,* Chicago, 1994, Dartnell. The FOG INDEX^{SM} Scale is a service mark licensed exclusively to RKCommunication Consultants by D. and M. Mueller.

Box 3-15 *Flesch Formula*

1. For short pieces, test the entire selection. For longer pieces, test at least three randomly selected samples of 100 words each. Do not use introductory paragraphs as part of the sample. Start each sample at the beginning of a paragraph.
2. Determine the average sentence length by counting the number of words in the sample and dividing by the number of sentences. Count as a sentence each independent unit of thought that is grammatically independent, that is, if its end is punctuated by a period, question mark, exclamation point, semicolon, or colon. In dialogue, count speech tags (e.g., "he said") as part of the quoted sentence.
3. Determine the word length by counting all the syllables in the sample as if reading the words aloud. Divide the syllables by the number of words in the sample and multiply by 100.
4. These indices are then applied to the formula to compute the reading ease,

$$RE = 206.835 - 1.015\ SL - .846\ WL$$

where *RE* is the reading ease score, *SL* is the average sentence length in words, and *WL* is the average word length measured as syllables per 100 words.

Interpretation of Flesch Reading Ease Score

READING EASE	GRADE	DESCRIPTION OF STYLE	NO. SYLLABLES/100 WORDS	AVERAGE SENTENCE LENGTH
90-100	5	Very easy	123	8
80-90	6	Easy	131	11
70-80	7	Fairly easy	139	14
60-70	8-9	Standard	147	17
50-60	10-12	Fairly difficult	155	21
30-50	College	Difficult	167	25
0-30	College graduate	Very difficult	192	29

From Flesch R: *The art of readable writing*, New York, 1974, Harper & Row, pp 184-186, 247-251.

---

individuals for the purpose of selecting appropriate teaching interventions. Of the available tests that have been commonly used in clinical settings, two are health specific. Table 3-2 describes the tests.[32] Signed informed consent before use may be required since this information may be embarrassing or be used in a biased way if confidentiality is broken. Results should not be recorded in medical charts. The tests can also be used in populations to identify the kinds of educational materials they could use.

Since functional literacy varies by context and setting, tests specific to health are likely to be more useful. Health literacy encompasses a constellation of skills including the ability to perform basic reading and numeracy tasks required to function in the health environment. Interest in it is sparked in part by the fact that health professionals and institutions have liability for adverse outcomes of patients who do not understand important health information. Literacy is not only a reading problem; because of limited vocabulary or difficulty following complex sentence structure, these patients are also likely to struggle with oral communication.

Further information on the Test of Functional Health Literacy in Adults (TOFHLA) may be obtained in Nurss and others.[42] It measures comprehension skills in the middle to low levels of literacy ability and takes up to 22 minutes to administer. TOFHLA incorporates common health tasks such as reading prescription vials, interpreting an appointment slip, using a chart describing eligibility for financial aid, understanding results from medical tests, following instructions for an upper gastrointestinal tract test, understanding the patient rights and responsibilities section of a Medicaid application form, and comprehending a standard hospital informed consent form. Baker and others[2] found that 19% of high school graduates in their study showed inadequate literacy and 11% marginal

---

Box 3-16   *SMOG Testing*

The SMOG formula was originally developed by G. Harry McLaughlin in 1969. It will predict the grade-level difficulty of a passage within 1.5 grades in 68% of the passages tested. That may be close enough for your purposes. It is simple to use and faster than most other measures. The procedure is presented below.

Instructions

1. You will need 30 sentences. Count out 10 consecutive sentences near the beginning, 10 consecutive from the middle, and 10 from the end. For this purpose, a sentence is any string of words punctuated by a period (.), an exclamation point (!), or a question mark (?).
2. From the entire 30 sentences, count the words containing three or more syllables, including repetitions.
3. Obtain the grade level from the table to the right, or you may calculate the grade level as follows: Determine the nearest perfect square root of the total number of words of three or more syllables and then add a constant of 3 to the square root to obtain the grade level.

Example

Total number of multisyllabic (3 or more syllables) words	67
Nearest perfect square	64
Square root	8
Add constant of 3	11—This is the grade level

Table A. SMOG Conversion Table

Word Count	Grade Level
0-2	4
3-6	5
7-12	6
13-20	7
31-42	8
43-56	9
57-72	10
73-90	12
91-110	13
111-132	14
133-156	15
157-182	16
183-210	17
211-240	18

Developed by Harold C. McGraw, Office of Educational Research, Baltimore County Public Schools, Towson, Maryland.

From McLaughlin GH: SMOG grading: a new readability formula, *J Reading* 12:639-646, 1969; Doak CC, Doak LG, Root JH: *Teaching patients with low literacy skills*, Philadelphia, 1985, JB Lippincott.

---

literacy as measured by TOFHLA. These patients were seeking medical care in the walk-in clinic of an emergency department.

Rapid Estimate of Adult Literacy in Medicine (REALM) is a 66-word reading recognition test that can be used to screen for low literacy in a few minutes. The word list and directions for administering and scoring may be found in Figure 3-4.[13]

One of five adult Americans is functionally illiterate, reading at or below the fifth-grade level. Concentrated in inner city populations, in minorities and among those older than 65 years of age, these individuals understand little if any of the written materials provided for them by health professionals. Five percent of the adult population cannot read. Even the use of audiotaped instructions taxes the language and thinking skills of these persons. These patients may also have problems with basic clinician-patient communication (such as three times a day) and lack the necessary vocabulary to ask pertinent questions.[13]

Many individuals who are illiterate have normal or above normal IQs. They will nearly always try to conceal their illiteracy and will use excuses such as not having time or having left their eyeglasses at home. They may be articulate and well dressed. Frequently, they "go along" and react positively even when they do not understand. However, illiterate persons cannot use reference documents or catalogs effectively, can-

---

Box 3-17 *Special Rules for SMOG Testing*

Hyphenated words are one word.

For numerals, pronounce them aloud and count the syllables pronounced for each numeral (e.g., for the number 573, five = 1, hundred = 2, seventy = 3, and three = 1, for a total of 7 syllables).

Proper nouns should be counted.

If a long sentence has a colon, consider each part of it as a separate sentence. However, if possible, avoid selecting that segment of the passage.

The words for which abbreviations stand should be read aloud to determine their syllable count (e.g., Oct. = October = 3 syllables).

SMOG on Shorter Passages

Sometimes it may be necessary to assess the readability of a passage of less than 30 sentences. You can still use the SMOG formula to obtain an approximate grade level by using a conversion number from Table B and then using Table A (see Box 3-16) to find the grade level.

First count the number of sentences in your material and the number of words with three or more syllables. In Table B, in the left-hand column, locate the number of sentences, and locate the conversion number in the column opposite. Multiply the word count found earlier by the conversion number. Use this number in Table B to obtain the corresponding grade level.

For example, suppose your material consisted of 15 sentences and you counted 12 words of three or more syllables in this material. Proceed as follows:

1. In Table B, left-hand column, locate the number of sentences in your material. For your material, the number is 15.
2. Opposite 15 in the adjacent column, find the conversion number. The conversion number for 15 is 2.00.
3. Multiply your word count, 12, by 2 to get 24.
4. Now look at Table A to find the grade level. For a word count of 24, the grade level is 8.

Table B. SMOG Conversion for Samples With Fewer Than 30 Sentences	
Number of Sentences in Sample Material	Conversion Number
29	1.03
28	1.07
27	1.10
26	1.15
25	1.20
24	1.25
23	1.30
22	1.36
21	1.43
20	1.50
19	1.58
18	1.67
17	1.76
16	1.87
15	2.00
14	2.14
13	2.30
12	2.50
11	2.70
10	3.00

From McLaughlin GH: SMOG grading: a new readability formula, *J Reading* 12:639-646, 1969; Doak CC, Doak LG, Root JH: *Teaching patients with low literacy skills*, Philadelphia, 1985, JB Lippincott.

---

not follow instruction sheets, or cannot comprehend simple road maps.[24] In focus groups, low-literacy patients did not know what "orally" meant and were not sure if medications for an ear infection should go in the mouth or in the ear.[36]

The consequences of this problem affect the patient and the caregiver responsible for the patient's well-being; the caregiver also faces the possibility of litigation initiated by a patient acting without knowledge that should have been provided. Thus techniques known to be most effective should be used to teach these individuals.[15]

1. Eliminate everything that is extraneous.
2. Build to complexity when it is necessary; break content into components; and build with review, feedback, and questions.
3. Require patients to demonstrate what they have learned.
4. Give more rewards to those who are

Text continued on p. 68

What is Pneumonia?

Pneumonia is a serious infection or inflammation of your lungs. The air sacs in the lungs fill with pus and other liquid. Oxygen has trouble reaching your blood. If there is too little oxygen in your blood, your body cells can't work properly and you may die.

Until 1936, pneumonia was the number one cause of death in the U.S. Then the use of antibiotics brought it under control. Now this deadly enemy is making a comeback, in part because some bacteria can resist antibiotics. Pneumonia and influenza combined have ranked as the sixth leading cause of death since 1979.

Pneumonia affects your lungs in two ways. *Lobar* pneumonia affects a section (lobe) of a lung (see diagram below).

Bronchial pneumonia (or bronchopneumonia) affects patches throughout both lungs (see diagram below).

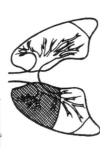

■ Affected area

©1996 American Lung Association

1

Pneumonia is not a single disease. It can have over 30 different causes. There are four main causes of pneumonia:

Causes of Pneumonia

1. Bacteria
2. Viruses
3. Mycoplasmas
4. Other causes, such as pneumocystis

Bacterial Pneumonia

Bacterial pneumonia can attack anyone from infants through the very old. Alcoholics, the debilitated, postoperative patients, people with respiratory diseases or viral infections, and people who have weakened immune systems are at greater risk.

Pneumonia bacteria are present in some healthy throats. When body defenses are weakened in some way—by illness, old age, malnutrition, general debility or impaired immunity—the bacteria can multiply and cause serious damage. Usually when a person's resistance is lowered, bacteria work their way into the lungs and inflame the air sacs.

The tissue of part of a lobe of the lung, an entire lobe, or even most of the lung's five lobes becomes completely filled with liquid (this is called "consolidation"). The infection quickly spreads through the bloodstream and the whole body is invaded.

The *pneumococcus* is the most common cause of bacterial pneumonia. It is one form of pneumonia for which a vaccine is available.

Symptoms: The onset of bacterial pneumonia can vary from gradual to sudden. In the most severe cases, the patient may experience shaking chills, chattering teeth, severe chest pain, and a cough that produces rust-colored or greenish mucus. A person's temperature often rises as high as 105 degrees F. The patient sweats profusely and breathing and pulse rate increase rapidly. Lips and nail beds may have a bluish color due to lack of oxygen in the blood. A patient's mental state may be confused or delirious.

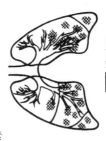

2

Viral Pneumonia

Half of all pneumonias are believed to be caused by viruses. More and more viruses are being identified as the cause of respiratory infection, and though most attack the upper respiratory tract, some produce pneumonia, especially in children. Most of these pneumonias are not serious and last a short time.

Influenza virus may be severe and occasionally fatal. The virus invades the lungs and multiplies, but there are almost no physical signs of lung tissue becoming filled with liquid. It finds many of its victims among those who have heart or lung disease or who are pregnant.

Symptoms: The initial symptoms of viral pneumonia are the same as influenza symptoms: fever, a dry cough, headache, muscle pain, and weakness. Within 12 to 36 hours, there is increasing breathlessness; the cough becomes worse and produces a small amount of mucus. There is a high fever and there may be blueness of the lips. In extreme cases, the patient has a desperate need for air and severe breathlessness. Other viral pneumonias are complicated by an invasion of bacteria—with all the typical symptoms of *bacterial* pneumonia.

Mycoplasma Pneumonia

Because of its somewhat different symptoms and physical signs, and because the course of the illness differed from classic pneumococcal pneumonia, mycoplasma pneumonia was once believed to be caused by one or more undiscovered viruses and was called "primary atypical pneumonia."

Identified during World War II, mycoplasmas are the smallest free-living agents of disease in man, unclassified as to whether they are bacteria or viruses, but having characteristics of both, they generally cause a mild and widespread pneumonia. They affect all age groups, occurring most frequently in older children and young adults. The death rate is low, even in untreated cases.

3

Symptoms: The most prominent symptom of mycoplasma pneumonia is a cough that tends to come in violent attacks, but produces only sparse, whitish mucus. Chills and fever are early symptoms, and some patients experience nausea or vomiting. The patient's heartbeat is often slow and in some extreme cases patients may suffer from breathlessness and have a bluish color to lips and nail beds.

Other Kinds of Pneumonia

Pneumocystis carinii pneumonia (PCP) is caused by an organism long thought of as a parasite but now believed to be a fungus. PCP is the first sign of illness in many persons with AIDS, and perhaps 80 percent of AIDS patients (four out of five) will develop it sooner or later. It can be successfully treated in many cases. It may recur a few months later, but treatment can help to prevent or delay its recurrence.

Other less common pneumonias may be quite serious and are occurring more often. Various special pneumonias are caused by the inhalation of food, liquid, gases or dust, and by fungi. Foreign bodies or a bronchial obstruction such as a tumor may promote the occurrence of pneumonia, although they are not causes of pneumonia. Rickettsia (also considered an organism somewhere between viruses and bacteria) cause Rocky Mountain spotted fever, Q fever, typhus, and psittacosis—diseases that may have mild or severe effects on the lungs. Tuberculosis pneumonia is a very serious lung infection and is extremely dangerous unless treated early.

Pneumonia Treatment and Recovery

If you develop pneumonia, your chances of a fast recovery are greatest under certain conditions: if you're young, if your pneumonia is caught early, if your defenses against disease are working well, if the infection hasn't spread, and if you're not suffering from other illnesses.

4

Continued

Figure 3-3 Sample instructional pamphlet to be used for the lay public. (Courtesy American Lung Association.)

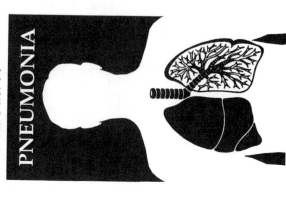

facts about...
PNEUMONIA

In the young and healthy, early treatment with antibiotics can cure bacterial pneumonia and speed recovery from mycoplasma pneumonia and a certain percentage of rickettsia cases. There is no effective treatment yet for viral pneumonia, which usually heals on its own.

The drugs used to fight pneumonia are determined by the germ causing the pneumonia and the judgment of the doctor. After a patient's temperature returns to normal, medication must be continued according to the doctor's instructions— otherwise the pneumonia may recur. Relapses can be far more serious than the first attack.

Besides antibiotics, patients are given supportive treatment: proper diet and oxygen to increase oxygen in the blood when needed. In some patients, medication to ease chest pain and to provide relief from violent cough may be necessary.

The vigorous young person may lead a normal life within a week of recovery from pneumonia. For the middle-aged, however, weeks may elapse before they regain their accustomed strength, vigor, and feeling of well-being. A person recovering from mycoplasma pneumonia may be weak for an extended period of time. In general, a person should not be discouraged from returning to work or carrying out usual activities but must be warned to expect some difficulties. Adequate rest is important to maintain progress toward full recovery and to avoid relapse. Remember—don't rush recovery!

Prevention is Possible

Because pneumonia is a common complication of influenza (flu), getting an influenza shot every fall is good pneumonia prevention.

Vaccine is also available to help fight pneumococcal pneumonia—one type of bacterial pneumonia. Your doctor can help you decide if you—or a member of your family—needs the vaccine against pneumococcal pneumonia. It is usually given only to people at high risk of getting the disease and its life-threatening complications.

5

The greatest risk of pneumococcal pneumonia is usually among people who:

• Have chronic illnesses such as lung disease, heart disease, kidney disorders, sickle cell anemia, or diabetes.

• Are recovering from severe illness.

• Are in nursing homes or other chronic care facilities.

• Are age 65 or older.

If you are at risk, ask your doctor for a pneumococcal pneumonia shot.

The vaccine is generally given only once. Ask your doctor about any revaccination recommendations. The vaccine is not recommended for pregnant women or children under age two.

Since pneumonia often follows ordinary respiratory infections, the most important preventive measure is to be alert to any symptoms of respiratory trouble that linger more than a few days. Good health habits—proper diet and hygiene, rest, regular exercise, etc.—increase resistance to all respiratory illnesses. They also help promote fast recovery when illness does occur.

If You Have Symptoms of Pneumonia

1. Call your doctor immediately. Even with the many effective antibiotics, early diagnosis and treatment are important.

2. Follow your doctor's advice. In serious cases, your doctor may advise a hospital stay. Or recovery at home may be possible.

3. Continue to take the medicine your doctor prescribes until told you may stop. This will help prevent recurrence of pneumonia and relapse.

4. Remember—even though pneumonia can be treated, it is an extremely serious illness. Don't wait, get treatment early.

6

To find out more about pneumonia and other types of lung disease, contact your local American Lung Association by dialing 1-800-LUNG-USA (1-800-586-4872).

We need your support to fight lung disease, the third leading cause of death in the U.S. Call your local American Lung Association to find out how you can help.

Call 1-800-LUNG-USA
(1-800-586-4872)

When You Can't Breathe, Nothing Else Matters®

AMERICAN LUNG ASSOCIATION®

0029   11/96

Figure 3-3, cont'd

Box 3-18	*Planning Home Care*

Dear Caregiver:

Taking care of a patient with Alzheimer's disease requires patience and understanding—and it requires you to look at the patient's environment with new eyes. Then you need to change that environment to help him function as well as possible.

Keeping these points in mind, read over the following tips to help you plan your daily care.

Reduce Stress

Too much stress can worsen the patient's symptoms—he can become combative and severely agitated. Try to protect him from the following potential sources of stress:
- A change in routine, caregiver, or environment
- Fatigue
- Excessive demands
- Overwhelming, misleading, or competing stimuli
- Illness and pain
- Over-the-counter medications

Establish a Routine

Keep the patient's daily routine stable so he can respond automatically; adapting to change may require more thought than he can handle. Even eating a different food or going to a strange grocery store may overwhelm him.

Also, make a schedule of the patient's daily activities:
- List the activities necessary for his daily care, and include ones that he especially enjoys (such as weeding in the garden). Designate a time frame for each activity.
- Establish bedtime rituals—especially important to promote relaxation and a restful night's sleep for both of you.
- Stick to your schedule as closely as possible (for example, breakfast first, then dressing) so the patient won't be surprised or need to make decisions.
- Keep a copy of the schedule for other caregivers. To help them give better care, include notes and suggestions about techniques that work for you; for instance, "Speak in a quiet voice" or "When helping Mitchell dress or bathe, take things one step at a time, and wait for him to respond."

Practice Reality Orientation

In your conversations with the patient, orient him to the day and the activity he'll perform. For instance,

say "Today is Tuesday and we're going to have breakfast now." Do this every day. The patient will be more aware of his immediate environment, and he'll know what to expect without being challenged to remember events.

Simplify the Surroundings

Eventually, the patient won't be able to correctly interpret what he sees and hears. Protect him by trying to decrease the noise level in his environment and by avoiding busy areas, such as shopping malls and restaurants.

Does the patient mistake pictures or images in the mirror for real people? If so, remove the photos and mirrors. Also, avoid rooms with busy patterns on wallpaper and carpets because they can overtax his senses.

To avoid confusion and encourage the patient's independence, provide cues. For example, hang a picture of a toilet on the bathroom door.

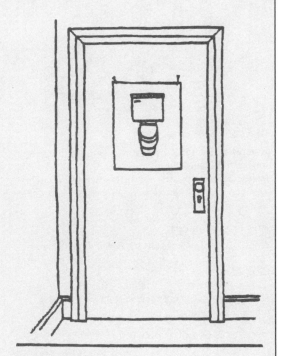

From A caregiver's guide: planning home care, *Nursing 92* 22(5):75-82, 1992.

Continued

Box 3-18	*Planning Home Care—cont'd*

Avoid Fatigue

The patient will tire easily, so plan important activities for the morning when he's functioning best; save less demanding ones for later in the day. Remember to schedule breaks. In the early stages of the disease, he'll need about 15 to 30 minutes of listening to music or just relaxing in the morning and in the afternoon. As the disease progresses, schedule longer, more frequent breaks (perhaps 40 to 90 minutes). If the patient naps during the day, have him sleep in a reclining chair rather than in a bed so he won't confuse day and night.

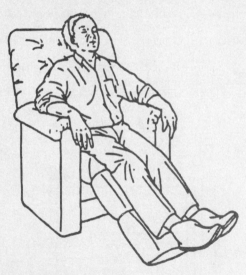

Don't Expect Too Much

Accept the patient's limitations. Don't demand too much from him—this forces him to think about a task and causes frustration. Instead, offer help when needed, and distract him if he's trying too hard. You'll feel less stressed too.

Prepare for Illness

If the patient becomes ill, his behavior will deteriorate. He'll have a low tolerance for pain and discomfort.

Never rely on the patient to take his own medicine. He may forget to take it or miscount what he's taken. Always supervise him.

Use the Sense of Touch

Because the patient's visual and auditory perceptions are distorted, he has an increased need for closeness and touching. Remember to approach him from the front—you don't want to frighten him or provoke belligerent or aggressive behavior.

Respect his need for personal space. Limit physical contact to his hands and arms at first, then move to more central parts of his body, such as his shoulders or head.

Using long or circular motions, lightly stroke the patient to help relieve muscle tension and give him a sense of his physical self. Physical contact also expresses your feelings of intimacy and caring.

Allowing the patient to touch objects in the environment can help relieve stress by providing information. Let him handle, poke, pull, or shake objects—for example, a handbag, a brush, or a comb. Make sure they're unbreakable and can't harm him.

Handle Problem Behavior

If the patient becomes restless or agitated, divert his attention with appropriate activity. Good choices include walking, rocking in a rocking chair, sanding wood, folding laundry, or hoeing in the garden. These repetitive activities don't require any particular sequence or planning. A warm bath, a drink of warm milk, or a back massage can also be calming.

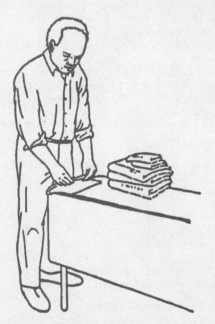

Although problem behavior can be taxing, try to remember that the patient can't help himself. Your understanding and compassion can increase his sense of security.

| TABLE 3-2 | Formal Literacy Screening Tests |

Test	Description	Advantages	Disadvantages
TOFHLA (Test of Functional Health Literacy in Adults)	50-item comprehension and 17-item numerical ability test based on tasks often required of patients seeking health care (e.g., reading prescription bottle or appointment slip).	Only test that evaluates numeracy skills Soon available in Spanish Assesses comprehension, not just word recognition	Not validated prospectively Not available for clinical use
WRAT-R (Wide Range Achievement Test-Revised)	Reading recognition test.	Takes 3-5 min More accurate than REALM in assessing degree of impairment	Not available in Spanish
SORT-R (Slosson Oral Reading Test-Revised)	Measures ability to pronounce words of varying difficulty.	Easy to administer and score	Patients dislike the small print and large number of items
PIAT-R (Peabody Individual Achievement Test-Revised)	Reading comprehension subset consists of 88 items. Patients read a sentence and choose from among 4 pictures the one that best represents the meaning of the task.	Assesses comprehension rather than word recognition	Long, takes 30-40 min to complete
REALM (Rapid Estimate of Adult Literacy in Medicine)	Reading recognition test that measures patients' ability to pronounce medical terms. This 66-item version is still valid; much faster than 125-item version. Patients read as many words aloud as possible. Words correctly pronounced scored as plus, nonattempted words scored as minus, and incorrectly pronounced ones as a check.	Items in test relevant to medicine Takes 3-5 min	Spanish version not valid

From Lasater L, Mehler PS: The illiterate patient: screening and management, *Hosp Pract* 33(4):163-170, 1998.

RAPID ESTIMATE OF ADULT LITERACY IN MEDICINE
(REALM)©

Terry Davis, PhD • Michael Crouch, MD • Sandy Long, PhD

Patient Name/
Subject # _____ Date of Birth _____

Reading
Level _____

Grade
Completed _____

Date _____ Clinic _____ Examiner _____

List 1		List 2		List 3	
fat	____	fatigue	____	allergic	____
flu	____	pelvic	____	menstrual	____
pill	____	jaundice	____	testicle	____
dose	____	infection	____	colitis	____
eye	____	exercise	____	emergency	____
stress	____	behavior	____	medication	____
smear	____	prescription	____	occupation	____
nerves	____	notify	____	sexually	____
germs	____	gallbladder	____	alcoholism	____
meals	____	calories	____	irritation	____
disease	____	depression	____	constipation	____
cancer	____	miscarriage	____	gonorrhea	____
caffeine	____	pregnancy	____	inflammatory	____
attack	____	arthritis	____	diabetes	____
kidney	____	nutrition	____	hepatitis	____
hormones	____	menopause	____	antibiotics	____
herpes	____	appendix	____	diagnosis	____
seizure	____	abnormal	____	potassium	____
bowel	____	syphilis	____	anemia	____
asthma	____	hemorrhoids	____	obesity	____
rectal	____	nausea	____	osteoporosis	____
incest	____	directed	____	impetigo	____

SCORE

List 1 _____
List 2 _____
List 3 _____
Raw
Score _____

Figure 3-4 Rapid Estimate of Adult Literacy in Medicine (REALM)©. (From Davis TL and others: Practical assessment of adult literacy in health care, *Health Educ Behav* 25: 613-624, 1998.)

Continued

RAPID ESTIMATE OF ADULT LITERACY IN MEDICINE

The Rapid Estimate of Adult Literacy in Medicine (REALM) is a screening instrument to assess an adult patient's ability to read common medical words and lay terms for body parts and illnesses. It is designed to assist medical professionals in estimating a patient's literacy level so that the appropriate level of patient education materials or oral instructions may be used. The test takes 2 to 3 minutes to administer and score. The REALM has been correlated with other standardized tests.

Correlation of REALM with SORT, PIAT-R, and WRAT-R			
	PIAT-R Recognition	SORT	WRAT-R
Correlation Coefficient	.97	.96	.88
P Value	p<.0001	p<.0001	p<.0001

Reliability Studies	
Test-Retest	Inter-Rater
(n = 100)	(n = 20)
.99	.99

DIRECTIONS:

1. Give the patient a laminated copy of the REALM and score answers on an unlaminated copy that is attached to a clipboard. Hold the clipboard at an angle so that the patient is not distracted by your scoring procedure. Say:

    "I want to hear you read as many words as you can from this list. Begin with the first word on List 1 and read aloud. When you come to a word you cannot read, do the best you can or say "blank" and go on to the next word."

2. If the patient takes more than five seconds on a word, say "blank" and point to the next word, if necessary, to move the patient along. If the patient begins to miss every word, have him/her pronounce only known words.

3. Count as an error any word not attempted or mispronounced. Score by marking a plus (+) after each correct word, a check (√) after each mispronounced word, and a minus (−) after words not attempted. Count as correct any self-corrected word.

4. Count the number of correct words for each list and record the numbers in the "SCORE" box. Total the numbers and match the total score with its grade equivalent in the table below.

GRADE EQUIVALENT	
Raw Score	Grade Range
0-18	**3rd Grade and Below** Will not be able to read most low literacy materials; will need repeated oral instructions, materials composed primarily of illustrations, or audio or video tapes.
19-44	**4th to 6th Grade** Will need low literacy materials; may not be able to read prescription labels.
45-60	**7th to 8th Grade** Will struggle with most patient education materials; will not be offended by low literacy materials.
61-66	**High School** Will be able to read most patient education materials.

Figure 3-4, cont'd

insecure in their ability to learn; they need more rewards than do others to accomplish small tasks.

5. To reduce the reading level and literacy demand, use a conversational style, active voice, short words, and short sentences.

6. Use visual aids, especially line drawings, with only one idea portrayed in each picture; use captions not longer than 10 words.

7. Show only correct behavior.

8. Organize material in the order patients will use it, and use words that are familiar to them.

9. Pretest all materials.

10. Use stories.

An example of a pamphlet for patients with limited literacy may be found in Figure 3-5. This is written at a lower reading level than the sixth-grade level recommended for instructional materials (75% of adult Americans are able to read at this level).[15] Other teaching approaches such as demonstration, group activities, and discussions may be more effective with these populations.

Computers

Computers are used for instructional purposes such as drill and practice in problem solving with feedback until a skill is mastered; for games; and as simulators in which one learns how, for example, to adjust insulin level with a program that models the body's blood glucose and responses to insulin, diet, and exercise. Based on an on-line assessment of what the patient understands, computers can provide highly individualized self-paced learning and can document the learning process. They can be used to elicit information from patients that can help tailor patient education and discharge planning. They can include photos and videos and narrated sound tracks for those with limited reading skills.

ComputerLink is a computer network that has been used to provide information and decision-support functions for caregivers of persons with Alzheimer's disease. A recent study[6] showed that this system enhanced the caregivers' confidence and decreased their sense of isolation, which is especially important in that other services are inaccessible because they require leaving home.

A behavioral treatment program for obesity uses an interactive microcomputer small enough to be carried by subjects during their normal daily routines. Learners make self-reports on consumption of food and exercise. If they forget to do so, they are reminded by the computer.

Computer games can help adolescents understand the responsibilities parents face, as well as the costs of childbirth and child rearing. Throughout the game, the teen's readiness for parenting is visually displayed on a thermometer gauge. The program simulates, for example, a 1-year-old with a fever who cries persistently at night or a 2-year-old with temper tantrums. A similar game called "Romance" addresses sex and birth control. It provides simulated outcomes and realistic information. After these games were introduced in clinics, teenage pregnancy rates declined by 15%. Computer-assisted instruction uses role-modeling and desensitization to raise teens' self-esteem. As teens gain new information, they are empowered with new ways to make decisions.[43]

Computers can generate individualized information leaflets. They incorporate new information easily. On-line, computer-based information systems can educate college students about topics such as acquired immunodeficiency syndrome (AIDS)—information that students might not seek at the health centers. Computer information systems can answer questions, offer recent research updates, and display guides to community services. They provide a useful and confidential source of information within a broader AIDS education program.[44]

Visual Materials

When one teaches about actual physical objects, it is often preferable to use the real thing. Nothing but a baby can act like a baby during a bath. However, models are useful when three dimensions must be retained but (1) the real thing is too small, large, complicated, or expensive;

(2) the real thing is unavailable; (3) the desired view cannot be exposed; or (4) the object cannot be manipulated. For example, for demonstrating the birth of a baby, a doll may be advanced through an actual-size model of the bony structure of the pelvis. Many times, anatomy and physiology cannot be adequately visualized with the use of a real person because other tissues are in the way or a body part, such as the eye, is too small and complex. A dummy can be useful for showing the position of a tracheostomy and how to remove and reinsert parts of the tube. It can also be used for practicing general movements with the suction tube. The dummy is clearly limited because it lacks functioning muscles and secretions. Some teachers would insist that it is better to start the learner working with a real tracheostoma. However, if a patient with one is not available, or if the available patient's tracheostoma is difficult to care for, early practice on a model may be helpful. Models in the form of dummies are used to teach resuscitation techniques because a person whose heart or breathing has stopped is not usually available.

Thus models may be used because they can teach better than real objects can or because they are more practical to use. At times they are absolutely essential. However, models frequently are expensive and may not be readily available in many places where patients are being taught.

The research literature on pictorial learning is sparse in comparison with that on verbal learning. The theory of how people learn from pictures is not completely developed. Pictorial learning is superior to verbal learning for recognition and recall. For example, pictographs (pictures that represent ideas and assist in their recall) attain meaning when they are explained and remind the person of the associated idea. A drawing of a toothbrush, teeth, three vertical lines, and the sun and moon are a reminder to brush teeth 3 times/day.[26] However, when the subject matter is abstract, it is difficult to communicate with pictures. Media used to convey pictures always distort the various visual dimensions—resolution, color fidelity, and size—to some degree. For example, paintings may eliminate or exaggerate various parts of an object. These distortions may or may not be important to a particular learning task.

Photographs and drawings lack the third dimension but are readily available or can be produced by the teacher. The third dimension is not imperative when the teacher is showing familiar objects or those in which shape and space are not the primary considerations. Examples that fall into these categories and are frequently not available include an infected finger or an abnormal stool in infants. However, the learner must be aware that odor can be important in recognizing abnormal stool. In both of these examples, photographs would be more desirable than diagrams because they more accurately portray the details of the real item.

Drawings are particularly pertinent for removing superfluous detail present in real objects. During an explanation to a patient about diverticulitis, visualization is obviously desirable. Whereas a photograph shows details of the tissue that the patient does not need to know, a simple line drawing can communicate the concept of a pouch in the intestinal wall. In other instances, drawings in the form of cartoons are used to create interest in a topic. Figure 3-5 presents instructions for hand injuries graphically enhanced and illustrated to improve patient understanding.[17]

Pictures may be presented in many ways, depending on the size of the audience and equipment available. For a single individual, visuals on paper 8½ by 11 inches can be used. For small groups, posters can be prepared. Drawings can be made with crayons or felt-tipped pens on flip charts (pads of paper approximately 32 by 26 inches) supported on an easel or chair back. Cutouts can be attached by magnets or flannel to metal or flannel boards. Drawings can be done on the chalkboard. Overhead projectors use transparencies (sheets of plastic) prepared with diagrams or drawn at the time of presentation and projected. More commonly, caregivers interact with an individual patient and use an easily obtained visual aid, such as a picture in the birth atlas, sketch the objects needed for a given lesson, or use a prepared teaching aid.

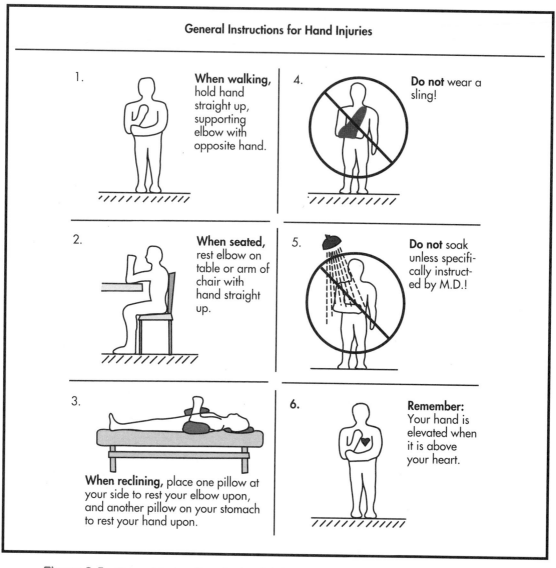

Figure 3-5 General instructions for hand injuries. (From Dooley AR: A collaborative model for creating patient education resources, *Am J Health Behav* 20(2):15-19, 1996.)

Teaching by television requires many of the same skills as doing an in-person demonstration. Videotapes can be used as "triggers," providing an instructional stimulus that can be followed by discussion groups. In addition, the teacher can use the film of the patient's own cardiac catheterization to teach both the patient and the family about the extent or the absence of cardiac problems. This approach eliminates generic information in other educational tools that may not be immediately useful to a particular patient. The information can be particularly helpful when a decision has to be made. Often, patients need concrete evidence to accept their diagnoses or to consider treatment options.[5]

Two reviews have summarized studies of television's power to produce an effect in patient education.[22,41] Use of videotapes is as effective as are other presentations. The most suitable educational applications of television are that (1) it presents powerful role models of particular behavior, attitudes, and values; (2) it presents vivid, active illustrative material not otherwise readily available; and (3) it provides direct feedback about a learner's performance of complex interpersonal and psychomotor skills (this assumes the person's performance is videotaped). From a practical point of view, videos are produced cheaply and can be tailor-made for a given patient population. Using video presentations ensures a standard level of teaching. They can be particularly effective now because of the high rate of functional illiteracy in the United States and because people probably are oriented more to viewing than to reading.

Screening, Preparing, and Testing Teaching Materials

All materials must be viewed and evaluated before they are used for teaching. Previewing is necessary to identify material that the teacher believes is incorrect or is contradictory to other sources being used. It may be necessary to reject an audiovisual aid because it is beyond the level of the learners' understanding or because the aid may be peripheral to the objectives. Materials must also be culturally relevant.

After preview, an instructional material or product should undergo two steps to improve its effectiveness as a teaching tool.

1. Product verification. Arrange a tryout of the materials under conditions approximating those in which the finally developed product will be used, using a pretest measure on each instructional objective; record time spent on program components, teacher-learner behavior, and other relevant measures of student use of the material; use a postassessment measure and release the materials for general use if performance is high on all objectives.
2. Product revision. Identify the objectives not well met; from data gathered in the verification step, propose revisions; test the revised version.

Learner data are most important in judging learnability. A more complete testing program should be used when there is no precedent for either the content or teaching method, when learning materials are more complex and expensive, when the materials seek to change attitudes rather than to increase knowledge, when materials are designed for long-term rather than short-term use; and when the target audience is large. This involves repetitive tryouts with individuals to identify major errors, repetitive tryouts with small groups, and a field test when the materials are well developed.

Sets of criteria for quality instructional materials, developed by two different authors, may be found in Box 3-19.[4] The criteria by Doak, Doak, and Root are scored into the Suitability Assessment of Materials and particularly incorporate literacy-relevant factors (Figure 3-6).[15]

Planning and Implementing Instruction

All items necessary for constructing a teaching plan have been introduced. Evaluation, which is also part of the plan, is discussed thoroughly in

Box 3-19   *Domain of Instructional Design Principles Survey*

1. Drawings/illustrations represent racial and ethnic groups.
2. The learning objectives are made clear to the target group.
3. The size of the patient education material (PEM) is one that is easily handled by the target group (5 × 8 inches is easy to handle; 8 × 10 inches is easy to file).
4. The learning objectives cover the main points to be learned from the PEM.
5. The learning objectives for the PEM and the procedures for accomplishing them are distinguishable.
6. The relevance of the educational content to the target group is clearly stated.
7. Only the most essential information is presented, using not more than 3-4 main points (i.e., what, where, when, and how).
8. Sentence parts are kept in logical order.
9. Titles and subtitles are clear and informative.
10. There is sufficient contrast between the ink and the paper to make reading easy.
11. Drawings/illustrations are labeled clearly.
12. The use of double (or multiple) negatives in sentences is avoided.
13. The content is presented in an unbiased manner that respects free choice on the part of the target group.
14. The content is presented in a way that relates and integrates the new information to what is already known and understood by the target group.
15. Mnemonic devices are used as retrieval cues for important information (e.g., ABC = Airway, Breaths, and Compressions for cardiopulmonary resuscitation [CPR].)
16. The material builds from the familiar to the unfamiliar.
17. The educational content is appropriate to community standards.
18. The focus of the PEM is on how to accomplish the learning task.
19. The educational content is written in a style that is patient-centered and specific.
20. The content includes descriptions of physical sensations that the target group is likely to experience during diagnostic and therapeutic procedures.
21. The vocabulary of the PEM comprises words commonly used by the target group.
22. Important ideas and points of content are repeated as reinforcement throughout the PEM.
23. Important information is organized as lists or categories.
24. The information most important to the target group is presented first.
25. One idea per paragraph is presented.
26. Short, simple sentences are used to convey one idea at a time.
27. Terms are used in a consistent manner throughout the PEM.
28. Supplemental information is separated from the main points and is provided as an appendix or other special section.
29. The PEM includes a space for patient-generated questions.
30. A listing of resources that provide additional information about the topic is included in the PEM.
31. Necessary health terms are defined.
32. Topic headings and advance organizers (e.g., topic outlines, introductory summaries) are used.
33. The content is presented in concrete terms rather than as abstract concepts and ideas.
34. The first sentence of each paragraph is the topic sentence.
35. Specific, precise instructions are given if the target group is expected to carry out some self-care activity.
36. The title of the PEM is short and conveys the meaning of the material.
37. Drawings/illustrations are recognizable to the target group with or without explanatory text.
38. A table of contents is provided for PEMs that are lengthy.
39. The table of contents is designed to match the readers' questions.
40. The PEM includes a space for patient-generated questions.
41. The content focuses on what the target group should do as well as what they need to know.
42. Drawings/illustrations accurately convey the content to improve understanding of the material.
43. Opportunities are provided in the text for the target group to use the new concepts just presented.

From Bernier MJ: Establishing the psychometric properties of a scale for evaluating quality in printed education materials, *Patient Educ Couns* 29:293-299, 1996.

Box 3-19 *Domain of Instructional Design Principles Survey—cont'd*

44. The main ideas of the PEM are divided into meaningful content units.
45. Drawings/illustrations present only essential content relevant to the educational purpose.
46. Specialized vocabulary lists are developed and placed at the front of the PEM for easy reader access.
47. Ideas are expressed using one- to two-syllable words as much as possible.
48. Drawings/illustrations are placed next to the text to which they refer.
49. The font or print size is easily read by the target group.
50. The second person, *you,* is used instead of the third person except in situations where the content may be emotionally charged (e.g., cancer or AIDS information).
51. The type style is easy to read.
52. The paper used in the PEM is of a nonglare (uncoated) type for ease of reading.
53. The lines of drawings/illustrations are heavy enough to be seen by the target group.
54. Questions are posed throughout the PEM as a means of engaging the reader in the content and highlighting the main points.
55. Contractions are used to make the text more personal (e.g., *you'll* instead of *you will*).
56. A positive writing style is used.
57. The content is verified as accurate by persons experienced in the content area.
58. Consideration is given to eye span of the text (e.g., 50-70 characters per line is most comfortable for reading).
59. The tone of the PEM is personal and nonthreatening.
60. Equal consideration to gender is given in the use of pronouns.
61. The content is respectful of the customs and traditions of the target group.
62. The writing style is one that engages the reader and stimulates active participation.
63. The PEM is written at a readability level that is appropriate to the target group (e.g., material intended for the general public should be written at the sixth- to eight-grade level).
64. The leading (space between each line of type) used facilitates reading (10-point type requires 2 points of leading; 11-point type requires 3 points, very small type requires more leading to make text less dense and more readable).
65. Color is used as a cuing agent to highlight materials and promote learning.
66. Drawings/illustrations represent gender equally where content is appropriate to both sexes.
67. Each drawing/illustration conveys a single idea or concept.
68. The purpose of the PEM is made clear to the target group of learners.
69. PEMs intended for long-term use are constructed of materials that will withstand handling and use.
70. The material moves from simpler to more complex content in a manner that is organized and logical.
71. The examples used in the PEM contain the central characteristics of the ideas and concepts under discussion.
72. Examples are used to bridge the gap between what the target group already knows and the content to be taught.
73. Both upper and lower case letters are used for ease of reading.
74. The information load of the material (amount of information and novelty/obscurity of information) is appropriate to the target group.
75. The most important information is highlighted in bold print.
76. The spacing and layout of text and drawings/illustrations are attractive and pleasing to the eye.
77. The lines of the text are justified for ease of reading.
78. The learning objectives and educational content of the PEM relate to one another.
79. The active voice is used.
80. The learning objectives of the PEM are related to the intended outcome.
81. Arabic numbers are used to facilitate ease of reading when numbers are included in the educational content.
82. The cover of the PEM is attractive and eye catching.
83. The PEM has aesthetic appeal.
84. The first lines of paragraphs are indented for ease of reading.
85. The margins surrounding the text are wide enough to provide ease of reading and space for note taking by the target group.
86. The educational content is current.
87. Accurate and coherent summaries/synopses of the message being delivered are included throughout the PEM.
88. Numbers are written as numbers rather than as text.
89. The ideas being presented in the PEM are logically related and present a coherent structure for the information being conveyed.
90. The colors used in the PEM should be in keeping with the mood of the topic.

2 points for superior rating
1 point for adequate rating
0 points for not suitable rating
N/A if the factor does not apply to this material

FACTOR TO BE RATED	SCORE	COMMENTS

1. CONTENT

(a)   Purpose is evident
(b)   Content about behaviors
(c)   Scope is limited
(d)   Summary or review included

2. LITERACY DEMAND

(a)   Reading grade level
(b)   Writing style, active voice
(c)   Vocabulary uses common words
(d)   Context is given first
(e)   Learning aids via "road signs"

3. GRAPHICS

(a)   Cover graphic shows purpose
(b)   Type of graphics
(c)   Relevance of illustrations
(d)   List, tables, etc., explained
(e)   Captions used for graphics

4. LAYOUT AND TYPOGRAPHY

(a)   Layout factors
(b)   Typography
(c)   Subheads ("chunking") used

5. LEARNING STIMULATION, MOTIVATION

(a)   Interaction used
(b)   Behaviors are modeled and specific
(c)   Motivation—self-efficacy

6. CULTURAL APPROPRIATENESS

(a)   Match in logic, language, experience
(b)   Cultural image and examples

Total SAM score: _____

Total possible score: _____ Percent score: _____%

Figure 3-6   SAM (Suitability Assessment of Materials) scoring sheet. (From Doak CC, Doak LG, Root JH: *Teaching patients with low literacy skills,* ed 2, Philadelphia, 1996, Lippincott.)

SAMPLE STANDARD TEACHING PLAN
Mutliple Sclerosis

Patient Learning Objectives	Content	Education Mode	Modifications/Comments	Objectives Met (Date/Initials)
Patient will define the remission/ exacerbation aspects of the disease process.	Infection, trauma, immunization, delivery after pregnancy, stress, climactic changes How remission/exacerbation is experienced	E D		
Patient will demonstrate how to use various community resources.	Local and national multiple sclerosis society chapters Public health nurse Visiting Nurse Association Community support groups Social workers, therapists Vocational rehabilitation agencies Home health agencies Extended and skilled care facilities Financial counseling	E P V RP		
Patient will specify the safety precautions associated with symptoms.	Decreased sensation Visual disturbances — Safety precautions Motor deficits	E R P		
Patient will take medications correctly and will recognize expected effects and side effects and interactions with over-the-counter medicines associated with each medication.	Corticosteroids How to take— Immunomodulators recognizing Cholinergics expected Anticholinergics effects and Muscle relaxants side effects	E R RP		
Patient will perform exercises to promote muscle strength and mobility.	Measures for preventing contractures and skin breakdown Transfer techniques and proper body mechanics Use of assistive devices and other measures to minimize neurological deficits	E R V M		
Patient will diagnose and self-manage constipation, urinary retention, or urinary tract infection (UTI), including proper self-catheterization technique or care of indwelling urinary catheters.	Constipation Urinary retention — How to UTI diagnosis and self-manage	E R		

Figure 3-7 Sample standard teaching plan.   *Continued*

Chapter 4. Because the purpose of a teaching plan is to force the teacher to examine the relationships among learner receptivity, objectives, content, teaching methods, tools, and evaluation, a plan should be written.

Teaching plans can be written in many formats. The major criterion for judging a format is whether it clearly states the various elements of the teaching process. Are the relationships among assessment-readiness, objectives, teaching actions, and content and evaluation clear? Is the format easy to follow in the urgent atmosphere of teaching in a busy clinical situation? When teaching and learning are a major intervention, it is usual to construct a separate teaching plan, possibly one that can be incorporated into the general nursing care plan. An example appears in Figure 3-7. Increasingly teaching is

Patient Learning Objectives	Content	Education Mode	Modifications Comments	Objectives Met (Date/Initials)
Patient will identify indications of upper respiratory infection and implementation of measures that help prevent regurgitation, aspiration, and respiratory infection.	Cough, increased nasal and respiratory secretions, inability to tolerate breathing of cold air, temperature 100.4° F (38° C), dysphagia How to manage these effects	E V		
Patient will alter diet as necessary.	A nutritious, well-balanced diet Soft food for patients with chewing difficulties High-fiber diet for patients experiencing constipation	E V P M		
Patient will relate the importance of follow-up care to achieve desired outcomes.	Visits to physician Visits to physical therapist Visits to occupational therapists Speech, sexual, or psychological counseling	E P V		

Resource Box (list available patient resources here):

Education Mode Key	Signature	Initial
P = Pamphlet B = Book R = Reciprocal demonstration D = Dialogue E = Explication V = Video RP= Role playing M = Modeling		

Figure 3-7, cont'd

being incorporated into clinical pathways. Figure 3-8 shows an example of a basic pathway. This format can be modified for any diagnosis and also used as a documentation tool.[19]

Availability of good protocols, teaching tools, and forms for recording teaching is essential to ensure that teaching is actually being delivered to patients.

In purposeful, planned teaching, the caregiver carries out the plan. It cannot work perfectly, but it can be used as a guide unless feedback from the patient indicates clearly that it is inappropriate or ineffective. If this happens, the planning process must be repeated, and new data must be added.

Experienced teachers can do that on the spot and move ahead. Others will need to stop the teaching session and, if possible, replan and reimplement.

Staff training is also important to implement programs. Traditional methods of teaching health professionals how to teach often focus only on the theoretical aspects of the teaching-learning process. Frequently, little help is offered to transfer this information into the practice setting. One approach involves apprenticing novice teachers to master teachers, allowing them to observe and participate and gradually do the teaching on their own with feedback from the

BASIC CLINICAL PATHWAY

Patient name _____ Admit _____

Primary diagnosis _____

Standard of care	Number of visits	Outcome	Initials
Physical and mental assessment Vital signs and blood pressure Mental and physical status Response to medications	Every visit	Temperature, pulse and blood pressure are within acceptable limits. Medication is producing desired effects.	

Educational assessment
Disease pathophysiology
  Definition
  Etiology
  Process/progression
  Causes of exacerbation
  Complications
	1-3	Patient/family comprehends information on disease pathophysiology.	

Medication teaching
  Use of drug
  Side effects
  Adverse reactions
	1-3	Patient/family is able to verbalize understanding of medications.	

Treatments/procedures	1-3	Patient is able to verbalize understanding of reason for treatment and able to perform treatment independently.	

Safety-related issues
  Emergency measures
  Universal precautions
  Safety in the home
	1
	1-2
	1-2
		Patient is able to access emergency care.
		Patient is able to protect self from safety or infection control related problems.	

Discharge planning Ongoing care needed for patient resource help	1-2	Patient/family understands discharge instructions. Patient verbalizes understanding for follow-up visits with physician.	

Quality management

Is pathway being followed?

Date ____Yes ____No ____   Date ____Yes ____No ____
Date ____Yes ____No ____   Date ____Yes ____No ____

If pathway is not followed, what is the variance and action plan?

Date _____Variance _____
Action plan _____
Date _____Variance _____
Action plan _____

Figure 3-8 Basic clinical pathway. (From Freeman SR, Chambers KA: Home health care: clinical pathways and quality integration, *Nurs Manag* 28(6):45-48, 1999.)

master teacher. Videotaping teaching interactions provides an opportunity for self-evaluation and critique from a master teacher.

SUMMARY

Educational objectives are based on assessment of a patient's readiness and need to learn; they are the framework for the instructional plan. Instructional forms and teaching materials are identified or constructed to provide the learning conditions necessary for meeting the objectives. Teaching plans put these elements together and guide implementation.

 Study Questions

1. A study of patients with lacerations who were treated in an emergency department found that those whose discharge instructional materials contained illustrations were 1.5 times more likely to choose correct responses than were those whose instructions did not contain illustrations.[1] Does this finding surprise you?
2. A mother comments to you, "My baby has clumsy fingers." You determine that the child's growth and development are normal for his or her age but that the child could profit from environmental stimulation to develop eye-hand coordination and prehension. What kinds of general teaching approaches might be used?

References

1. Austin PE and others: Discharge instructions: do illustrations help our patients understand them? *Ann Emerg Med* 25:317-320, 1995.
2. Baker DW, Parker RM, Williams MV, Clark WS: Health literacy and the risk of hospital admission, *J Gen Intern Med* 13:791-798, 1998.
3. Basara LR, Juergens JP: Patient package insert readability and design, *Am Pharm* NS34(8): 48-53, 1994.
4. Bernier MJ: Establishing the psychometric properties of a scale for evaluating quality in printed education materials, *Patient Educ Couns* 29: 283-299, 1996.
5. Billiard SJ, Beattie S: A nontraditional approach to cardiac education: the use of cardiac catheterization films, *Prog Cardiovasc Nurs* 5:21-25, 1990.
6. Brennan PF, Moore SM, Smyth KA: The effects of a special computer network on caregivers of persons with Alzheimer's disease, *Nurs Res* 44:166-172, 1995.
7. Bulechek GM and others: Nursing interventions used in practice, *Am J Nurs* 94(10):59-64, 1994.
8. Busselman KM, Holcomb CA: Reading skill and comprehension of the Dietary Guidelines by WIC participants, *J Am Diet Assoc* 94:622-625, 1994.
9. Buxton T: Effective ways to improve health education materials, *J Health Educ* 30(1):47-50, 61, 1999.
10. Colagiuri R, Colagiuri S, Naidu V: Can patients set their own educational priorities? *Diabetes Res Clin Pract* 30:131-136, 1995.
11. Crowe L, Billingsley JI: The rowdy reactors: maintaining a support group for teenagers with diabetes, *Diabetes Educ* 16:39-43, 1990.
12. Davis TC and others: Reading ability of parents compared with reading level of pediatric patient education materials, *Pediatrics* 93:460-468, 1994.
13. Davis TL and others: Practical assessment of adult literacy in health care, *Health Educ Behav* 25: 613-624, 1998.
14. DeBasio N, Rodenhausen N: The group experience: meeting the psychological needs of patients with ventricular tachycardia, *Heart Lung* 13: 597-602, 1984.
15. Doak CC, Doak LG, Root JH: *Teaching patients with low literacy skills*, ed 2, Philadelphia, 1996, Lippincott.
16. Dollahite J, Thompson C, McNew R: Readability of printed sources of diet and health information, *Patient Educ Couns* 27:123-134, 1996.
17. Dooley AR: A collaborative model for creating patient education resources, *Am J Health Behav* 20(2):15-19, 1996.
18. Freda MC, Damus K, Merkatz IR: Evaluation of the readability of ACOG patient education pamphlets, *Obstet Gynecol* 93:771-774, 1999.
19. Freeman SR, Chambers KA: Home health care; clinical pathways and quality integration, *Nurs Manag* 28(6):45-48, 1999.
20. Fry E: A readability formula that saves time, *J Reading* 11:513-516, 1968.
21. Fry E: A readability formula for short passages, *J Reading* 33:594-597, 1990.
22. Gagliano ME: A literature review on the efficacy of video in patient education, *J Med Educ* 63:785-792, 1988.

23. Graber MA, Roller CM, Kaeble B: Readability levels of patient education material on the World Wide Web, *J Fam Pract* 48:58-61, 1999.

24. Greene VL, Monahan DJ: The effect of a professional guided caregiver support and education group on institutionalization of care receivers, *Gerontologist* 27:716-721, 1987.

25. Gronlund NE: *How to write and use instructional objectives*, ed 5, Englewood Cliffs, NJ, 1995, Prentice-Hall.

26. Houts PS and others: Using pictographs to enhance recall and spoken medical instructions, *Patient Educ Couns* 35:83-88, 1998.

27. Iowa Intervention Project: Validation and coding of the NIC taxonomy structure, *Image* 27:43-49, 1995.

28. Jacobs MK, Goodman G: Psychology and self-help groups, *Am Psychol* 44:536-545, 1989.

29. Kilmon C: A taxonomy of pediatric primary care nursing interventions, *Nurs Health Care* 15:150-156, 1994.

30. Kozma RB: Learning with media, *Rev Educ Res* 61:179-211, 1991.

31. Kulik JA, Mahler HIM: Effects of preoperative roommate assignments on preoperative anxiety and recovery from coronary bypass surgery, *Health Psychol* 6:525-543, 1987.

32. Lasater L, Mehler PS: The illiterate patient: screening and management, *Hosp Pract* 33(4):163-170, 1998.

33. Ley P and others: A method of increasing patients' recall of information presented by doctors, *Psychol Med* 3:217-220, 1973.

34. Madhumitan, Kumar KL: Twenty-one guidelines for effective instructional design, *Educ Technol* 35(3):58-61, 1995.

35. Massett HA: Appropriateness of Hispanic print materials: a content analysis, *Health Educ Res* 11:231-242, 1996.

36. Mayeaux EJ and others: Improving patient education for patients with low literacy skills, *Am Fam Physician* 53:205-211, 1996.

37. Meade CD, Howser DM: Consent forms: how to determine and improve their readability, *Oncol Nurs Forum* 19:1523-1528, 1992.

38. Meade CD, Smith CF: Readability formulas: cautions and criteria, *Patient Educ Couns* 17:153-158, 1991.

39. Meade CD, Wittbrot R: Computerized readability analysis of written materials, *Comput Nurs* 6:30-36, 1988.

40. Murphy PW and others: Rapid Estimate of Adult Literacy in Medicine (REALM): a quick reading test for patients, *J Reading* 37:124-130, 1993.

41. Nielsen E, Sheppard MA: Television as a patient education tool: a review of its effectiveness, *Patient Educ Couns* 11:3-16, 1988.

42. Nurss JR, Parker RM, Williams MV, Baker DW: *Test of functional health literacy in adults*, Atlanta, 1995, Center for the Study of Adult Literacy, Georgia State University.

43. Starn J, Paperny DM: Computer games to enhance adolescent sex education, *MCN Am J Matern Child Nurs* 15:250-253, 1990.

44. Wolitski RJ, Rhodes F: AIDS info on-line: a computer-based information system for college campuses, *J Am Coll Health* 39:90-93, 1990.

Chapter 4

Evaluation and Research in Patient Education

Evaluation determines the worth of something by judging it against a standard, usually stated as a learning objective and defined by a field of practice or study. Evaluation can serve several purposes. It can direct and motivate learning because it provides evidence about patients' accomplishments or skills that they need to develop. Evaluation can also be used to judge whether someone ought to be selected or certified for having met a particular level of expertise. Patient education generally has not been used to provide a formal certification; however, evaluative judgments about learning commonly provide the basis for allowing a patient to progress to another setting, such as home. Evaluation also reinforces correct behavior on the part of learners and helps teachers determine the adequacy of their teaching. In each situation it is important to think through the purpose of the evaluation first.

Once the standard is clear, the next step is to assign evaluative tasks to the learners. Ambiguous tasks produce faulty evidence and lead to faulty conclusions concerning how much the patient has learned. As a result the learner is confused. Evidence is compared with criteria or standards of adequate performance, and a judgment of adequacy or inadequacy is made. The teaching that follows a judgment of inadequate

learning can correct errors in the patient's performance, present correct behavior, and explain the errors and correct behavior, as well as improve teaching.

Evaluating programs of patient education is also necessary for teaching groups of patients over a period of time. Program evaluation provides direction for improvement of learning in individual patients and leads to judgments about how to improve the program.

Research in patient education is very important to evaluation because it establishes the kind of learning goal that can be attained and what is known about how best to attain it. The research base for patient education is currently large, with some of it summarized through review articles or meta-analyses (a statistical approach to summarizing the results from multiple studies on the same question). A summary of reviews and meta-analyses on patient education is presented in Appendix C.

In the current state of patient education practice, purposive evaluation is not routinely carried out; indeed, learning goals (which are the base for evaluation) are frequently not clearly articulated. In addition, the most useful outcomes from patient education (problem solving in real life situations) are frequently not used. For example, the most common outcome measures from diabetes education are patient knowledge and glycosylated hemoglobin. Knowledge appears to be necessary but not sufficient to produce adequate patient self-management skills and functioning; therefore measures of knowledge may more properly be thought of as process measures on the way to other outcomes.[8]

Clinical success has traditionally been appraised in terms of mortality and physiological measures such as blood pressure, laboratory tests, x-ray study findings and definable clinical events. Increasingly, patients' perceptions of symptoms, their ability to function in everyday life, their satisfaction with care, and their ability to make health care decisions are seen as important and predictive of future use of health care services.[4] A taxonomy of nurse-sensitive outcomes of patient care more closely related to outcomes of patient education is available.[10] Outcomes relevant to patient education include anxiety control, caregiver performance, perceived ability to perform, and participation in health care behaviors. Lorig and others[11] define a set of outcomes from self-management education for chronic diseases which include: self-management behaviors (e.g., exercise, cognitive symptom management, mental stress management, use of community services, and communication with providers) and self-efficacy for self-management behaviors for disease management in general, and to achieve outcomes such as management of depression and symptoms, and health states such as disability, and social role limitations.

Although many formally developed measurement tools are available, they are not routinely used in clinical practice. Those with appropriate psychometric characteristics should be used—this is the only way clinical practice judgments will become more objective and reliable. Increasingly, disease management programs form the organizational structure in which outcomes are assessed and care processes improved. Review of a hospitalization may show that it was precipitated by lack of self-management skills. In reviewing the case, the nurse case manager determines that self-management education is needed. After the education is accomplished, the patient's recovery is tracked to see if the education was effective.

OBTAINING MEASURES OF BEHAVIOR

All measurement involves observation of behavior. Such observation is more or less direct. Observations are more direct if the method of measurement involves viewing actual behavior as it occurs in natural settings and having access to its intended meaning. They are less direct if the method of measurement involves the subject's response to substitute situations that may be largely verbal and requires much inference of intended meaning. Each method contains certain weaknesses that can produce error in measurement.

Because one of the major purposes of measurement and evaluation activities is to predict how the individual will behave in the future, it is best to base this prediction on observation of actual behavior (direct measurement).

What people say they will do and what they actually do may be different. People often respond in ways that are socially acceptable. Behavior in the affective domain is perhaps the most difficult to measure because the individual can easily control the expression of feelings. Direct observation of behavior when the individual is unaware of being observed is the best opportunity for accurate assessment.

Although indirect measurements contain error, they also possess advantages that can contribute greatly to accurate assessment. Natural behavior is often inaccessible because it occurs in private—in family interactions. Natural behavior might occur infrequently and in various places. For example, it might surface in response to emergencies that require resuscitation measures, such as insulin shock, diabetic coma, or ingestion of poisons by a child.

Natural behavior might also occur infrequently, that is, at times when the observer may not be present. The strategy behind most tests used in indirect measurement is to present the situation in such a way that the provider can elicit the desired behavior in a written, oral, or performance response to a mock situation. Test results for complex behaviors are more accurate if the learner responds to situations on videotape rather than responding to written test situations.

Thus far in this chapter several major sources of error in measurement have been identified. One source of error is the constant possibility that indirect measures may present a false picture of an individual's behavior. A second source of error lies in the complexity of behavior. An observer may be unable to identify the causes of a particular behavior or be unable to measure thought patterns and attitudes even by direct observation. A third source is the bias of human observers. Observers cannot attend to or record all stimuli. They tend to assign meanings according to their own views. A fourth source of error is sampling. It is often not feasible in terms of time and effort expended to observe an individual's or a group's behavior repeatedly to account for the variation in performance from day to day and from situation to situation. It is not possible to inventory all aspects of an individual's knowledge about a particular subject. Obtaining samples over a period of time and in general areas of subject matter decreases error to an acceptable level.

The degree of error allowable depends on the predictions and decisions made and on the precision of the best measuring tool available. The provider should be more concerned with the person who needs to know how to care for a child's tracheostomy at home than with the person who needs to know how to do prenatal exercises. In both cases observing the learner engaged in the behavior would provide appropriate data for evaluation. However, for tracheostomy care the teacher should observe many times, measuring the learner's behavior against objective criteria agreed on by experts. To evaluate the learner's understanding, the caregiver can supplement the observation with oral or written questions, asking the learner what to do if the tube becomes dislodged or why suctioning is done a particular way. All methods of measure-

ment are prone to particular errors. To arrive at a decision, the best information often can be gained by using a combination of methods.

Measurement involves obtaining a record of pertinent behavior. Not only is it difficult to record all that occurs, but also this mass of information is not useful. The guideline for the pertinence of recording behavior is the statement of objectives. If the statement has met all the specifications for preciseness and clarity outlined in Chapter 3, it is much easier to decide which information is useful to record. Envision the difference in trying to evaluate these two patient objectives: (1) to know injection sites; (2) to draw on his or her own skin five areas suitable for injection of insulin. It is difficult to identify and measure the content and behavior of objective number one. Note that no time is stipulated in this objective. Tests limiting time are appropriate only if the learned behavior requires speed.

Rating Scales and Checklists

The most complete recording of behavior is obtained from videotape. This method offers the added advantage that it can be reviewed with the learner to offer feedback on performance. A videotape, however, does not provide access to the learner's thinking unless he or she verbalizes it while recording. By itself it does not summarize the kind of behavior seen or identify its meaning in relation to objectives. To fill this need, a rating scale that describes pertinent behavior in words (anchored) can be constructed.

To reduce error in measurement, these words must be precise so that misinterpretation is avoided. For example, the rating scale (Box 4-1) can be refined so that several teachers who are observing a learner's behavior can independently classify it at one of the three points (shown in Box 4-1) with little variation. If the raters cannot agree, the wording probably needs to be clarified. After the scale is refined, individual caregivers can use it by themselves.

Of course, it is possible for an individual to display behavior from two different levels of functioning (see descriptions of behavior in

---

Box 4-1   *Sample Rating Scale*

Subobjective: To obtain 1 ml of aqueous fluid for injection from a 2-ml vial with a 2-ml syringe, 22-gauge needle, using sterile technique.

Consistently uses contaminated syringe, needle, or top of vial. Cannot push needle through diaphragm. Is rarely aware of erring and if so usually does not know how to correct the error.	Occasionally contaminates. Can push needle through diaphragm. Has difficulty withdrawing all the fluid and obtaining accurate measurement (within 0.1 ml). Can usually diagnose errors while doing the procedure and correct them.	Rarely contaminates. Can obtain last few drops out of vial without damaging needle. Can measure within 0.1 ml even if bubbles are present. Can change needle or syringe if defective or contaminated. Corrects errors by self.

(Other scales can be developed for other subobjectives of the skill of giving an injection.)

Box 4-1). For example, the patient may contaminate the syringe and needle fairly often (lowest level) but be quite skilled at removing bubbles from the syringe and measuring accurately (highest level). Behaviors are usually at adjacent levels on the rating scale because certain skills involve comparable levels of coordination. The difference may be that the learner is careless about contaminating. Checks can be made beside individual statements at various levels of the description. This will ensure that the teacher does not lose information about the learner's performance by checking just one of the categories on the line.

Another alternative is construction of several scales for this particular subobjective, each dealing with one set of behaviors—maintenance of sterility, obtaining and measuring fluid, or handling errors. Space is usually left below each rating scale for comments. A well-developed scale includes all pertinent points and rarely requires extra written comments. The form is developed to preclude recording behavior by writing it out at great length.

Other factors in the construction of a rating scale, besides preciseness of the descriptions, contribute to its quality as a measuring instrument. One factor is the number of levels of achievement represented in the behavior descriptions. The sample rating scale given here uses three levels of achievement because it is

difficult for an observer to discriminate among more than five levels of achievement. Four or five steps could have been used. Note that the kinds of behaviors described in the scale are those that are crucial to the success of the skill as described in the objective: asepsis, accuracy of measurement, and ability to perceive and correct errors. Concerns such as inserting the needle precisely through the center of the rubber stopper or the particular manner in which the syringe is grasped are not considered crucial. The following is an example of a checklist that could be used in lieu of the sample rating scale in Box 4-1.

❑ Scrubbed top of vial with disinfectant sponge
❑ Punctured rubber vial with needle without contaminating
❑ Withdrew all fluid from vial
❑ Expelled excess air from syringe without losing fluid
❑ Measured fluid to within 0.1 ml of the correct dose

Boxes 4-2, 4-3, and 4-4 provide examples of rating scales—for breast self-examination, for patient satisfaction, and for rating the umbilical cord of a newborn. Do these instruments elicit critical data? Are the most important elements included? Are some more crucial than others? If so, should they be marked so that patients who

Box 4-2 Breast Self-Examination Proficiency Rating Instrument

Inspection

Arms at sides
Arms over head
Hands on hips
Leaning forward:
 Looks for symmetry, size, shape
 Looks for puckering, dimpling
Examines skin for color, texture, lesions
Inspection Total

Palpation

Hand behind head
Begins exam at 12 o'clock
Examines all parts of breast
Closely examines upper outer quadrant
Uses circular motion for each palpation
Uses pads of fingers
Presses firmly and deeply
Squeezes nipple
Inspects axilla
Palpation Total

Total

From Wood RY: Reliability and validity of a breast self examination proficiency rating instrument, *Eval Health Prof* 17:418-435, 1994.

Box 4-3 Satisfaction with Decision Instrument

You have been considering whether to consult your health care provider about hormone-replacement therapy. Answer the following questions about your decision. Please indicate to what extent each statement is true for you AT THIS TIME.

Use the following scale to answer the questions.
 1 = strongly disagree
 2 = disagree
 3 = neither agree nor disagree
 4 = agree
 5 = strongly agree

1. I am satisfied that I am adequately informed about the issues important to my decision.
2. The decision I made was the best decision possible for me personally.
3. I am satisfied that my decision was consistent with my personal values.
4. I expect to successfully carry out (or continue to carry out) the decision I made.
5. I am satisfied that this was my decision to make.
6. I am satisfied with my decision.

From Holmes-Rovner M and others: Patient satisfaction with health care decisions, *Med Decis Making* 16:58-64, 1996.

Box 4-4 Cord Rating Scale

Score	Redness	Discharge	Odor	Dryness	Other/Comments
0	None	None	None	Hard	
1	Within 1/8" of cord		Yes	Drying	
2	Within 1/4" of cord	Reddish discharge		Soft, moist	
3	Within 1/2" of cord	Yellowish discharge		Wet	

NB: It is normal to have a scant amount of bleeding from the cord site if the cord stump sticks to the diaper.

MUST have a score of 7-10 for infection.

Pustules present?
 _____ Yes
 _____ No
 If yes, how long have they been present? _____
 Where located? _____

From Ford LA, Ritchie JA: Maternal perceptions of newborn umbilical cord treatments and healing, *J Obstet Gynecol Neonatal Nurs* 28:501-506, 1999.

cannot do critical steps are identified? Would two health care providers watching a patient perform this procedure give him or her the same number of points? Might it help to include further descriptors of correct performance for each step?

Oral Questioning

Oral questioning is a flexible form of measurement often used in combination with techniques such as observation. It attempts to reach those behaviors that cannot be easily observed. For example, a caregiver may ask patients questions to determine if they understand the basis for their actions in performing a psychomotor skill. Oral questioning also allows construction of hypothetical situations that are not present in the actual teaching environment. Examples of these practices include asking a man learning to irrigate his colostomy why he is preparing the equipment as he is or asking a mother what she would do if her baby turned blue, which may include a demonstration of resuscitation techniques.

The method of oral questioning can be expensive in terms of the time it takes, particularly if it is done in a one-to-one teacher-learner relationship. The strength of oral questioning over written testing is that the teacher knows immediately whether the learner understands the question and the teacher can let the learner know immediately whether the answer is right. In a group-teaching situation this kind of direct interchange is limited—although the reaction of one learner responding to another learner's answer can be very educational. In large groups the advantages of oral questioning are somewhat lost because every individual cannot respond to an oral question unless that response is in writing.

The verbal nature of both oral and written questioning may handicap individuals who have difficulty expressing themselves. Many individuals probably find it easier to express themselves orally than in writing. In addition, those who are verbally fluent may seem to know more. For these reasons combinations of methods, such as observation of behavior and oral questioning, can often provide a truer picture than a single method can.

It is a common misconception that oral questioning does not require much preparation on the part of a teacher. Questions must be very carefully phrased so that (1) a learner can understand them and (2) they test the objective. With knowledge of an individual's previous exposure to an idea, questions can be phrased to stimulate thinking at any level of the cognitive domain. Box 4-5 shows sample objectives and questions that should test various levels of thinking. Questions need to be carefully phrased to avoid leading a patient to the socially desirable answer or to "the answer" the provider wants, which may be an inappropriate reiteration of the information just presented by the provider. Such a circumstance may indicate that a patient has not comprehended the material well enough to express the idea in alternative ways.

Written Measurement

Written measurement is indirect and demands at least some reading skill and knowledge of test taking on the part of a learner. Well-constructed tests offer an excellent opportunity to measure learning at all levels of the cognitive domain, with efficient use of teacher time.

Tests are prepared by individuals or groups of teachers in a particular institution and are used within that institution. They may be adapted to and published by other institutions, or they may be developed by test experts and sold. Tests sold commercially should provide a manual with information that explains the purposes of the test. Also, the manual should give evidence that the test accurately measures the goals it claims to measure and that it does so reliably. Evidence should include information that describes how well the test covers the subject matter. If, for example, the test is meant to evaluate knowledge of nutrition, it should include items on all the major concepts in nutrition today. This quality of a test is called content validity. Additional information should describe how closely the test score is related to actual patient behavior in the present (concurrent validity) or the future (predictive validity). For example, if a patient with diabetes scores high on the test, is he or she giving good

Box 4-5	*Sample Objectives and Oral Questions for Evaluation*

Objectives	Questions
To state what effect worry in the mother may have on her breast milk (level of knowledge)	"What effect can worry have on a mother's breast milk?" (This question presumes that the learner has read or been told of this relationship.)
To translate instructions for time and route on a medicine bottle into appropriate action (level of comprehension)	Present to learners several medicine bottles with directions for time and route different from those on their own bottles. "How and when should these be taken?"
Given general knowledge of safety, to plan how to rid a house of safety hazards (level of application)	"How would you make your kitchen safer?" Repeat the question for bathroom and other rooms, being certain that areas covered include fire safety, electrical hazards, safety from poisons, safety from falling.
To distinguish how an uninformed opinion differs from scientific reasoning (level of analysis)	This can be analysis only if the individual has not been told or has not discussed the difference. Otherwise, he or she will repeat thoughts that are not original thoughts and will be at the level of knowledge or comprehension. Several examples of quack and scientific reasoning may be presented and the learner asked to state differences based on those samples.
To assess the health care one is receiving in terms of its completeness, one's satisfaction with it, and the results obtained (level of evaluation)	"What quality of care would you say you have received? Consider its completeness, your satisfaction with it, and the results that have occurred."

self-care now? Will he or she be giving good self-care in the future? A similar kind of statement about future self-care would be needed for those doing less well on the test. If a test contains a high degree of validity, its value for decision making is greater than that of a test with a low degree of validity.

Only rarely are locally developed tests studied this carefully. Teachers who use their own tests and have continuing contact with the same patients gain a feeling for how closely the test relates to their patients' actual behavior. However, these teachers rarely perform studies that provide them with accurate test-validity information. Measurement characteristics of more than 50 tools used in patient education may be found in Redman.[13] Several sample tools may be found on the following pages. The Chicago Lead Knowledge Test can be used to evaluate lead education programs (Box 4-6). (One group of

parents in Chicago knew the answers to about half of these questions.)[12] The Methotrexate Knowledge Questionnaire[3] was used in one quality improvement study to increase patient understanding of methotrexate toxicity and inadvertent unsafe use (Box 4-7). Half of patients taking this medication experience symptoms, and although knowledge scores generally improve after a teaching intervention, data about how safely patients actually take this medication should also to be gathered.

Sample items from a scale to measure the performance and frequency of self-care actions specific to patients with chronic obstructive pulmonary disease (COPD) may be found in Box 4-8. Reported self-care actions are another example of outcomes that may be achieved by patient education. A final example of a written instrument is one that measures perceived personal control, an outcome central to coping with health

Box 4-6	*Chicago Lead Knowledge Test: Questions and Responses**				

		RESPONSES (PERCENTAGE)		
QUESTION	**CORRECT ANSWER**	**CORRECT**	**INCORRECT**	**DON'T KNOW**
General Information				
1. Lead paint chips can be poisonous when eaten.	True	95	1	4
2. High blood lead level can affect a child's ability to learn.	True	92	1	7
3. Most children have symptoms right away if they have an elevated blood lead level.	False	58	7	35
4. Apartment owners are required to tell renters about known lead-containing paint in the apartment when a lease is signed.	True	43	14	43
5. A child's highest blood lead level generally occurs around 5 years of age.	False	18	12	70
Exposure				
6. Lead paint is more likely to be found in newer homes than in older homes.	False	88	5	7
7. Living in a building during renovation/remodeling can increase a child's exposure to lead.	True	87	2	11
8. One way for children to get lead poisoned is by having lead dust on their hands and then putting their hands in their mouth.	True	86	2	12
9. A child can become lead poisoned during exposure to lead-containing dust.	True	85	1	14
10. Some pottery imported from Mexico or other countries is not safe to use for cooking or eating because it contains lead.	True	73	2	25

*In the survey, questions were ordered as follows: 6, 2, 1, 5, 3, 7, 17, 20, 23, 8, 19, 14, 18, 4, 11, 13, 10, 9, 12, 16, 15, 21, 24, 22.

From Mehta S, Binns HJ: What do parents know about lead poisoning? *Arch Pediatr Adolesc Med* 152:1213-1218, 1998.

threats including those addressed in genetic counseling (Box 4-9).[2]

In some instances, no appropriate instrument will be available, and items to measure patient progress and outcomes must be constructed. Although multiple-choice, true-false, and matching items can be used, they may not provide accurate assessments for persons with marginal literacy. Short questions may be asked in oral or written form. An example is: "What should be done if your child eats poison, and why should it be done?" Note that this question, whether oral or written, requires recall of information. However, the response will elicit a different behavior than does discriminating among answers that are already present in multiple-choice, true-false, and matching items.

The ability to recall is desirable for information used frequently. It is essential for emergency situations, such as child poisoning, diabetic coma, or seizures. The objective is to be able to recall the information and then act on it. A person must be able to produce the information from memory, not just recognize it among several alternatives. Periodic self-testing of memory for specific information will strengthen retention of

| Box 4-6 | *Chicago Lead Knowledge Test: Questions and Responses—cont'd* |

QUESTION	CORRECT ANSWER	RESPONSES (PERCENTAGE)		
		CORRECT	INCORRECT	DON'T KNOW
11. Parents who work with lead at their jobs can bring lead home on their clothes.	True	69	5	26
12. The lead a pregnant woman takes into her body can be transferred to the unborn baby.	True	67	2	31
13. Lead in soil cannot harm children.	False	65	4	31
14. Most cases of childhood lead poisoning are caused by drinking water that contains lead.	False	40	20	40
15. Most children get lead poisoning by breathing in lead, rather than by eating or swallowing lead.	False	30	24	46
16. Some herbal or traditional home remedies contain lead.	True	16	7	77
Prevention				
17. Washing a child's hands often helps prevent lead poisoning.	True	47	27	26
18. Warm tap water usually contains less lead than cold tap water.	False	39	6	55
19. Lead in water can be removed by boiling.	False	32	20	48
20. Cleaning a home with soap and water decreases the lead in the home more than dusting or sweeping.	True	32	34	34
Nutrition				
21. The human body needs a small amount of lead for good nutrition.	False	27	17	56
22. Less lead is taken up by the body if a child eats a balanced diet, without too many fatty foods.	True	13	26	61
23. A diet with a good amount of iron-containing foods will help decrease a child's chance of becoming lead poisoned.	True	12	39	49
24. A diet with enough calcium helps prevent lead poisoning.	True	9	29	62

infrequently used material. The strength of the recognition item is that it can enable learners to discriminate between ideas—ideas they might not otherwise consider—thus helping them test their depth of understanding.

As in Box 4-10, items can be written to test various levels of cognitive behavior. The level measured by a particular question depends on the information the learner has received. The true-false item form is used to test knowledge or comprehension. The multiple-choice form is more flexible and can be used at all levels. Synthesis requires independent thought; therefore it is tested

by methods that suggest no answers. At all levels visual materials can be incorporated into written questions. For example, the provider can show a mother photos of umbilical cords and ask her to indicate the one(s) that need(s) to be called to the attention of the nurse midwife and which one(s) will probably drop off soon.

Numerous possible errors in the construction of single test items and groups of items can prevent an accurate assessment of an individual's cognitive skills.

For open-ended questions the provider can develop criteria for correct responses. For example,

Box 4-7	*Methotrexate Knowledge Questionnaire and Item Values for Correct and Incorrect Answers*

PLEASE CIRCLE THE CORRECT ANSWER(S)	CORRECT RESPONSE	ITEM VALUE	
		CORRECT	WRONG
1. Methotrexate is usually taken HOW MANY TIMES PER WEEK?			
a. Once a day		—	−1
b. One day per week	b	+1	—
c. Three days per week		—	−1
2. When you are taking methotrexate, HOW MUCH ALCOHOL are you allowed to drink?			
a. Five drinks per week		—	−1
b. One drink per week		—	−1
c. No limit on the amount of alcohol I can drink		—	−1
d. None	d	+1	—
3. When is the best time to get your BLOOD TESTS done?			
a. One to two days after you take methotrexate		—	0
b. One to two days before you take methotrexate	b	+1	—
c. The day you take methotrexate		—	0
4. Methotrexate may cause BIRTH DEFECTS if either parent is taking it during the time the woman can become pregnant, or if a woman takes it during pregnancy _____ True _____ False	T	+1	−1
5. Which of the following are possible SIDE EFFECTS of methotrexate? (circle all that apply)			
a. Nausea	T	+1	0
b. Low blood counts	T	+1	−1
c. Mouth sores	T	+1	−1
d. Ingrown toenails	F	+1	0
e. Liver problems	T	+1	−1
6. You should CALL YOUR DOCTOR IMMEDIATELY if you experience which of the following? (circle all that apply)			
a. A temperature of greater than 101°F	T	+1	−1
b. Shortness of breath	T	+1	−1
c. Nausea and vomiting	T	+1	0
d. Constipation	F	+1	0

From Burma MR and others: Methotrexate patient education study: a quality improvement study, *Arthritis Care Res* 9:216-222, 1996.

Box 4-8	*Sample Questions from the COPD Self-Care Action Scale*

	FREQUENCY*				
ITEM	NEVER	RARELY	SOMETIMES	OFTEN	VERY OFTEN
How often do you cut down on things you usually do because of shortness of breath?	_____	_____	_____	_____	_____
How often do you get enough sleep and rest?	_____	_____	_____	_____	_____
If you develop signs of an infection, how often do you report it to your doctor?	_____	_____	_____	_____	_____
How often do you keep up with the air quality index or air pollution count report?	_____	_____	_____	_____	_____
When you become suddenly short of breath, how often do you change your position?	_____	_____	_____	_____	_____
When you are short of breath, how often do you sit on the edge of a chair, leaning forward?	_____	_____	_____	_____	_____

*Responses are assigned numeric values: 0 = *never*, 1 = *rarely*, 2 = *sometimes*, 3 = *often*, 4 = *very often*.
From Riley P: Development of a COPD self-care action scale, *Rehabil Nurs Res* 5(1):3-8, 1996.

Box 4-9	*Perceived Personal Control Questionnaire*

To what extent do you agree with the following statements?

0 = Do not agree;
1 = Somewhat agree;
2 = Completely agree.

_____ I think I understand what problem brought me to genetic counseling.
_____ I feel I know the meaning of the problem for my family's future and me.
_____ I think I know what caused the problem.
_____ I feel I have the tools to make decisions that will influence my future.
_____ I feel I can make a logical evaluation of the various options available to me in order to choose one of them.
_____ I feel I can make decisions that will change my family's future.
_____ I feel there are certain things I can do to prevent the problem from recurring.
_____ I feel I know what to do to ease the situation.
_____ I think I know what should be my next steps.

From Berkenstadt M and others: Perceived personal control (PPC): a new concept in measuring outcome of genetic counseling, *Am J Med Genet* 82:53-59, 1999.

Box 4-10	*Test Items on Various Levels of the Cognitive Domain*

Knowledge   T F   The hospital is required by law to use isolation with certain diagnoses.

Comprehension   T F   A patient will not be retained in isolation after a diagnosis is made.

Application   Isolation is a means of containing the spread of microorganisms. How can these methods be used with a person at home who has a cold?

Analysis   The basic principle(s) of our society that relate(s) to the reason isolation is used is (are):
a. Certain institutions have the right to carry out certain functions for the society.
b. An individual has certain rights.
c. The majority rules.
d. a and b.
e. a, b, c.

Synthesis   Suggest a set of rules for isolation that will maximize the well-being of staff, visitors, and patients.

Evaluation   It seems necessary to isolate persons with communicable disease to varying extents to protect others from the disease. Which one of the following policies would best achieve protection of the public and the welfare of the ill individual?
a. After diagnosis allow the individual and family a choice of sites for care.
b. Have a team of health personnel to enforce the proper degree of isolation in a hospital and the reporting of communicable disease.
c. Allow individual physicians and health agencies considerable latitude in establishing such policies.
(NOTE: The answer must not be in terms of opinion but must show evidence of judgment in terms of particular criteria, such as safety and psychological and sociological well-being.)

the following questions were asked of parents in one study: (1) What would you do if you just saw your child drinking a poison? (2) What would you do if your child just drank some toilet bowl cleaner? (3) What would you do if your child just drank some Drano or Liquid Plumr? Criteria for evaluating the answers to these questions are described as follows[5]:

Response	Action
Incorrect	Immediately make child vomit.
	Use ipecac without medical clearance.
	Give home remedy without seeking medical advice.
	Call ambulance.
	Miscellaneous response without therapeutic merit.
	No answer.
Partially correct	Rush child to emergency department or physician's office (for question 1).
	Follow directions on label of product ingested.
	Check a home reference for instructions.
Partially correct —cont'd	Neutralize poison, then call physician or poison control center.
Correct	Call physician immediately.
	Call poison control center immediately.
	Rush to emergency department (for questions 2 and 3 only).

Box 4-11 lists guidelines for writing multiple-choice test items.

Testing for trivia or for irrelevant material is an error to avoid. Consider the nurse who shows a film in conjunction with infant care classes. The following question is irrelevant to the objectives of most infant care classes:

The name of the movie you saw about your baby's bath was

a. "Your Baby's Bath"
b. "Bathing Baby"
c. "Morning Adventure"
d. "Mother Loves Baby"

Box 4-11	*Guidelines for Writing Multiple Choice Test Items*

1. Make all distractors plausible.
2. Avoid "None of the above" as an option.
3. Make all the options approximately the same length.
4. Avoid negatively stated items, especially double negatives.
5. Randomly vary the position of the correct answer.
6. Avoid grammatical mistakes. Each option should fit grammatically with the stem.
7. Avoid using "All of the above" as an option.
8. Put as much of the item as possible into the stem. Do not repeat words in the options.
9. The stem should present a definition problem and not lead into a series of unrelated true/false statements.
10. There should be only one correct or best answer.
11. Avoid superfluous wording and irrelevant material.
12. Attempt to measure higher order learning by using novelty.
13. Use three to five options, depending on how many can be logically created for each item.
14. Do not give irrelevant clues to the correct answer.
15. Avoid specific determiners, such as always, never, all, none.

From Ellsworth RA, Dunnell P, Duell OK: Multiple-choice test items: What are textbook authors telling teachers, *J Educ Res* 83:289-293, 1990.

Clues in the language of an item may give away the correct answer to someone who is test-wise. The following example, based on a pamphlet explaining isolation care, gives one clue—it uses exactly the same terminology as that used in the teaching presentation:

T F   Your illness may be transmitted to others.

In such a case an individual learns to recognize the words without necessarily knowing what they mean. Grammatical clues, such as a plural subject used in the stem, can make some choices in a multiple-choice question grammatically incorrect. An example, using a plural subject and a plural verb, follows:

Areas under the scalp where bone has not yet filled are known as

a. Meconium
b. An umbilicus
c. Fontanels
d. All of the above

The following matching item illustrates several problems with clues, ambiguity, and vocabulary level:

Directions: Match the body part with the action that best describes how to wash it.

Body part	Washing action
_____ 1. Vulva	a. With a pointed object
_____ 2. Neck	b. With a soft washcloth
_____ 3. Soft spot	c. Vigorously but gently
_____ 4. Ear	d. With a twisted piece of cotton

Mothers may not know the term "vulva" unless it has been specifically introduced to them. Some learners would eliminate choice *a* because they would know that no one washes the body with pointed objects. The fact that choice *a* is so obviously a less plausible answer is a clue.

True-false items are notorious for having clues, and they can also be ambiguous. Statements containing absolute terms such as "all," "always," "certainly," and "entirely" are more often false than true. Statements with words that qualify, such as "generally," "sometimes," "as a rule," or "may," are more often true than false. Uncertainty about the correct answer ensues when part of a question is true and part of it is false, as in the following example:

T F   The umbilical cord may be swabbed with alcohol to dry it and sterilize it.

Many times true-false items that are long in text are true.

For all kinds of items, the best distractors (incorrect choices) are misconceptions that are common among learners. It is easy to learn about these misconceptions by listening to patients talk among themselves, with visitors, or with nurses or by watching them perform certain skills. The following is an example:

T F   The soft spot should not be touched when the baby is being bathed.

Multiple-choice items may have high complexity and readability levels. The goal in test construction is to produce items that will assess learners' knowledge accurately. Clues and implausible distractors help learners choose the correct answer by guessing, and thus they appear to know more than they do. By contrast, ambiguity makes it difficult for learners to demonstrate the knowledge they actually have. Testing for trivia may reliably provide information, but it is information about unimportant learning. Such errors should be avoided.

Test theorists suggest generating a number of items representing a domain (an objective) and randomly drawing a sample of items from each domain. For example, a major objective for instruction about bathing infants might be to cleanse the infant safely. First of all, much of the evaluation of learning in this situation should be accomplished by observing the caregiver's motor skills. For evaluation of cognitive skill a group of written items may be collected that test the objectives. Table 4-1 presents a summary of the advantages and disadvantages of various measures in evaluating patient education.

Earlier chapters emphasized the emerging importance of self-efficacy as an outcome measure of patient education. Two examples of measures of self-efficacy in particular areas and for particular tasks are shown Boxes 4-12 and 4-13.

EVALUATIVE JUDGMENTS

Measurement is carried out so that the teaching-learning process can be evaluated more accurately than it could be by general impressions. Evaluation must go beyond measurement. It requires a value judgment about learning and teaching. Evaluation must summarize the evidence and determine how well the objectives are being met.

Measurement and evaluation occur continuously during teaching, serving to redirect the activities of teachers and learners. Information about learners' progress is gathered by having learners respond to questions or perform periodically, or both. The expressions of boredom, interest, confusion, or enlightenment on learners' faces give clues about their understanding of the material being taught.

Some individuals are able to tell a teacher that they do not understand. Others cannot identify or express their uncertainty. To identify material that is not clear to learners, the provider can retrace the explanation or the skill demonstration, can ask questions at intervals, or can observe and critique the performance of a skill by a learner. This technique will point out terms used by the teacher that learners may not understand, or it may reveal that learners are overloaded with complex instructions. Trying to reteach without determining the nature of the learning problem may cause a caregiver to make the same error again. It is unwise to teach for a long time (or even one lesson period) without requiring learners to respond so that teaching and learning errors can be corrected.

Adequacy of learning must eventually be evaluated in terms of meeting the final objectives and commonly accepted outcomes. Of course, if satisfactory evaluation takes place as the teaching is going on, the degree of attainment of final objectives or the time needed to meet the final objectives can be quite accurately predicted (Box 4-14).

Critical paths (examples are provided in other chapters) provide a structure of expected outcomes within particular time frames that guide all care, including patient education.

Crucial decisions regarding patients, such as whether they can live alone, rest on the outcome of learning. The minimum performance necessary for an individual to function must be identified. Certain basic information and skills must be learned because they are essential to the performance of a particular task. Other information and skills may also be crucial, depending on how independently the individual will be functioning.

TABLE 4-1	Types of Measurement	
Technique	**Advantages**	**Disadvantages**
Direct Observation	Performance under real or simulated conditions can be assessed Task is credible to patient Measure has good content validity	Awareness of the observer may affect performance Training, supervising, using observers are costly Number of patients who may be studied and their locale may be restricted because of the high per-patient cost of observing
Observational Checklist	Simple, objective task to record observations Observer error low	Checklist may be long if a multifaceted behavior is measured
Anchored Rating Scale	Simple, objective task to record observations Observer error low More gradations of judgment allowed than typical of an observational checklist	Difficult to write behavioral descriptions that differ by equal amounts over an ordered scale Descriptions may introduce several dimensions into a single rating
Observational Record	Permits routine recording of simple, repetitive behaviors	Inferences depend on sample of time and fineness of recording unit
Anecdotal Notes	May provide unique insights, illustrations	May be irrelevant to outcomes of interest
Critical Incidents	Characterize adaptive and maladaptive behavior May serve as the basis for more structured measurement	Time-consuming to collect and analyze Focus on behavioral extremes; ignore typical behavior that is not outstandingly adaptive or maladaptive
Physiological Measures	Measure is accurate Measure is a good indicator of health status Measure is responsive to compliance with health care regimen	Measure may be multiply determined; not affected by teaching outcomes alone Measure may depend on patient's willingness and ability to perform routine self-testing and recording Measurement may be costly to obtain and analyze Measurement may be invasive
Self-Report	Provides data and insights not available from other sources Measures cognitive, affective, and performance outcomes directly	Subject to faking, socially desirable response set Requires skill in construction of instrument
Oral Self-Report	Little reading and no writing required of patient Contingent questions, probing, and question clarification possible Cheap, group administration of instruments is possible	Recording burden for interviewer Responses may be biased by interviewer Data collection individualized and costly

From McSweeney M: Measuring the effect of patient education. *Diabetes Educ* 7(3):9-15, 1981.　　*Continued*

TABLE 4-1	Types of Measurement—cont'd	
Technique	**Advantages**	**Disadvantages**
Written Self-Report	Cheap, group administration of instruments is possible	Reading and recording burdens are placed on patient
		Questions are fixed; probes and clarifications cannot be introduced
		Possible reduction in response rate or quality resulting from respondent burden
Open-Ended Questions	Respondent free to shape reply	Extent of reply depends on verbal fluency of respondent
		Heavy recording burden for respondent or interviewer
		Inconsistent dimensions of response across patients
		Responses difficult to code and analyze
Closed, Fixed-Alternative Questions	Easy recording, coding, processing of data	Construction of instrument is time-consuming
	Limited dimensions for replies	Dimensions on which choices will vary must be anticipated
	Relative insensitivity to verbal fluency	Choices may be forced among nonsalient options
Single Questions Per Topic	Speed, ease of response	Instability of response
Scales of Questions Per Topic	Stability of response	Increased length of instrument
Self-Monitoring	Recording occurs concurrently with behavior	Recording process may be reactive
	Access to all behaviors, covert and overt, is possible	Quality of record is dependent on patient's cooperation
		Self-monitored data may differ from externally observed data
Records	*Noninvasive*—supply data without added demands on patients	May not be organized to permit easy access retrieval
	Nonreactive—relatively insensitive to external manipulation to claim desired outcomes	Incomplete and/or inconsistent records
		Indirect measures; may not be directly relevant to teaching outcomes
Patient Charts, Physician Records	Relatively low cost of collection	May require health care professional to record and interpret relevant data
		Privacy considerations may restrict access to records or require hierarchy of obtained consents
Agency Service Records, Public Records and Reports	Data may be collected by relatively unskilled workers	Data come from a variety of sources with varying degrees of accessibility, reporting standards, and variable conceptualization

Box 4-12	*COPD Self-Efficacy Scale*

Read each numbered item below, and determine how confident you are that you could manage breathing difficulty or avoid breathing difficulty in that situation. Use the following scale as a basis for your answers:

    (a) = Very confident
    (b) = Pretty confident
    (c) = Somewhat confident
    (d) = Not very confident
    (e) = Not at all confident

1. When I become too tired.
2. When there is humidity in the air.
3. When I go into cold weather from a warm place.
4. When I experience emotional stress or become upset.
5. When I go up stairs too fast.
6. When I try to deny that I have respiratory difficulties.
7. When I am around cigarette smoke.
8. When I become angry.
9. When I exercise or physically exert myself.
10. When I feel distressed about my life.
11. When I feel sexually inadequate or impotent.
12. When I am frustrated.
13. When I lift heavy objects.
14. When I begin to feel that someone is out to get me.
15. When I yell or scream.
16. When I am lying in bed.
17. During very hot or very cold weather.
18. When I laugh a lot.
19. When I do not follow a proper diet.
20. When I feel helpless.
21. When I drink alcoholic beverages.
22. When I get an infection (throat, sinus, colds, the flu, etc.).
23. When I feel detached from everyone and everything.
24. When I experience anxiety.
25. When I am around pollution.
26. When I overeat.
27. When I feel down or depressed.
28. When I breathe improperly.
29. When I exercise in a room that is poorly ventilated.
30. When I am afraid.
31. When I experience the loss of a valued object or a loved one.
32. When there are problems in the home.
33. When I feel incompetent.
34. When I hurry or rush around.

From Wigal JK, Creer TL, Kotses H: The COPD self-efficacy scale. *Chest* 99:1193-1196, 1991.
COPD, Chronic obstructive pulmonary disease.

When measuring learning, teachers focus on the element they have identified as crucial. In a test, a learner should probably be able to answer or perform 94% of all crucial behaviors. This figure allows for some error in the measurement tool. Patient education must be followed by questioning and the reteaching of crucial items when patients give incorrect responses. In giving a written test, the teacher may easily lose sight of the difference between essential learning and other items. The scores may be added up, and the observer may decide that any learner who has answered half the items correctly has learned adequately. The question may never be asked: Exactly what does the learner know? Observers of motor skills are more likely to realize intuitively that an individual who is not placing crutches in the proper position will have difficulty learning to walk with them.

The person constructing a series of teaching items must be sure that the plan measures an individual's ability to transfer knowledge and skills gained in the instructional situation to other situations described or suggested by the objectives. Thorough testing of transfer is necessary because knowledge about ways to produce and verify transfer without careful measurement is insufficient. Initial learning must be established well enough to allow for transfer. Stimulus variation

Box 4-13   *Arthritis Self-Efficacy Scale**

Self-Efficacy Pain Subscale

In the following questions, we'd like to know how your arthritis pain affects you. For each of the following questions, please circle the number which corresponds to your level of certainty that you can now perform the following tasks.

1. How certain are you that you can decrease your pain quite a bit?
2. How certain are you that you can continue most of your daily activities?
3. How certain are you that you can keep arthritis pain from interfering with your sleep?
4. How certain are you that you can make a small-to-moderate reduction in your arthritis pain by using methods other than taking extra medication?
5. How certain are you that you can make a large reduction in your arthritis pain by using methods other than taking extra medication?

Self-Efficacy Function Subscale

We would like to know how confident you are in performing certain daily activities. For each of the following questions, please circle the number that corresponds to your certainty that you can perform the tasks as of now, without assistive devices or help from another person. Please consider what you routinely can do, not what would require a single extraordinary effort.

AS OF NOW, HOW CERTAIN ARE YOU THAT YOU CAN:

1. Walk 100 feet on flat ground in 20 seconds?
2. Walk 10 steps downstairs in 7 seconds?
3. Get out of an armless chair quickly, without using your hands for support?
4. Button and unbutton 3 medium-size buttons in a row in 12 seconds?
5. Cut 2 bite-size pieces of meat with a knife and fork in 8 seconds?
6. Turn an outdoor faucet all the way on and all the way off?
7. Scratch your upper back with both your right and left hands?

8. Get in and out of the passenger side of a car without assistance from another person and without physical aids?
9. Put on a long-sleeve front-opening shirt or blouse (without buttoning) in 8 seconds?

Self-Efficacy Other Symptoms Subscale

In the following questions, we'd like to know how you feel about your ability to control your arthritis. For each of the following questions, please circle the number that corresponds to your level of certainty that you can now perform the following activities or tasks.

1. How certain are you that you can control your fatigue?
2. How certain are you that you can regulate your activity so as to be active without aggravating your arthritis?
3. How certain are you that you can do something to help yourself feel better if you are feeling blue?
4. As compared with other people with arthritis like yours, how certain are you that you can manage arthritis pain during your daily activities?
5. How certain are you that you can manage your arthritis symptoms so that you can do the things you enjoy doing?
6. How certain are you that you can deal with the frustration of arthritis?

---

*Each question is followed by the scale:

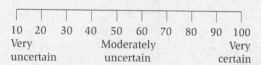

Each subscale is scored separately, by taking the mean of the subscale items. If one-fourth or less of the data is missing, the score is a mean of the completed data. If more than one-fourth of the data is missing, no score is calculated. (The authors invite others to use the scale and would appreciate being informed of study results.)

From Lorig K and others: Development and evaluation of a scale to measure perceived self-efficacy in patients with arthritis, *Arthritis Rheum* 32:37-44, 1989.

Box 4-14	*Possible Errors in Teaching-Learning Process if Goals Are Not Being Met*

Readiness/Motivation Goals

1. Did the learner ever accept the goals, or were you teaching only what you believed to be important?
2. What evidence do you have that the goals were appropriate?
3. Were the goals clearly written and understood by teacher and learner?
4. Were the goals broken into sufficient intermediate steps to provide guidance?

Teaching-Learning

1. Had teaching materials previously been tried with persons of ability similar to your patient and found successful?
2. If previous experience with the materials was not available, in what ways did their characteristics match the patient's readiness?
3. Were evaluative data gathered often during teaching, to give evidence of areas of success and lack of success?
4. Was teaching continued for sufficient time for learning to be thorough?
5. Were the data gathered for evaluation sufficiently valid and reliable to form an adequate basis for the evaluative decision?
6. Were baseline data obtained for measuring change? People rarely start with no knowledge or skill.

(a variety of situations and tasks) in the initial learning produces transfer and determines how much time instruction and learning difficult tasks should take at various stages in the process of learning.

Suppose that the following are related objectives:

- To take a diuretic in the prescribed dosage and at the prescribed time
- To recognize the desired and undesired effects of the medication
- To contact the nurse practitioner when undesired effects occur

Instruction for such objectives would no doubt include information about the purpose of the medication, skills needed to take it, monitoring of desired and undesired effects, behavioral reinforcements for adherence, and practice in problem situations related to taking the medication correctly. It is not feasible to give instruction that represents all possible situations an individual will encounter. If representative situations are used for teaching, most individuals can transfer information to similar situations. To check the amount of transfer a patient actually can make, questions should be constructed to deal with variations or combinations of themes already presented that represent situations a patient might encounter. With a series of questions it is possible to map the areas that a patient does and does not know. The following questions should require transfer (if they have not been used in the original instruction):

1. Suppose you have intestinal flu with vomiting and diarrhea for several days. How would this affect the taking of your diuretic?
2. If the belts on your clothes feel tighter over a period of 3 days, what should you do?
3. You are visiting friends for a few days, and you find that they do not have any citrus fruit. What should you do?

The interpretation of evaluation by teacher and learner is of utmost importance. Learners will have varying degrees of insight into their progress. Allowing for teacher bias, teachers and learners will agree more or less on the amount of progress that has been made. Learners should assess their progress and should discuss differences and similarities with regard to the teacher's assessment. This kind of interchange will help each party. However, when differences of opinion persist, the caregiver must maintain responsibility.

For example, a home health nurse may be teaching a daughter to give bed care to her older adult mother. After several sessions, the daughter believes that she is performing adequately. However, the nurse observes that the daughter is careless about regular turning and that foot support is not being used—lessons that have been taught. Whatever the daughter's reason, emotional or otherwise, for not giving essential care, the nurse is faced with a choice. One alternative is to find the basis for the lack of learning and reteach the learner, weighing the likelihood that the learner will change against the relative adequacy of the care. The other is to suggest that the learner make other arrangements for care because the nurse is responsible for supervision of care. Sometimes the learner becomes hostile, which may be a way of expressing a desire to get out of the situation. Evidence of positive change in learners is rewarding for teachers as well as learners.

The relationship between a learner's competence and a teacher's competence is entangled in evaluation. To some extent this relationship depends on which person is regarded as more responsible for learning. Sometimes it is obvious that a teacher cannot communicate or does not understand the subject matter. In this case the teacher needs to be helped to develop teaching skill. Teaching has the potential for being both harmful and ineffective, and professional incompetence exists in this area of nursing or medicine as in any other area. Possible harmful effects of ineffective teaching include leaving a patient with incapacitating confusion, a loss of self-confidence, or an inability to accomplish necessary reintegration into a family or other social group.

Evaluation of teaching and learning also includes a perspective of the known limitations of teaching today—particularly in the area of motivating individuals. Knowledge of the determinants of behavior at the present time is both limited and fragmented, and practical means of assessing the relative influence of each factor are virtually nonexistent. Therefore in a particular situation it is difficult to estimate how each factor that is already present is influencing particular behavior and how new factors might affect behavior. In many of the complex situations that require learning, reality factors, such as poverty, health, and family crisis, limit the effect that

teaching can have. In such situations small, but important, effects are characteristic even of the "good" programs.

One solution has been to use several complementary kinds of interventions (teaching may be one) to maximize the effect. Sometimes nothing seems to have an effect, and an individual or family does not recover from illness or achieve high-level wellness. Explanation may be sought through inquiry into a patient's perceptions, motives, values, intelligence, and grasp of relevant knowledge. It has also been suggested that a patient's situation might reflect a condition such as powerlessness, and his or her ability to learn may be only one of the behaviors affected.

Thus evaluation during and at the conclusion of a segment of teaching-learning is a summation and interpretation of the results of measurement. It reinforces successful behaviors of learners and teachers. It also provides a time to analyze progress and to redirect activities.

PROGRAM EVALUATION

Increasingly, patient education services are organized into programs of common goals: teaching and evaluation approaches for patients with similar conditions and learning needs. The remainder of this book provides many examples of such programs.

Several preconditions must be met to evaluate an educational program. If they are not met, proceeding may not be worthwhile. For example, an instructional program must have a reasonable design that can produce observable effects. If the goals are not clearly defined, or if the teaching intervention will not yield the goals, the program should be redesigned before an institution spends the resources that a thorough evaluation requires. For example, if (1) the outcome of a program is to ensure patient adherence to a drug regimen, (2) needs assessment shows low adherence in the target group, yet (3) the program's design involves only a pharmacist who hands out drug information sheets when he or she has time, it is unlikely that the program as designed can meet its goals. Effecting adherence requires more than drug information, and a delivery system that is haphazard, diffuse, or unclear will not be effective.

Evaluation is especially important in the initial implementation of a recently designed program, when problem areas have been identified in a refined program or when the program is introduced at a new site. It is also becoming increasingly necessary to justify offering the program or to support accreditation or reimbursement requests. Unfortunately, regular collection of evaluative data occurs rarely in patient education; instead, judgments are made on impressions, or teaching is assumed to be effective.

Ruzicki[16] outlines a series of steps to conduct an evaluation and illustrates this process with the evaluation of a cardiac rehabilitation program at her hospital as an example. The target audiences for the evaluation were identified as the hospital's patient education committee, the administration, cardiologists, and cardiac surgeons. Six evaluative questions were formulated:

1. Does the program meet stated objectives for patient learning?
2. Does it have an impact on changes in risk-factor behaviors after discharge?
3. As a result of their participation in the program, do patients believe that they can manage their own care after discharge?
4. Which teaching techniques are viewed as most helpful by patients?
5. Are physicians satisfied with the program, and do they notice differences after discharge in patients who have participated?
6. Are teaching staff members satisfied with the program, and do they implement it consistently?

It is essential to focus an evaluation through the development of questions. Because resources for evaluation in this example were limited, questionnaires were used, and sample patients were studied.

Results of the evaluation showed that the program was functioning as it should overall. However, the evaluation revealed that there was a lack of documentation and that the nurses were not familiar with some of the information they were expected to teach or with the closed-circuit television films available. The evaluation clearly served as a management tool for improvement of the program.[16]

Some of Ruzicki's questions relate to evaluation of the outcomes of the program and some to process. Administrators are frequently interested in the cost per infection averted after a patient education program and in whether the program could be more cost efficient. Costs usually include personnel, equipment and depreciation, materials, other operating expenses, and sometimes a portion of overhead costs. The easiest way to get a sense of efficiency is to compare one program with another that shows the same outcomes and utilization. Administrators also are interested in statistics such as unplanned readmissions that can be traced to inadequate or prematurely terminated care, including incomplete patient learning. Readmission data have been used by many payers to screen for quality of care. Ashton and others[1] developed readiness-for-discharge criteria covering clinical stability, education of the patient and family, and follow-up medical care among patients with diabetes, heart failure, and obstructive lung disease. Use of these criteria to time discharge appropriately will diminish costly early readmission, a significant financial concern in today's payment climate.

RESEARCH IN PATIENT EDUCATION

Reference to the research base that strengthens patient education practice is made throughout this book. In addition, Appendix C presents meta-analyses and research reviews of bodies of studies in patient education. This work, which began to appear in the literature in 1979, continues to accumulate. Overall these research summaries show that patient education or psychoeducational interventions (which imply a strong behavioral focus) studied in this research were effective for a wide variety of patient outcomes and contributed significantly to patient welfare.

This body of work shows limitations in the research base for patient education. Few studies have addressed the costs of patient education and the savings it produces; this is a serious omission. Study designs frequently do not provide evidence about what mechanisms in the educational interventions were effective, and sometimes whole bodies of work do not appear to include educationally relevant elements, such as feedback, in their interventions. In addition, studies of culturally diverse populations tend to be limited, thus providing little guidance for educational interventions for these groups.

Summaries of research, particularly meta-analyses, allow us to determine when enough attention has been paid to particular research questions, so that available resources are used for more relevant questions. In general, simple tests of the efficacy of educational interventions have been well studied; attention should rather be turned to more direct comparisons of different kinds of educational interventions.

An example of process, outcome, and, to a certain extent, efficiency outcome in a public health setting has been reported by Dignan and others.[6] The Forsyth County Cervical Cancer Prevention Project is a community-based health education program designed to encourage African-American women in the target population to obtain Papanicolaou (Pap) smears on a regular basis and to return for follow-up care when necessary. Process monitoring is done to ensure documentation of program activities, such as distribution of printed materials and coverage of the target population. Those monitoring the process discovered that leaflets distributed in grocery stores were not reaching low-income women often enough. Thereafter distribution of the leaflets was timed to coincide with receipt of Social Security payments. Interviews with members of the target population provided perspective about which materials and activities were having the greatest impact in raising awareness of the importance of cervical screening. In addition, morbidity and mortality data were used. Evaluation served to redirect and improve the campaign as it progressed at a cost of 7% of the project's annual expenditures.

SUMMARY

Although evaluation is the final step in the process of teaching-learning, it is forward-looking because its message redirects activity (Box 4-14). Information necessary for an evaluation of how well objectives have been met is gathered by various measurement techniques. A concerted effort is made to gather reliable information by perfecting measuring tools and by using them in conjunction with one another. This method provides a sounder basis for decisions about the competence of the learner to behave in the manner specified in the objectives. A large body of research results have accumulated that support the efficacy of the patient education interventions tested in those studies.

 Study Questions

1. You observe a nurse who has been teaching a patient how to give himself an injection. The nurse asks the patient the following questions as he goes through the procedure: Is it all right to give the injection with the same syringe and needle you used yesterday? Review why you are wiping the skin a particular way. What would you do if the tip of the needle touched the table as you were picking up the syringe? What would you do if you touched the skin now (after it has been cleansed with the alcohol sponge and before the injection is given)? State the subobjective that the nurse is evaluating.

2. How is the notion of transfer of learning used in evaluation?

3. You are trying to teach a mentally disabled youngster self-dressing skills, and he is inattentive and rebellious. It is obvious that he is showing lack of motivation to learn. List

three possible factors that might be producing this behavior, and indicate the action a caregiver might take in response to each.

4. You are the teacher in a class for patients with diabetes who make the following comments. What evidence does each question or comment give about the individual's understanding?

   a. "Would blood sugar be the same for man, woman, or child?"

   b. "I don't feel I'm really a diabetic because I don't have to take insulin." (The patient is a 19-year-old woman in whom pregnancy precipitated signs and symptoms of diabetes. The physician has ordered that her diabetes be controlled by diet.)

   c. Father whose 8-year-old son has newly diagnosed diabetes, talking to a college student who has been insulin-dependent for 2 years: "Are you able to hunt?"

5. Read the article by Frances Taira on individualized medication sheets,[17] and study Table 3, Medication Knowledge Tool: Interview and Assessment. Do the test items adequately test the objectives? Would two different providers using this test come to the same conclusion about the patient's knowledge?

6. Read the article by Margaret Reuter on parenting needs of abusing parents.[14] Focus on the evaluation tool reproduced in the Appendix to the article. Is this tool a measure of feelings, as indicated in the directions?

References

1. Ashton CM and others: The association between the quality of inpatient care and early readmission, *Ann Intern Med* 122:415-421, 1995.

2. Berkenstadt M and others: Perceived personal control (PPC): a new concept in measuring outcome of genetic counseling, *Am J Med Genet* 82:53-59, 1999.

3. Burma MR, Rachow JW, Kolluri S, Saag KG: Methotrexate patient education study: a quality improvement study, *Arthritis Care Res* 9:216-222, 1996.

4. Clancy CM, Eisenberg JM: Outcomes research: measuring the end results of health care, *Science* 282:245-246, 1998.

5. Dershewitz RA, Posner MK, Paichel W: The effectiveness of health education on home use of ipecac, *Clin Pediatr* 22:268-270, 1983.

6. Dignan MB and others: Use of process evaluation to guide health education in Forsyth County's Project to Prevent Cervical Cancer, *Public Health Rep* 106:73-77, 1991.

7. Ford LA, Ritchie JA: Maternal perceptions of newborn umbilical cord treatments and healing, *J Obstet Gynecol Neonatal Nurs* 28:501-506, 1999.

8. Glasgow RE: Outcomes of and for diabetes education research, *Diabetes Educator* 25(6, suppl):74-88, 1999.

9. Holmes-Rovner M and others: Patient satisfaction with health care decisions, *Med Decis Making* 16:58-64, 1996.

10. Johnson M, Maas M, editors: *Classification of nursing outcomes*, St Louis, 1997, Mosby.

11. Lorig K and others: *Outcome measures for health education and other health care interventions*, Thousand Oaks, CA, 1996, Sage.

12. Mehta S, Binns HJ: What do parents know about lead poisoning? *Arch Pediatr Adolesc Med* 152:1213-1218, 1998.

13. Redman BK: *Measurement tools in patient education*, New York, 1998, Springer.

14. Reuter MM: Parenting needs of abusing parents: development of a tool for evaluation of a parent education class, *Community Health Nurs* 5:129-140, 1988.

15. Riley P: Development of a COPD self-care action scale, *Rehabil Nurs Res* 5(1):3-8, 1996.

16. Ruzicki DA: Evaluation: it's what you do with what you've got that counts, *Promot Health* 6(4):6-9, 1985.

17. Taira F: Individualized medication sheets, *Nurs Econ* 9:56-58, 1991.

18. Wood RY: Reliability and validity of a breast self examination proficiency rating instrument, *Eval Health Prof* 17:418-435, 1994.

Part II

The Infrastructure for Delivery of Patient Education

Introduction to Part II

DELIVERY OF PATIENT EDUCATION

Patient education is currently defined as an essential part of practice in state practice acts for most health professionals, in various federal and state regulations, and in accreditation criteria (see Appendix D for hospital accreditation criteria). Because patient education has not usually been a reimbursable service and does not bring in revenue, the degree of formalization of a structure for delivery of these services seems to have fluctuated and may not be at a lower ebb than it was during the 1980s.

The health care system in the United States has moved significantly to managed care and capitated arrangements. This situation creates more positive incentives to use education to teach people how to manage their own self-care and avoid use of expensive institutional services. In spite of these changed incentives, it is not clear how many patients who are in need of appropriate patient education actually receive it. Apparently no data about the availability of patient education services in nonhospital sectors of the health care industry are available.

Very limited data are available about patient education services. The American Hospital Association reports that 52% of hospitals in the United States have a patient education center and 40% a health information center.[1] Large surveys of patients' perceptions of their experiences in hospitals show significant lack of satisfaction with the educational and supportive aspects of care. Many patients believed hospitals did not do well at providing emotional support and alleviating fears and anxieties or in preparing patients to go home. They saw a confusing, expensive, unreliable, and often impersonal disassembly of health professionals and institutions. Patients talk about how assertive they must be to get answers and the frustrations of trying to coordinate care among many different specialists. About one third of hospital patients indicated that they had not been told about danger signals to watch for after they went home, side effects of medicines they were to take, when they could expect to resume normal activities, or not having enough say regarding their treatment. Patients often expressed the fear that information about their illness or prognosis was being withheld from them.[2]

Several kinds of initiatives in which patient education is central can be cited.

- Patient learning centers are sometimes available in health care institutions. The center is a laboratory-like environment for learning, practicing, and demonstrating self-care skills such as blood pressure and pulse monitoring, self-administration of insulin and monitoring blood glucose, breastfeeding, well newborn care, and caring for a person recovering at home.

Many centers focus as well on building self-efficacy among patients and their families for managing their own care. Insurance companies may cover the fees charged for use of the patient learning center.[3,4]

- The Planetree model[12] operates on a philosophy of compassion, dignity, shared knowledge, coordination and integration of care, emotional support and the alleviation of fear and anxiety, and the freedom of informed choice. The first unit was established in 1981. The physical space for the unit reflects its philosophy with a homelike, healing environment and a schedule set by patient needs. Patients are assisted in understanding their illness and therapy, and they are guided toward achieving wellness through resources such as a library of printed and videotaped materials. A recent randomized clinical trial studying the effectiveness of the Planetree model hospital unit compared with other medical-surgical units in that hospital found few differences in health behaviors of patients and no differences in length of stay. However, Planetree patients reported more satisfaction and better mental health status and functioning after discharge.[7]

- Nurse-managed clinics or programs frequently provide education. An example is a hospital-based smoking cessation program for noncardiac patients. During hospitalization the nurse provided 1 hour of instruction including videotape, workbook with audiotape, and counseling about how to avoid high-risk relapse situations. Ten-minute nurse-initiated phone contacts after discharge found those who had relapses and needed additional instruction. Patients in such a nurse-managed program showed a significantly higher 12-month cessation rate than patients who got a standardized message from the physician and a booklet.[11] For programs in which ceasing a behavior like

smoking is the goal, behavioral techniques and self-monitoring are important.[9]

- Nurse-managed clinics providing self-care education are useful for many diseases such as asthma. Lorig and others[5] have shown that it is possible to teach patients with a variety of chronic illnesses (heart or lung disease, stroke, or arthritis) in one group. Common self-management skills that need to be learned include recognizing and acting on symptoms, using medications correctly, managing emergencies, maintaining nutrition and diet and adequate exercise, using stress reduction techniques, interacting effectively with health care providers, managing relationships with significant others, adapting to work, and managing psychological responses to illness such as depression.

- Practice guidelines, which define the standard of practice based on research, are now widely used in health care settings to improve the quality of care and to minimize undue variability in care. They frequently contain information to help patients understand the area of treatment and how to determine the quality of the treatment they are receiving. The Agency for Health Care Policy and Research (AHCPR) has developed many research-based guidelines, including those for management of acute pain. One institution attempting implementation of these guidelines found a number of problems; for example, parents had a significant lack of knowledge about the role they could take in assisting with their child's pain control. Relevant information frequently was not included in preoperative teaching. This finding prompted the institution to develop the standard of care statement shown in Box 1.[10] Note that these are process-oriented standards of care; one would hope for standards that also require attainment of an established level of patient outcome—in this case, in level of pain control.

| Box 1 | *Illustrative Standard of Care for Pediatric Pain Management* |

Education of the Patient and Family

- The patient and family will receive written and verbal information about pain management preoperatively in the clinic, or on admission to the hospital.
- The nurse will document the goals and expectations identified by the patient and family.

Assessment of Pain

- Assessment of pain on the nursing unit will be done immediately on admission and at least every 4 hours for the first 24 hours postoperatively.
- The same pain scale will be used consistently with the patient and family throughout the hospital stay.
- Patients will be reassessed for pain within 30 to 60 minutes after all pain interventions.

Intervention for Pain

- Pain control intervention will be provided around-the-clock (e.g., every 4 hours) for at least the first 24 postoperative hours, unless refused by the patient. Interventions can be moved to an as-needed schedule at the discretion of the nurse after 24 hours.
- Intervention will be offered on an as-needed basis if the child reports a pain rating of 3 or above on the Wong and Baker faces scale or the numeric scales, or if physiological or behavioral indicators of pain are present.
- Equianalgesic conversion charts will be used when converting a patient from IV medications to oral medications.

From Schmidt K and others: *J Nurs Care Qual* 8(3): 68-74, 1994.

- Delivery systems for pharmaceutical care have been significantly affected by regulations for patient education. Although a 1990 federal law requires pharmacists to counsel patients on Medicaid about their prescriptions, many states have adoped

laws requiring the counseling of all patients.[8] In addition, pharmacy benefit managers (PBMs) now serve as more than purchasing and dispensing agents; they monitor drug use and practice disease state management, focused at keeping the disease under control and saving resources. PBMs usually start with diabetes and asthma, two of the most costly conditions for plan sponsors. If the medical claims and test results data suggest that a patient's diabetes may not be controlled adequately, a letter is sent to the primary care physician noting that the health maintenance organization will provide special educational services and coverage of diabetes-specific tests and monitoring devices. If the database indicates that a person with asthma reorders a bronchodilator too often, chances are that the individual does not know how to use it correctly. The plan will alert and pay a pharmacist to counsel the patient on correct use.[6]

- The infrastructure described in the preceding discussion seems scattered, incoherent, and lacking in data. It is accurate to say that there is no concerted direction for patient education or even an organizational structure under which those committed to its development come together. Rather, patient education services have developed in separate practice areas, associated with disease or health states. Although there are some commonalities in their development, it is best to understand each of them in some detail. The chapters in Part II describe in depth many areas of practice.

AREAS OF PATIENT EDUCATION PRACTICE

Of the areas in which patient education is practiced, perhaps the oldest are diabetes education and pregnancy and parenting education. The field of diabetes education has developed a more formal structure than have most other fields; it includes advanced practice specialists who are certified, accreditation of diabetes education programs, and a large research base on which to base practice. Development of other areas of practice, such as education of patients and families with mental health needs, is much newer. For example, exploration of the educational structure on which to base programs for persons with schizophrenia and depression is ongoing.

References

1. American Hospital Association: *Hospital statistics,* Chicago, 1999, The Association.
2. American Hospital Association, Picker Institute: Eye on patients: excerpts from a report on patients' concerns and experiences about the health care system, *J Health Care Finance* 2(4):2-11, 1997.
3. Goldstein NL and others: Comparison of two teaching strategies, *Clin Nurs Res* 5:150-166, 1996.
4. Kantz B and others: Developing patient and family education services, *J Nurs Adm* 28(2):11-18, 1998.
5. Lorig KR and others: Evidence suggesting that a chronic disease self-management program can improve health status while reducing hospitalization, *Med Care* 37:5-14, 1999.
6. Mandelker J: The expanding role of PBMs, *Business and Health* Special Report, 1995.
7. Martin DP and others: Randomized trial of a patient-centered hospital unit, *Patient Educ Couns* 34:125-133, 1998.
8. Meade V: OBRA '90: how has pharmacy reacted? *Am Pharm* NS35(2):12-16, 1995.
9. Mullen PD and others: A meta-analysis of trials evaluating patient education and counseling for three groups of preventive health behaviors, *Patient Educ Couns* 32:157-173, 1997.
10. Schmidt K and others: Implementation of the AHCPR pain guidelines for children, *J Nurs Care Qual* 8(3):68-74, 1994.
11. Taylor CB and others: A nurse-managed smoking cessation program for hospitalized smokers, *Am J Pub Health* 86:1557-1560, 1996.
12. Weber DO: Planetree transplanted, *Healthcare Forum J* 35(5):30-37, 1992.

Chapter 5

Cancer Patient Education

GENERAL APPROACH

Education helps individuals detect their own cancer and aids in treatment and rehabilitation. Perhaps the greatest effort in cancer education has been placed on teaching self-assessment techniques such as breast self-examination and on persuading individuals to seek other screening techniques such as Papanicolaou (Pap) smears or colon cancer screening. Because minority women are more likely to seek medical care when breast and cervical cancers are in an advanced stage,[1] special attention is being paid to cultural models for assessing how individuals from these populations understand cancer and how interventions can best be delivered to them. Because cancer is a chronic disease, the needs of families and home caregivers and the use of cancer support groups have also received attention, as has the education necessary to adequately manage pain associated with the disease. Americans' knowledge about major risk factors and survival after early detection for common cancers (breast, cervical, and colon) is poor for all ages and races. Those at greatest risk—the oldest—have the least knowledge.[2]

EDUCATIONAL APPROACHES AND RESEARCH BASE

Two rigorous reviews of the effects of psychosocial interventions on adults with cancer are available. In 1995, Meyer and Mark[27] published a meta-analysis of 45 studies of nonpharmacological interventions intended to improve the quality of life of patients in whom one of the neoplastic diseases was diagnosed (see Appendix C). Outcomes of interest included emotional and functional adjustment, symptoms, and medical status. The interventions were broader than what are usually considered to be aspects of patient education and included progressive muscle relaxation, meditation, hypnotherapy, systematic desensitization, biofeedback, behavior modification or reinforcement, psychotherapy, and counseling. Most studies focused on white women in the United States. The summary found relatively small effect sizes: 0.31 for emotional adjustment, 0.32 for functional adjustment, and 0.41 for symptoms, with no difference among the various kinds of interventions (behavioral, counseling and therapy, informational and educational methods, or organized social support).[27] An effect size is the change (in standard deviation units) attributable to the experimental intervention.

Also in 1995, Devine and Westlake[8] published a meta-analysis of 116 studies of the effects of psychoeducational care for adults with cancer and found statistically significant beneficial effects of this care for anxiety, depression, mood, nausea, vomiting, pain, and knowledge. Differentiating among the effectiveness of various types of psychoeducational care was problematic. This constitutes a strong research base.

Concerns that teaching self-screening and encouraging its practice will raise anxiety were not supported in a study of testicular self-examination in young men.[39] More complex relationships among anxiety and skill, confidence, and adherence to breast self-examination (BSE) are documented in recent literature. As many as half of women with a family history of breast cancer have persistent distress related to their increased risk, with these feelings beginning as early as adolescence. Some overestimate their risk by as much as four times their actual risk. Lower rates of self-screening were found in women who were more distressed. Coming to terms with this risk requires information and support.[5,24] Not doing BSE or doing it irregularly can allow women to maintain control over their feelings of threat.

Demonstration as a method of teaching BSE is insufficient. Actual practice in developing tactile skill in detecting abnormalities must lead to competence and confidence. For women who did not feel competent of their ability to detect lumps, self-examination served to increase their feelings of being "out of control" with a resultant increase in anxiety. Women who rate their ability to self-examine highly have been found to be more likely to carry out regular BSE and to act on abnormalities they may find.[4]

In addition, Janz and others[23] summarized more than 33 intervention studies of BSE, which showed that more than 90% of women were aware of recommendations to practice BSE, yet only 25% to 35% did so on a monthly basis. Although the profusion of BSE information has gained women's attention, it has not encouraged many to practice or to become proficient at BSE. Most women have not been taught to detect lumps in a silicone breast model, which is believed to be a very useful method. BSE education can be augmented if the learner practices the technique on her own breasts while the provider stands ready to monitor and correct. Although this review is nearly a decade old, current research describes the same issues of a low percentage of women practicing BSE with competence and confidence issues remaining.[36]

Prompts and reminders seem to contribute to frequent long-term use of BSE. Reassessment and retraining (which takes 5 to 8 minutes) are also necessary and must be incorporated into events such as annual physical examinations and mammograms. Although researchers have developed an effective technology for training in these skills (use of silicone breast models for lump detection), the actual maintenance of such skills remains questionable. Evidence suggests that performance deteriorates after only one training session, returning to near pretraining levels after 6 months. From a learning perspective it can be understood that BSE skills are not typically performed often, and there is limited opportunity for corrective feedback and reinforcement.[31]

A related issue is education to persuade women to follow up on abnormal screening results. Stewart and others[35] note that there are clear and consistent findings that women with abnormal Pap smear results are more likely to complete recommended treatment and follow-up and to be less emotionally distressed by fear of cancer if they receive appropriate and reassuring educational materials.

Education to support patients in making decisions about their treatment is also of great importance. For example, women need information to choose from alternative treatments for breast cancer—the one most consistent with their own values. For obvious reasons many women have greater difficulty concentrating just before having a breast biopsy. A computer-based system contains information, referrals, and decision-making and social support programs for women with breast cancer. It allows them to talk anonymously with peers, to question experts, to learn where to obtain help, to read stories about people who have survived similar crises, to read relevant articles, to monitor their health status, to consider difficult decisions, and to plan how to regain control of their lives. This kind of system is especially important for those who live in rural areas where there may be less access to state-of-the-art treatment options, libraries, and social support groups. Because health crises are often protracted, an information and support service must be available when and where people need it, not just at a clinic.[19]

In addition, when there are many equivalent options for a single problem, formal decision aids have been found to be useful for establishing patient preferences. Figure 5-1 shows an example of a decision board to assist women with lymph node-positive breast cancer to choose between two adjuvant chemotherapy treatments. The clinician reads the written material aloud and explains the graphical material contained

on seven cards and placed on the board in sequence.[22] A similar approach can be used for men considering screening for prostate cancer. A recent study found well-educated men to be not well informed about the natural history of prostate cancer, the benefits of treatment or the predictive value of prostate specific antigen (PSA) tests—all important factors to understand before they can participate meaningfully in a decision about screening. Participation is particularly important because personal preferences of well-

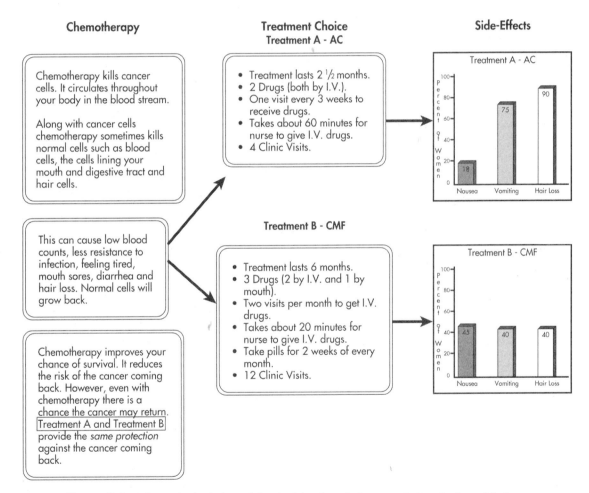

Figure 5-1 Schematic depiction of the decision board. (From Irwin E and others: Offering a choice between two adjuvant chemotherapy regimens: a pilot study to develop a decision aid for women with breast cancer, *Patient Educ Couns* 37:283-291, 1999.)

informed men have been found to be evenly divided between accepting or forgoing screening.[15]

Family support in dealing with cancer is also necessary. Several longitudinal studies of patients and spouses indicate that the stressful effects of cancer extend as long as 1 to 2 years after the initial diagnosis. For the most part spouses report receiving little information about their partner's illness, and their attempts to request information or to contact the physician by telephone were often unsuccessful. It is believed that families need a framework of expectations about the emotional aspects of recovery that can serve as a measure against which they can monitor progress and receive encouragement to view their concerns as a normal part of the recovery process.[29] A study of home caregivers[18] found significant needs that were not satisfied (barrier needs); these are identified in Box 5-1.[20] Note how many of these barrier needs are amenable to instruction. Both the importance and the satisfaction of most caregiver needs change over time and should be reassessed.

Part of the self-care that patients and families give at home consists of monitoring for signs and symptoms of progression of the disease or side effects of treatment. For example, in one study[26] patients with lymphoma were taught self-diagnosis and self-referral for on-demand treatment for herpes zoster, which can leave painful long-term effects if not treated. In patients who remembered receiving pamphlets with color photos of typical cutaneous zoster lesions, long-term complications were less prevalent.[26] Another example is teaching patients to detect early signs of spinal cord compression (frequently caused by vertebral metastases), a treatable oncological emergency that can lead to permanent neurological deficits.[30] Unexplained back pain, followed by weakness of the lower extremities, is the usual pattern of symptoms; such symptoms can easily confuse a patient, who might attribute this pain to other sources.

Educational interventions for pain management are important because pain affects 50% to 80% of cancer patients, and is poorly controlled in an estimated 80%. The content for a pain education program is shown in Box 5-2.[12] Al-

though it would have been helpful if behavioral objectives had also been included, evaluation of the outcome of the program found it effective in decreasing pain intensity and severity, decreasing perception of addiction, decreasing anxiety, increasing use of pain medications, and helping

---

Box 5-1 | *Top 25 Barrier Needs by All Subjects in Phase I (N = 492)*

1. Information about the underlying reasons for symptoms
2. Information about what symptoms to expect
3. Information about what to expect in the future
4. Information about treatment of side effects
5. Information about community resources
6. Honest and updated information
7. Ways to reassure my patient
8. Ways to deal with my patient's decreased energy
9. Ways to deal with the unpredictability of the future
10. Information about medications (side effects and scheduling)
11. Ways to encourage my patient
12. Information about my patient's psychological needs
13. Methods to decrease my stress
14. Ways of coping with my patient's diagnosis of cancer
15. Information about the type and extent of my patient's illness
16. Ways to cope with role changes
17. Information about the physical needs of my patient
18. Activities that will make my patient feel purposeful
19. Ways to be more patient and tolerant
20. Ways to deal with my depression
21. Ways to maintain a normal family life
22. Ways to discuss death with my patient
23. Ways to deal with my fears
24. Ways to combat fatigue
25. Ways to provide my patient with adequate nutrition

From Hileman JW, Lackey NR, Hassanein RS: Identifying the needs of home caregivers of patients with cancer. *Oncol Nurs Forum* 19:771-777, 1992.

to improve sleep.[11] Patient and professional education about pain relief is so important that 28 states have established initiatives to deal with cancer pain. Inadequate assessment of pain and fear of addiction are two strong educational needs that must be addressed.[17]

Rimer, Kedziera, and Levy[33] note that few systematically developed and carefully evaluated patient education programs on cancer pain control have been reported. Although cancer pain can be controlled, it frequently is not, and fear of pain is a common concern of persons with cancer and their families. During the educational assessment process, it is important to assess not only knowledge and cultural beliefs but also the meaning of pain—perceptions of what is causing it and how it affects life. Often patients use pain as an indicator of advancing disease or resistance to cancer therapy. To set common goals, patients and their families should be encouraged to verbalize expectations, and providers must help them understand what can reasonably be accomplished. Well-ingrained attitudes and beliefs about addiction must be addressed. Addiction refers to psychological dependence and is rare in the cancer patient population.

In addition to instrumental learning such as information about pain management, persons with cancer and their families struggle to establish meaning about what is happening to them. In life-threatening illness, meaning affects coping behavior, has an impact on psychosocial well-being, and is important in the struggle to obtain a sense of mastery. Meaning refers to an individual's understanding of the implications an illness has for his or her identity and for the future—perceptions of the ability to accomplish future goals, to maintain the viability of interpersonal relationships, and to sustain a sense of personal vitality, competence, and power. The constructed meaning scale, shown in Box 5-3, is a measure of

---

Box 5-2 *Pain Education Program Content*

Part I. General overview of pain
  A. Defining pain
  B. Understanding the causes of pain
  C. Pain assessment and use of pain rating scales to communicate pain
  D. Using a preventive approach to controlling pain
  E. Involvement of the family in pain management
Part II. Pharmacological management of pain
  A. Overview of drug management of pain
  B. Overcoming fears of addiction
  C. Fear of drug dependence
  D. Understanding drug tolerance
  E. Understanding respiratory depression
  F. Talking to the doctor about pain
  G. Controlling other symptoms, such as nausea and constipation
Part III. Nondrug management of pain
  A. Importance of nondrug interventions
  B. Use of nondrug modalities as an adjunct to medications
  C. Review of previous experiences with nondrug methods
  D. Demonstration of heat, cold, massage, relaxation/distraction, and imagery

From Ferrell BR, Rhiner M, Ferrell BA: Development and implementation of a pain education program, *Cancer* 72(suppl):3426-3432, 1993.

Box 5-3 *Constructed Meaning Scale*

1. I feel cancer is something I will never recover from.
2. I feel cancer is serious, but I will be able to return to life as it was before my illness.
3. I feel cancer has changed my life permanently so it will never be as good again.
4. I feel I have made a complete recovery from my illness.
5. I feel that I am the same person as I was before my illness.
6. I feel that my relationships with other people have not been negatively affected by my illness.
7. I feel that my experience with cancer has made me a better person.
8. I feel that having cancer has interfered with my achievement of the most important goals I have set for myself.

From Fife BL: The measurement of meaning in illness, *Soc Sci Med* 40:1021-1028, 1995.

such meaning. Each statement allows a response on a scale of 1 to 4: strongly disagree, disagree, agree, strongly agree. The lowest test score, 8, indicates a very negative sense of the meaning the illness holds for one's self and for one's future life. The authors discuss the validity and reliability in the text of their article.[13]

A number of measurement tools that may be used in clinical practice or research are presented and reviewed in Redman.[32] Instruments are available to assess informational needs of patients with breast cancer and colorectal cancer.

COMMUNITY-BASED EDUCATION AND EDUCATION OF SPECIAL POPULATIONS

Much education for the patient with cancer is community-based, as the preceding examples indicate. Particularly important are programs aimed at the issues of continuing care and remission, with its requirement for self-monitoring.

Patients must be taught how to communicate their pain to their health care teams, including the use of common pain-rating scales, and to describe pain site, quality, intensity, aggravating factors, and amount of relief current measures give as well as how long the relief lasts. They should also be able to participate in pain management, including use of medications and adjunctive strategies such as self-hypnosis, relaxation, and imagery. Pain control is an active process that requires frequent fine tuning to be successful. Whenever possible, the designated caregiver should be involved because this person may eventually need to manage the patient's care and can inadvertently undermine a well-designed teaching plan. The teaching plan is focused on a more recently accepted view that patients have a right to pain control, allowing them to optimize their quality of life.[33] A brief test of pain knowledge and experience that can be used in clinical settings may be found in Box 5-4. It will help to identify misunderstandings that can be corrected and establish an expectation for adequate pain relief.

At least two other groups of patients with considerable educational needs are consistently neglected. Women whose breast biopsies are benign still require education to answer questions such as: What is fibrocystic disease? Will benign breast disease turn into cancer?[7] Likewise, long term survivors of breast cancer frequently are confused about what is adequate follow-up once their cancer treatment ends. They want information about how to monitor their own bodies and how to manage symptoms such as lymphedema.[16]

Teaching tools for the education of patients with cancer are widely available from national voluntary and government agencies. As with other areas of practice, there are very few materials written at lower reading levels. Teaching tools are published regularly in professional journals, such as *Oncology Nursing Forum*, *Journal of the American Medical Association*, and *Nurse Practitioner*, which serve to educate the professional nursing community so that practitioners can fulfill their patient education roles. Figures 5-2 and 5-3 and Box 5-5 illustrate several examples of teaching tools. The leaflet on prostate cancer is an example of what is available in each issue of the journals noted above (Figure 5-2). The pamphlet describing the Pap test is written for populations of marginal literacy (Figure 5-3). The final example (Box 5-5) provides sensory information for colposcopy. Sensory as well as procedural information has in general been found to improve preparation for a procedure and to speed recovery.

The educational needs of a number of special populations with cancer require attention. For example, more than 50% of all cancers occur in the 11% of the population older than 65 years of age; yet very little attention has been paid to the educational needs of this population. Mortality caused by cancer is higher in minority groups, partially because some ethnic groups are less aware of the signs and symptoms of cancer and may have beliefs that are divergent from the mainstream of the health care system. Each major ethnic population serves as an umbrella for several diverse populations. It is important to look at cancer knowledge, beliefs, and attitudes by socioeconomic status as well as by cultural group. In addition, research has shown

---

Box 5-4 *Pain Knowledge and Experience*

STATEMENT	CORRECT RESPONSE
Cancer pain can be effectively relieved.	Agree
Pain medicines should be given only when pain is severe.	Disagree
Addiction refers to a person's desire to use drugs for their psychic effects rather than for the medical use of relieving pain. Most patients with cancer on pain medicines will become psychologically addicted to the medicines over time.	Disagree
Drug dependence means that a person would go through withdrawal if a pain medicine was stopped. Most patients with cancer receiving pain medicine will become physically dependent on the medicines over time.	Agree
It is better to give the lowest amount of medicines possible early on so that larger doses will be available later if the pain increases.	Disagree
It is better to give pain medicines around-the-clock (on a schedule) rather than only when needed.	Agree
Treatments other than medications (such as massage, heat, and relaxation) can be effective for relieving pain.	Agree
Pain medicines often interfere with breathing.	Disagree
Patients often are given too much pain medicine.	Disagree

Pain Experience Scale—Patient

Below is a statement about cancer pain and pain relief.
Please make an "X" on the line to indicate your response.

1. Cancer pain can be effectively relieved.

disagree _____ agree

From Ferrell BR, Ferrell BA, Rhiner M: Development and implementation of a pain education program, *Cancer* 72 (suppl):3426-3432, 1993.

---

that different ethnic groups have different styles of learning. Most efforts to meet the educational and informational needs of different ethnic groups have revolved around translated materials, focus groups conducted to ensure cultural relevance, and community leadership involvement. Past experiences with difficulties in an institutional or a learning environment may make it difficult for any individual to ask questions or seek assistance.[37]

A study of low-income African-American women older than 40 years of age in Atlanta, Georgia, found that their cancer models differed significantly from those held by clinicians.[18] The women attending these clinics endured cancer-screening tests that to them seemed to serve only as heralds of a disease that would ultimately kill them and that was outside the realm of physicians' abilities. Many women preferred to remain ignorant of the existence of cancer. Many believed that cancer originates as a bruise or sore that will not heal. Almost 60% believed that surgery just makes the cancer worse by exposing the tumor to air and thereby spreading the disease. Faith in God seemed to be one of the few completely benign and truly powerful treatment alternatives available to an individual with cancer. Given the explanatory models of this group of women, the question to ask is why any women in this group would undergo screening.

Two excellent examples of culturally relevant educational programs appeared in *Oncology Nursing Forum.*[9] In an effort to reach African-American adolescents, a video was made setting

Text continued on p. 122

PATIENT EDUCATION

Prostate Cancer

What is the prostate?
The prostate is a golf-ball-size gland that lies at the base of your urinary bladder (see illustration). The prostate aids in providing the fluid that carries sperm.

Are there different kinds of prostate disease?
Yes, there are. One type of prostate disease is prostate cancer, and two noncancerous (benign) conditions are benign prostatic hypertrophy (BPH) and prostatitis. BPH is a common condition in men over 50 years of age. In fact, the majority of men over 60 have some degree of BPH. Prostatitis refers to any inflammation of the prostate gland and may occur from bacterial infections or other causes of inflammation. Nonbacterial prostatitis is common in aging men.

Prostate cancer is the most common cancer in men; the average man has a 15.4% risk of developing this disease. The risk increases if a close relative has had prostate cancer. Other risk factors include being African-American, eating a high-fat diet, and being exposed to environmental toxins.

What are the symptoms of prostate disease?
The symptoms are similar for prostate cancer, BPH, and prostatitis. However, most men do not experience symptoms until the disease is advanced. Possible symptoms include

- frequent urge to urinate
- discomfort urinating
- difficulty emptying bladder
- difficulty starting a stream of urine

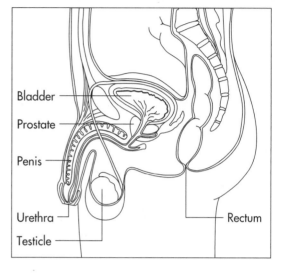

Bladder
Prostate
Penis
Urethra
Testicle
Rectum

- nighttime urination
- groin-area discomfort
- extreme lower abdominal pain.

Are there any tests for prostate disease?
Methods used to examine the prostate and to screen for cancer include the digital rectal exam (DRE), prostate specific antigen (PSA) test, and transrectal ultrasound (TRUS). These methods are most effective when used in combination.

An elevated PSA or an abnormal DRE can occur with benign conditions such as BPH and prostatitis, so a further evaluation by a urologist may be warranted to screen for cancer. The urologist may review the medical records, obtain a medical history, and repeat lab tests. The urologist will also examine the prostate. Based on the findings, you may be scheduled for an ultrasound and/or biopsy of the prostate.

Figure 5-2 Sample of leaflet on prostate cancer as appears in a professional journal. (From Patient education: prostate cancer, *Nurse Practitioner* 23[3]:35-36, 1998.)

Prostate Cancer

PSA
When the prostate is injured, its leaks PSA into the bloodstream. The level of PSA can be measured with a simple blood test and is very helpful for screening prostate cancer. The PSA rises slightly with age, so your age is one of the factors considered when the PSA results are interpreted.

DRE
The prostate is located just in front of the rectum, so it can be felt through the wall of the rectum, with a lubricated, gloved finger, during a DRE. The prostate has been described as feeling like an eraser or the tip of your nose. The DRE is used to estimate the size of the prostate and its general texture, and to locate any areas of irregularity or lumps. The exam is very brief. Because only the back portion of the prostate can be felt, the DRE does not always accurately detect changes.

Ultrasound
TRUS is usually performed in the urologist's office. While lying on your side, a probe is inserted into the rectum and pressed toward the prostate. The probe sends out "sound waves" that bounce off the prostate, giving a "picture" of its shape and consistency.

Biopsy
A biopsy (sample of prostate tissue) may be obtained with the ultrasound. If so, a biopsy instrument that holds a very small hollow needle is attached to the probe and positioned to take at least three samples

from each side of the prostate. You may experience some soreness or stinging each time a sample is taken. After the procedure is completed, the samples are sent to a lab, where the sample is carefully screened for cancerous cells.

If you need to have a biopsy, a laxative and an antibiotic may be prescribed, and you should not take aspirin for several days prior to the procedure. After the procedure, it is normal to see some blood in the urine, stool, and/or semen for several days.

What happens if the results show I have prostate cancer?
Your clinician will discuss which treatment option is best for you. Treatment options include "watchful waiting," surgery, radiation therapy, hormone therapy, and chemotherapy.

RESOURCES

American Foundation for Urologic Disease
1-800-242-2383

American Urologic Association
(410) 223-4310

American Cancer Society
1-800-ACS-2345

National Cancer Institute
1-800-4-CANCER

This teaching aid may be photocopied by health care professionals for use in their clinical practice. Hospitals and other institutions that wish to photocopy this material must first contact the Copyright Clearance Center at (508) 750-8400.

Figure 5-2, cont'd   For legend see opposite page.

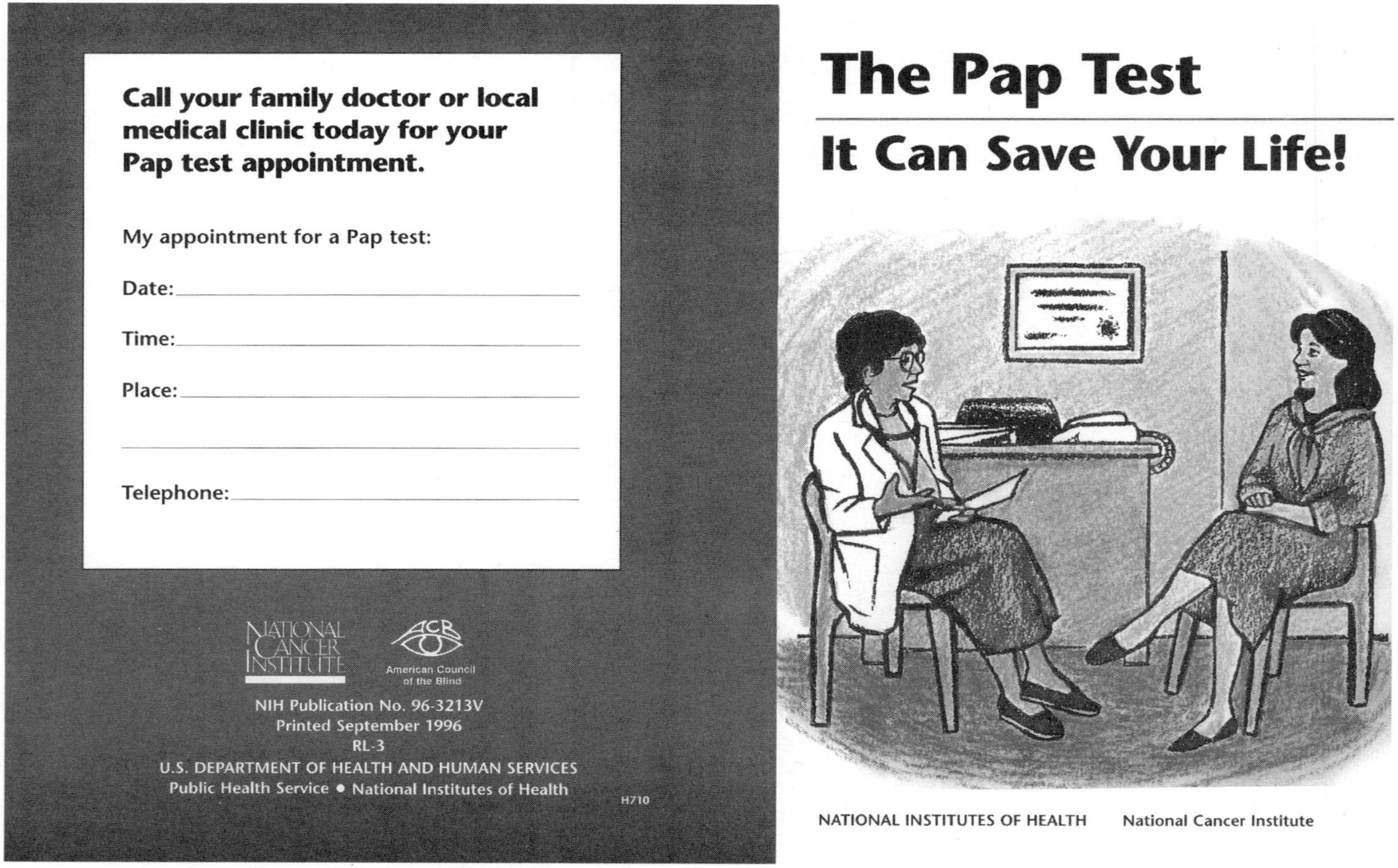

Figure 5-3 Sample Pap test pamphlet. (Courtesy The National Cancer Institute.)

Get your appointment for a Pap test today!

1. Could I have cancer of the cervix and not know it?

Yes—often there is no pain.

And this kind of cancer kills many women every year.

2. What does that mean for me?

It means get a Pap test.

A Pap test can find cancer early.

If it's found early, it's easier to cure.

3. How often should I get a Pap test?

Get a Pap test every year.

4. How is the Pap test done?

The nurse or doctor wipes a swab on the cervix in your vagina.

This takes only a few seconds.

5. Where do I get a Pap test?

▶ Family doctor
▶ OB/GYN
▶ Medical clinic
▶ Local health department

6. Who needs to have a Pap test?

You do if:

▶ You are **over 18**, or
▶ You are **18 or under** and have sex

There is no upper age limit for the Pap test.

Even women who have gone through the change of life (menopause) need a Pap test every year.

7. Why is a Pap test important to me?

Because it can tell if you have cancer of the cervix early—while it's still easier to cure.

It can save your life!

For more information on the Pap test, call the National Cancer Institute's Cancer Information Service at **1-800-4-CANCER** (1-800-422-6237). Persons with TTY equipment, dial **1-800-332-8615.**

☎ **Turn Page** →

Figure 5-3, cont'd   For legend see opposite page.

Box 5-5	*Sensory Information Message for Colposcopy*

Once you have changed into a hospital gown for the procedure, you will be taken to the colposcopy room. In the room, you will notice an examining table with stirrups, a cart holding instruments, and the colposcope (a piece of equipment that looks like a microscope). You will be asked to get up on the examining table and to slide down on the table so that your feet are in the stirrups. A clinician will explain the procedure to you either before it is done or as it is being done.

The clinician may perform a pelvic examination. Then, he/she inserts a speculum, which will feel cool and uncomfortable. Once the speculum is in place, the clinician will clean and examine your cervix. He/she also will apply vinegar to your cervix. The vinegar helps the clinician to see any abnormal area(s) better. The vinegar will feel cool.

The clinician may take a sample of secretions from your cervical canal. This means that he/she would quickly move a probe in and out of the cervix. If this is part of your examination you will feel a cramping sensation that will last as long as it takes to obtain the sample.

The clinician will take a biopsy specimen of any abnormal area(s) on the cervix. You will likely hear a snipping sound as the clamps come together and feel a pinch as the biopsy is being taken. The pinching sensation lasts only seconds.

The clinician will remove the speculum, which will give you a sense of relief. It may seem as though the speculum is being removed more slowly than it is when you have a Pap test. The reason for the difference is that the clinician can use the colposcope to take a good look at the top part of your vagina.

The clinician may also examine your external genitals. If this is part of your examination, he/she will spray vinegar on this area so that any abnormal area(s) are seen more easily. The vinegar will feel cool.

The procedure is now completed. You are asked to sit up on the side of the examining table. You will be given information about how and when you will receive the biopsy results.

From Nugent LS, Clark CR; Colposcopy: sensory information for client education, *J Obstet Gynecol* 25:225-231, 1996.

BSE instruction to rap music. Participants responded to the rap music with laughter, moving their arms in the air and their hands around their breasts in circular motions as directed in the song. A second excellent example gives information about cervical health in a game format called Loteria, which is familiar to many adult Hispanic women of Mexican descent.[34] As in the traditional Loteria game, pictures are matched with written text that instructs them about the risk factors for cervical cancer, screening guidelines for cervical cancer, and the increased rate for invasive cervical cancer found in adult Hispanic women. Because many members of the target population did not have transportation outside their community, the educational programs were presented in churches, clubs, and clinics, with gifts of cosmetics supplied to participants. The importance of staying well by undergoing regular Pap testing was highlighted as allowing the women to continue to perform their roles as mother and wife, important in the Hispanic culture.

Another example of a special population is the mildly handicapped or disabled adolescent girl, instructed in the performance of BSE.[40] Because the population taught was capable of second- to fifth-grade achievement, active participation, imitation, and reinforcement were used as learning principles. Behavioral objectives included demonstrating knowledge of the seven warning signals of cancer and the symptoms of breast cancer; knowing the American Cancer Society's recommendations for screening for breast cancer; demonstrating proper technique for BSE as evidenced by ability to find the lumps in the silicone breast and by answering questions correctly; and knowing where to go for a professional examination if they found suspicious lumps in their breasts.

A program to increase prostate cancer screening in African-American men found that a peer educator method (testimony by African-American men in support of prostate cancer screening) and phone calls aimed at removing screening barriers or reminders for screening were more effective than was "standard education." This population can often be more easily recruited into work sites, churches, housing projects, or barbershops than into health care settings. The men in this study needed to understand the absence of symptoms in early stages of prostate cancer, and the various treatment options available.[38]

"Witnessing," in which role models who have survived cancer tell of their experiences in groups at churches and community organizations, is well matched to certain cultures. These women did not know that mammography was associated with cancer, confused it with a Pap smear, and believed that the test was not necessary if their breasts were smaller or felt fine.[6,10] Cervical cancer screening education culturally acceptable for Native American women used talking circles, in which each member provides a 5- to 10-minute story, sharing information and support.[21] This culture has a strong oral tradition and a strong sense of privacy. Table 5-1 provides a list of breast cancer educational materials useful for this population.[3]

NATIONAL STANDARDS AND TESTED PROGRAMS

The Oncology Nursing Society has for some time had national standards of oncology education, including patient and family education, as well as public education (see Appendix D).

SUMMARY

Goals in education for patients with cancer include helping the patient adjust to the course of the disease, carry out self-care and prescribed regimens, recognize and control side effects, achieve a sense of participation in and control over care, and normalize lifestyle and interactions—all discussed in the preceding examples of educational interventions in institutional and community settings and with varied

populations. It is important to note that far more research and educational program development seem to be focused on breast and, to a lesser extent, cervical cancer than on other equally important neoplastic diseases, although the general principles of screening, self-care, coping, and family support are applicable to all.

 Study Questions

1. A breast and cervical cancer screening program was set up at several sites to serve low-income African-American women attending public clinics in Chicago. Part of the intervention was an educational program aimed at increasing knowledge about screening, which was evaluated by the classroom survey instrument that appears in Box 5-6. Provide a critique of this instrument.

2. The following questions were found on an instrument to measure patient knowledge about cancer: "Do you know how to examine your breasts?" "Do you know where your prostate gland is located in your body?"[14] Will these items yield valid answers?

3. An educational session on BRCA1/2 testing addresses the following topics: (1) inheritance of susceptibility to breast-ovarian cancer, (2) cancer risks associated with BRCA1 or BRCA2 mutations, (3) genetic linkage studies, gene identification, and tests for mutation status, (4) benefits of genetic testing including the potential for early detection and reduction of uncertainty, (5) limitations of genetic testing including incomplete penetrance and etiological heterogeneity, (6) risks of genetic testing including the potential for loss of insurance or employment and adverse psychosocial consequences for oneself and one's family, (7) options for prevention and surveillance and their limitations, and (8) assurance of confidentiality of test results and related information.[25] How would you judge this as a plan for the educational session?

4. A diagram for doing BSE may be found in Figure 5-4.[28] How would you use this diagram to teach low-income women?

TABLE 5-1	Native American and Low Literacy Breast Cancer Education Materials	
Educational Materials	**Description**	**Availability**
Native American		
"Circle of Life: A Breast Cancer Awareness Project for Native American Women" educational kit	This train-the-trainer kit includes Native American designs and artwork on flip charts, brochures, and a teacher's and trainer's manual.	American Cancer Society, Oklahoma Division
"How to Examine Your Breasts" poster	The poster depicts a Native American shield with a step-by-step illustration of breast self-examination.	National American Women's Health Education Resource Center, Lake Andes, S.D.
"Malam Nau Yahiwapo: Women's Gathering Place" folder and fact sheets	The decorative folder contains fact sheets about breast health, clinical breast examination, breast self-examination, and mammography (ninth-grade reading level).	Arizona Disease Prevention Center, Tucson, Ariz.
"We are the Circle of Life: Pass on the Gift of Health" poster	The poster depicts an artistic drawing of four Native American women, with the caption "Get yearly mammograms and Pap screenings."	American Indian Health Care Association, St. Paul, Minn.
"Continue the Circle: Enjoy the Gift of Health" mammogram poster	The poster depicts three Native American women from three generations, with the caption "Please get a mammogram."	American Cancer Society, Minneapolis, Minn.
"What Women Should Know About Cancer" brochure	The brochure discusses the early signs of breast and other cancers and contains seven easy-to-read comics.	American Cancer Society, Eureka, Calif.
"Breast Cancer: Know the Facts—A Situation No Woman Wants to Face" brochure	The brochure contains information about breast cancer and recommended screening guidelines, with Native American art on the cover (ninth-grade reading level).	Native American Women's Health Education Resource Center, Lake Andes, S.D.
Low Literacy		
"A Mammogram Could Save Your Life" brochure	The brochure stresses the importance of mammography and answers questions about the procedure.	National Cancer Institute, Bethesda, Md.
"Take Care of Your Breasts" brochure	The brochure defines mammography and provides guidelines for mammography screening.	National Cancer Institute, Bethesda, Md.
"Breast Cancer Questions and Answers" pamphlet	The pamphlet answers nine basic questions about breast cancer.	American Cancer Society, Atlanta, Ga.
"Woman to Woman: Straight Talk About Mammography" video	The video depicts older women of all races voicing their concerns about mammography.	American Cancer Society, Atlanta, Ga.

From Bront JM, Fallsdown D, Iverson ML: The evolution of a breast health program for plains Indian women, *Oncol Nurs Forum* 26:731-739, 1999.

| **Box 5-6** | *Classroom Survey Instrument (Requires true or false answers)* |

1. Women who have had multiple sexual partners increase their risk of cervical cancer.
2. Bumping or bruising your breasts can cause breast cancer.
3. Shortness of breath is not a warning sign for breast cancer.
4. A chest x-ray exam cannot help discover breast cancer early.
5. Women over 40 should have a breast exam about once every 3 years.
6. All women, regardless of age, should have an annual mammogram.
7. All women, regardless of age, should have an annual Pap smear.
8. Diets high in fat may increase a woman's risk for breast cancer.
9. If you have a lump in your breast, it is likely to be cancer.
10. Pain is usually a symptom of early breast cancer.
11. Pain in both breasts which comes and goes is normal for women even after menopause.
12. An experienced physician can diagnose breast cancer by feeling a lump.
13. When you are examining your breasts, you should always use the palms of your hands.

From Ansell D and others: A nurse-directed intervention to reduce barriers to breast and cervical cancer screening in Chicago inner city clinics, *Pub Health Rep* 109:104-111, 1994.

How To Do Breast Self-Examination

Do breast self-examination (BSE) every month. Become familiar with how your breasts usually look and feel. Do BSE to find any change from what is normal for you.

If you still menstruate, the best time to do BSE is 2 or 3 days after your period ends. These are the days when your breasts are least likely to be tender or swollen.

If you no longer menstruate, pick a certain day—such as the first day of each month—to remind yourself to do BSE.

If you are taking hormones, talk with your doctor about when to do BSE.

Here's what you should do to check for changes in your breasts.

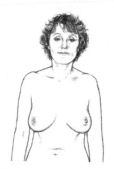

1 Stand in front of a mirror that is large enough for you to see your breasts clearly. Check each breast for anything unusual. Check the skin for puckering, dimpling, or scaliness. Look for a discharge from the nipples.

Do steps 2 and 3 to check for any change in the shape or contour of your breasts. As you do these steps, you should feel your chest muscles tighten.

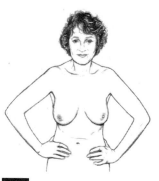

3 Next, press your hands firmly on your hips and bend slightly toward the mirror as you pull your shoulders and elbows forward.

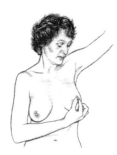

4 Gently squeeze each nipple and look for a discharge.

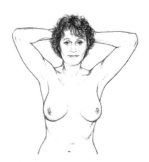

2 Watching closely in the mirror, clasp your hands behind your head and press your hands forward.

Figure 5-4   Technique for breast self-examination. (From The National Cancer Institute.)

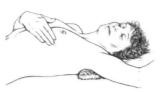

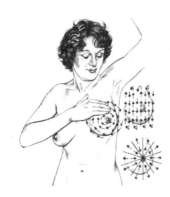

5 Raise one arm. Use the pads of the fingers of your other hand to check the breast and the surrounding area—firmly, carefully, and thoroughly. Some women like to use lotion or powder to help their fingers glide easily over the skin. Feel for any unusual lump or mass under the skin.

Feel the tissue by pressing your fingers in small, overlapping areas about the size of a dime. To be sure you cover your whole breast, take your time and follow a definite pattern: lines, circles, or wedges.

Some research suggests that many women do BSE more thoroughly when they use a pattern of up-and-down lines or strips. Other women feel more comfortable with another pattern. The important thing is to cover the whole breast and to pay special attention to the area between the breast and the underarm, including the underarm itself. Check the area above the breast, up to the collarbone and all the way over to our shoulder.

Lines: Start in the underarm area and move your fingers downward little by little until they are below the breast. Then move your fingers slightly toward the middle and slowly move back up. Go up and down until you cover the whole area.

Circles: Beginning at the outer edge of your breast, move your fingers slowly around the whole breast in a circle. Move around the breast in smaller and smaller circles, gradually working toward the nipple. Don't forget to check the underarm and upper chest areas, too.

Wedges: Starting at the outer edge of the breast, move your fingers toward the nipple and back to the edge. Check your whole breast, covering one small wedge-shaped section at a time. Be sure to check the underarm area and the upper chest.

6 It's important to repeat step 5 while you are lying down. Lie flat on your back, with one arm over your head and a pillow or folded towel under the opposite shoulder. This position flattens the breast and makes it easier to check. Check each breast and the area around it very carefully using one of the patterns described above.

7 Some women repeat step 5 in the shower. Your fingers will glide easily over soapy skin, so you can concentrate on feeling for changes underneath.

If you notice a lump, a discharge, or any other change during the month—whether or not it is during BSE—contact your doctor.

Figure 5-4, cont'd   For legend see opposite page.

References

1. Ansell D and others: A nurse-delivered intervention to reduce barriers to breast and cervical cancer screening in Chicago inner city clinics, *Pub Health Rep* 109:104-111, 1994.

2. Breslow RA and others: Americans' knowledge of cancer risk and survival, *Prev Med* 26:170-177, 1997.

3. Bront JM, Fallsdown D, Iverson ML: The evolution of a breast health program for Plains Indian women, *Oncol Nurs Forum* 26:731-739, 1999.

4. Chalmers KI, Luker KA: Breast self-care practices in women with primary relatives with breast cancer, *J Adv Nurs* 23:1212-1220, 1996.

5. Chalmers K, Thomson K, Degner LF: Information, support and communication needs of women with a family history of breast cancer, *Cancer Nurs* 19:204-213, 1996.

6. Davis TC and others: Knowledge and attitude on screening mammography among low-literate, low-income women, *Cancer* 78:1912-1920, 1996.

7. Deane KA, Degner LF: Determining the information needs of women after breast biopsy procedures, *AORN J* 65:767-776, 1997.

8. Devine EC, Westlake SK: The effects of psychoeducational care provided to adults with cancer: a meta-analysis of 116 studies, *Oncol Nurs Forum* 22:1369-1381, 1995.

9. Ehmann JL: BSE rap: intergenerational ties to save lives, *Oncol Nurs Forum* 20:1255-1259, 1993.

10. Erwin DO and others: Increasing mammography and breast self-examination in African American women using the Witness Project model, *J Cancer Educ* 11:210-215, 1996.

11. Ferrell BR, Ferrell BA, Rhiner M, Grant M: Family factors influencing pain, *Postgrad Med J* 67(suppl 2):S64-S69, 1991.

12. Ferrell BR, Rhiner M, Ferrell BA: Development and implementation of a pain education program, *Cancer* 72(11 suppl):3426-3432, 1993.

13. Fife BL: The measurement of meaning in illness, *Soc Sci Med* 40:1021-1028, 1995.

14. Fitch MI and others: Health promotion and early detection of cancer in older adults: assessing knowledge about cancer, *Oncol Nurs Forum* 24:1743-1748, 1997.

15. Flood AB and others: The importance of patient preference in the decision to screen for prostate cancer, *J Gen Intern Med* 11:342-349, 1996.

16. Gray RE and others: The information needs of well, long-term survivors of breast cancer, *Patient Educ Couns* 33:245-255, 1998.

17. Greene PE: America responds to cancer pain; a survey of state pain initiatives, *Cancer Pract* 1:65-71, 1993.

18. Gregg J, Curry RH: Explanatory models for cancer among African-American women at two Atlanta neighborhood health centers: the implications for a cancer screening program, *Soc Sci Med* 39:519-526, 1994.

19. Gustafson D and others: Development and pilot evaluation of a computer-based support system for women with breast cancer, *J Psychosoc Oncol* 11(4):69-93, 1993.

20. Hileman JW, Lackey NR, Hassanein RS: Identifying the needs of home caregivers of patients with cancer, *Oncol Nurs Forum* 19:771-777, 1992.

21. Hodge FS, Fredericks L, Rodriguez B: American Indian women's talking circle: a cervical screening and prevention project, *Cancer* 78(7 suppl):1592-1597, 1996.

22. Irwin E and others: Offering a choice between two adjuvant chemotherapy regimens: a pilot study to develop a decision aid for women with breast cancer, *Patient Educ Couns* 37:283-291, 1999.

23. Janz NK and others: Interventions to enhance breast self-examination practice: a review, *Public Health Rev* 17:89-163, 1991.

24. Kash KM and others: Psychological counseling strategies for women at risk of breast cancer, *Monogr Natl Cancer Inst* 7:73-79, 1995.

25. Lerman C and others: What you don't know can hurt you: adverse psychologic effects in members of $BRCA_1$-linked and $BRCA_2$-linked families who decline genetic testing, *J Clin Oncol* 16:1650-1654, 1998.

26. Maung ZT and others: Patient education for self-referral and on-demand treatment for herpes zoster in lymphoma patients, *Leuk Lymphoma* 11:447-452, 1993.

27. Meyer TJ, Mark MM: Effects of psychosocial interventions with adult cancer patients: a meta-analysis of randomized experiments, *Health Psychol* 14:101-108, 1995.

28. Nettina SM: *The Lippincott manual of nursing practice*, ed 6, Philadelphia, 1996, Lippincott.

29. Northouse LL, Peters-Golden H: Cancer and the family: strategies to assist spouses, *Semin Oncol Nurs* 9:74-82, 1993.

30. Peterson R: A nursing intervention for early detection of spinal cord compressions in patients with cancer, *Cancer Nurs* 16:113-116, 1993.

31. Pinto BM: Training and maintenance of breast self-examination skills, *Am J Prev Med* 9:353-358, 1993.

32. Redman BK: *Measurement tools in patient education,* New York, 1997, Springer.
33. Rimer BK, Kedziera P, Levy MH: The role of patient education in cancer pain control, *Hospice J* 8:171-191, 1992.
34. Sheridan-Leos N: Women's Health Loteria: a new cervical cancer education tool for Hispanic females, *Oncol Nurs Forum* 22:697-701, 1995.
35. Stewart DE and others: The effect of educational brochures on follow-up compliance in women with abnormal Papanicolaou smears, *Obstet Gynecol* 83:583-585, 1994.
36. Strickland CJ and others: Improving breast self-examination compliance: a Southwest Oncology Group randomized trial of three interventions, *Prev Med* 26:320-332, 1997.
37. Villejo L, Meyers C: Brain function, learning styles, and cancer patient education, *Semin Oncol Nurs* 7:97-104, 1991.
38. Weinrich SP and others: Increasing prostate cancer screening in African American men with peer-educator and client-navigator interventions, *J Cancer Educ* 13:213-219, 1998.
39. West MD, Finney JW: Training in early cancer detection and anxiety in adolescent males: a preliminary report, *Dev Behav Pediatr* 17:98-99, 1996.
40. Whitaker VB, Aldrich L: A breast self-examination program for adolescent special education students, *Fam Community Health* 16(2):30-40, 1993.

Chapter 6

Cardiovascular and Pulmonary Patient Education

CARDIOVASCULAR PATIENT EDUCATION

Educational Approaches and Research Base

Approximately 58 million persons in the United States (20% of the total population) have one or more types of cardiovascular disease, which includes high blood pressure, coronary heart disease, stroke, rheumatic fever or disease, or other forms of heart disease.[45] Reported educational programs in the cardiovascular area deal with topics that involve alteration of risk factors, management of congestive heart failure, decrease in time delay until treatment for myocardial infarction (MI) and for stroke, implementation of cardiac rehabilitation after MI or cardiac surgery, regimen maintenance, and management of sickle cell disease. Data gathered in 1995 showed that a high portion of office visits did not include counseling for prevention of cardiovascular disease. Physicians cited as reasons a lack of time or reimbursements and a lack of professional training, particularly for providing dietary counseling.[45]

In the 1970s and 1980s several countries, including the United States, invested in large-scale clinical research trials designed to decrease cardiovascular risk factors—high blood pressure, smoking, high blood cholesterol levels, excess weight, and lack of exercise—by facilitating adoption of health practices in entire communities. The interventions lasted 5 to 8 years and frequently used a theoretical framework based on principles of behavioral change. Interventions focused on changing the community environment, training indigenous leaders, educational self-help, and diffusion of the innovation through social networks in the community, in part to provide people with social support to maintain the initial action.

Multimedia campaigns were aimed at large audiences and were carefully segmented to influence individuals to change behavior by using clear, repetitive messages. The impact of these programs was modest, with improvement in behavioral risk factors but equivocal effects on biological risk factors such as blood pressure and blood cholesterol. Effects on actual cardiovascular heart disease risk are yet to be shown.[57]

Although the popularity of large community studies has waned, community-based education is still used to decrease risk factors and patient delay of treatment and is very important for population subgroups that have not been reached successfully (e.g., ethnic minority groups, adults with low literacy levels, older women).

The National Cholesterol Education Program is a national campaign using mass media to promote lowering of the blood cholesterol distribution in the entire population. It has used two strategies: a patient-based or clinical approach for those with hypercholesterolemia and a population-based approach. The campaign cites as evidence of success the fact that from 1983 to 1995 the percentage of the public who had heard of high blood cholesterol rose from 77% to 93%, from 1986 to 1995 the proportion who knew a desirable blood cholesterol was below 200 mg/dl jumped from 16% to 69%, from 1983 to 1995 the percentage of U.S. adults who had ever had their cholesterol level checked climbed from 35% to 75%, and the percentage who knew their own level increased from 3% to 49%.[13] In 1991 the National Heart Attack Alert Program was launched to educate health care providers, patients, and the general public about the importance of rapid and appropriate response to symptoms and signs of acute MI.[21]

The research base for educational and psycho-educational interventions in cardiovascular disease is growing. One meta-analysis[48] summarizes 18 controlled studies of cardiac patient education. The programs provided in these studies demonstrated a measurable impact on blood pressure (effect size 0.51), mortality (effect size 0.24), exercise (effect size 0.18), and diet (effect size 0.19). An effect size can be interpreted as the change (in standard deviation units) attributable to the experimental intervention. Stated another way, the subjects participating in patient education interventions in these studies showed a 28% increase over control subjects in effect on blood pressure and a 19% improvement in survival. Many of the interventions were relatively intensive, with frequent contact and high total contact. Exploration of less intensive interventions

would be helpful to assess the amount of investment in education that is required to obtain optimal outcomes. No significant difference was found between didactic and behaviorally focused interventions.

A review (not a meta-analysis) of 46 studies of cognitive, educational, and behavioral strategies to improve compliance with cardiovascular disease risk reduction found that successful strategies included signed agreements, self-efficacy enhancement, behavioral skill training, and telephone-mail contact. The comparative efficacy of these approaches was generally not tested.[8] A meta-analysis of 102 studies testing the effects of patient education and psychosocial support on blood pressure found statistically significant large treatment effects on knowledge and compliance and small to medium-sized statistically significant beneficial effects on blood pressure.[18] A meta-analysis of 37 studies of health education and stress management programs for patients with coronary heart disease found that these programs yielded a 34% decrease in mortality from cardiac disease, a 29% decrease in recurrence of MI, and significant effects on blood pressure, cholesterol, body weight, smoking behavior, physical exercise, and eating habits.[22] In addition, a meta-analysis of 23 randomized controlled trials of the addition of psychosocial treatments to traditional exercise-based cardiac rehabilitation regimens found that they decreased mortality and morbidity, psychological distress, and some biological risk factors, especially during the first 2 years after the intervention.[40]

Understanding patient delay in seeking care after symptoms of acute myocardial infarction (AMI) or stroke has long been a high priority. Since the mid-1980s, several large-scale studies have demonstrated that thrombolytic therapy can significantly reduce mortality from AMI: the shorter the interval, the better the outcome. Yet over the past three decades, there has been little success in reducing delay time, including that for second MIs.

The phenomenon of delay needs to be understood before education and counseling strategies to reduce delay can be designed. Approximately one third of patients do not report an abrupt onset of symptoms and frequently have difficulty identifying the time of onset. These patients may report vague symptoms or symptoms that wax and wane over time, sometimes disappearing completely. Knowledge of the symptoms of AMI does not ensure that a patient will recognize or acknowledge his or her own AMI symptoms and does not reduce delay in seeking health care.[20] Many subjects reported that they had expectations about the symptoms of heart disease that focused on location, intensity, associated symptoms, and quality. Expectations did not match the symptom experience of 74% of subjects, and these individuals delayed significantly longer before seeking treatment than did subjects whose expectations did match their experience. The longest phase is the time it takes individuals to interpret their symptoms as cardiac and decide to seek medical attention.[37]

Thus despite widespread educational campaigns through public media, patient delay may not be affected because there is no uniform presenting syndrome for patients with AMI[37]; therefore the educational content provided to patients may not be accurate for them. Although knowledge of chest pain as an important heart attack symptom is high and relatively uniform, knowledge of arm pain or numbness, shortness of breath, sweating, and other important symptoms is less common, especially among those of lower socioeconomic status and racial and ethnic minority groups. Risk factor status has not been found to be associated with knowledge of heart attack symptoms.[27] A number of instructional approaches have been suggested but as yet are untested, including the use of role model stories based on the real experiences of patients with heart attacks. The wall poster shown in Figure 6-1 provides a very specific protocol, which can also be made into a wallet card. Patients may not follow such instructions because they are made to feel foolish when their judgment about presenting themselves in emergency rooms is questioned.

Zapka and others[65] find that a substantial portion of providers questioned the appropriateness of 911 use; some primary care physicians preferred that patients call them before 911, even though this approach frequently creates delays in treatment. Some physicians believed that telling patients about symptoms would stimulate their feeling these symptoms. Many nurses believed physicians were not well prepared to teach patients and at the same time were not supportive of nurses doing so.

About 20% of eligible patients attend cardiac rehabilitation programs after an MI. Originally designed in the 1960s to focus on exercise, some now have incorporated secondary prevention programs to teach patients how to decrease risk factors, such as smoking cessation, control of dietary cholesterol, and management of anxiety and depression. Payment for these risk factor prevention programs has generally not been supported by insurance.

Congestive Heart Failure Self-Management Education

This field of patient education and the dramatic results that can be attained have recently been discovered. Congestive heart failure is the most common indication for hospital admission among older adults with up to 40% being readmitted in 6 months, often because of inadequate self-management skills. Half of these rehospitalizations are believed to be preventable. Patients must feel confident to carry out instructions for the prescribed diet and medical management and to monitor weight and symptoms for worsening of their disease (weight gain, edema, orthopnea, and fatigue). Patients often have no idea what heart failure is and know only about heart attack and fat rather than sodium and fluids.

Intervention approaches (sometimes called disease management) shown to effectively prevent hospital readmission include case management, telemanagement, multidisciplinary teams, and nurse-run clinics. In all of these approaches, patient education and intensive follow-up are central. Some interventions are as minimal as sending packets of information and videotapes to a patient's home. Heidenrich and others[32] report results of a randomized controlled trial in which

Chest Pain Can Be An Emergency

If you feel any of the following
- Chest pain or discomfort that is very bad and lasts longer than 15 minutes,
- Chest discomfort along with weakness, feeling sick to your stomach, feeling faint or dizzy, and sweating,
- Chest discomfort that feels like tightness, pressure, burning, or heaviness that lasts for about 15 minutes,
- Sudden shortness of breath with no other cause . . .

CALL 911

A Heart Attack can also feel like . . .
- A mild chest discomfort, that may go on and off even when you are at rest,
- Or it may feel like regular heartburn, or indigestion.
  - Note the time the chest discomfort starts.
  - If it feels like heartburn, take some antacid like TUMS, Mylanta, or whatever it is you usually take for heartburn.
  - Note how long your discomfort lasts.
  - IF THE "MILD CHEST DISCOMFORT" OR "HEARTBURN" LASTS FOR 15 MINUTES OR MORE,

CALL 911

ASK TO BE TAKEN TO THE EMERGENCY ROOM.
Have it checked out. Better safe than sorry.

If you already have prescription for nitroglycerin
- When the discomfort starts, sit down, and take 3 nitroglycerin one at a time - 5 minutes apart.
- IF AFTER THE THIRD ONE, THE PAIN OR DISCOMFORT IS STILL THERE (even if it's mild),

CALL 911

ASK TO BE TAKEN TO THE EMERGENCY ROOM.

DO NOT DRIVE YOURSELF TO THE HOSPITAL!
- If your community emergency number is not 911, the number to call is _____
- If your community does not have an emergency number, your driver's name and phone number are _____
  _____

- Your doctor's name and phone number are _____
_____

- I will keep my EKG in my wallet.
- I will bring it with me every time I go to the hospital or doctor.

- I will call **The Professionals** at any time if I have questions about what to do in cases where I am unsure.

The Professionals 784-2255 or 1-800-377-HEALTH

Figure 6-1   A sample wall poster/handout. (From Blank FSJ and others: Development of an ED teaching program aimed at reducing prehospital delays for patients with chest pain, *J Emerg Nurs* 24:316-319, 1998.)

patients at home received a digital scale and an automatic blood pressure cuff and were taught to use them. Each day the patient called a toll-free number and entered the blood pressure, pulse, weight, and symptoms into a computerized voice answering system. A computer algorithm checked them with an acceptable range and if the readings were outside this range or there were new symptoms, the computer paged a nurse who called the patient and faxed the results to the physician. In this intervention patients received weekly educational mailings providing instruction on diet, exercise, and common therapies and a 10-minute call from the nurse discussing these topics. Intervention programs are often very cost effective with an 8:1 return on investment.[60]

Few data are available about how many patients receive heart failure education and how effective it is. Table 6-1 provides an example of a critical pathway used to structure home health care for these patients. Most patients with congestive heart failure are candidates for the kinds of programs described above.

Hypertension and Stroke

Management of hypertension is a major reason for using ambulatory care facilities. Patients must play a significant role in monitoring their own blood pressure, resulting in improved management of the hypertension, a decrease in body weight, and diminished use of antihypertensive drugs. In one model a structured treatment and patient education program was introduced into primary care practice after careful education of the physician and office staff.[29] In another,[58] patients were trained to measure their own blood pressure and return readings by mail, and they were given a standard procedure to follow in case of unusually high or low readings at home. For men in this study, management of uncomplicated hypertension through physician visits and periodic home blood pressure measurement was equal or superior to management by more frequent office visits alone and at a lower cost. A final study of education in decreasing dietary sodium and brisk walking showed lower blood pressure readings and less use of antihypertensive medications than in a control group.[36]

Stroke is the third leading cause of death and the leading cause of adult disability.[50] Stroke prevention and self-management patient education has been less common than has similar education for MI. Statistics show that only 5% of patients seek treatment for stroke in less than 3 hours, symptoms are not recognized, and patients and family think nothing can be done or that the situation is not an emergency.[14] As for MI, knowledge of stroke symptoms is not associated with early presentation to the emergency department; neither is having had a prior stroke.[63]

Education has been shown to be important in three respects. Morrison and others[46] show significantly lower anxiety and depression among patients with acute strokes who were educated with a self-help workbook. Wiles and others[62] find that caregivers for persons with stroke needed information about coping with daily care activities of bathing and dressing; the significance of symptoms such as memory loss, swallowing difficulties, irritability, and depression; how these symptoms could be managed; and how long they might last. Finally, a decision aid can be used to assist patients with atrial fibrillation, and therefore an increased risk of stroke, to choose between warfarin and aspirin therapy for stroke prevention. Like hormone replacement therapy and benign prostatic hypertrophy, the relative values of the benefits and risks are a matter of patient choice.[41]

Teaching tools for cardiovascular patient education are commonly available. Unlike teaching tools, tools for assessment and evaluation are far less available and tend to be focused on simpler learning activities. A knowledge questionnaire for hypertension is shown in Box 6-1. Evaluate this tool. Should the score on this tool predict compliance with the regimen for treating hypertension?[10] Remember that true/false tests can give inaccurate scores because guessing, by itself, gives a 50% success rate.

A similar questionnaire for knowledge about cholesterol is presented in Table 6-2. Inasmuch as most Americans can reduce their serum

Text continued on p. 141

TABLE 6-1	**Critical Path for Follow-up Care of the Patient with CHF**		
Visit/Week #1	**Visit/Week #2**	**Visit/Week #3**	**Visit/Week #4**
Medications	Medications	Medications	Medications
Patient:	Patient:	Patient:	Patient:
1. Verbalizes knowledge of meds—drug dosage, frequency, desired effect, and 2 side effects of 2-3 meds.	1. Shows compliance with med schedule.	1. Refills prescriptions as prescribed.	1. Continues same behaviors.
2. Agrees to follow med schedule.	2. Recalls action and side effects of 1-3 additional meds (if needed).	Nurse:	Nurse:
Nurse:	3. Shows correct use/avoidance of OTC meds.	1. Continues to instruct and reinforce patient learning as required.	1. Evaluates patient learning and provides reinforcement as needed.
1. Reviews hospital discharge med schedule.	Nurse:		
2. Assesses for adequate supply of meds and supplies.	1. Assesses patient compliance with med schedule.		
3. Develops plan for self-administration of meds.	2. Identifies barriers to compliance.		
4. Reinforces importance of compliance.	3. Problem solves with patient.		
5. Provides info about 2-3 meds leaving written info if indicated.	4. Assesses patient knowledge of medications.		
6. Assesses use of OTC meds.	5. Assesses for medication side effects.		
	6. Assesses use of incompatible OTC meds.		

From Lasater M: The effect of a nurse-managed CHF clinic on patient readmission and length of stay. *Home Healthcare Nurs* 14(5):351-356, 1996.
CHF, congestive heart failure; *OTC,* over the counter.

TABLE 6-1	Critical Path for Follow-up Care of the Patient with CHF—cont'd

Visit/Week #1	Visit/Week #2	Visit/Week #3	Visit/Week #4
Activity Patient: 1. Performs ADLs without signs or symptoms of activity intolerance. 2. Takes frequent rest periods and spaces activity throughout the day. Nurse: 1. Assesses and documents baseline activity level. 2. Instructs in-home walking program (intensity, frequency, and duration). 3. Teaches patient to take own pulse. Interventions Physical Exam Labs Treatments	Activity Patient: 1. Follows home walking program as instructed and tolerated. 2. Takes own pulse accurately. Nurse: 1. Assess for changes in patient's baseline activity level. 2. Reviews home walking program to include target pulse range, duration, frequency, and symptoms of intolerance.	Activity Patient: 1. Continues home walking program. Nurse: 1. Assesses for misconceptions of appropriate exercise.	Activity Patient: 1. Continues same behaviors. Nurse: 1. Evaluates patient learning and provides reinforcement as needed.

ADLs, activities of daily living.

Continued

TABLE 6-1 Critical Path for Follow-up Care of the Patient with CHF—cont'd

Visit/Week #1	Visit/Week #2	Visit/Week #3	Visit/Week #4
Consults			
Patient:	Patient:	Patient:	Patient:
1. Records daily weights.	1. Is compliant with scheduled MD office visit.	1. Continues same behaviors.	1. Continues same behaviors.
2. Uses TED hose correctly if indicated.	Nurse:	Nurse:	Nurse:
Nurse:	1. Reviews data from last visit.	1. Reviews data from last visit.	1. Reviews data from last visit.
1. Reviews H&P and hospital discharge form.	2. Performs cardiopulmonary assessment.	2. Performs cardiopulmonary assessment.	2. Performs cardiopulmonary assessment.
2. Performs complete cardiopulmonary assessment.	3. Reports significant weight gain, new onset rales, edema to MD.	3. Reports significant weight gain, new onset rales, edema to MD.	3. Reports significant weight gain, new onset rales, edema to MD.
3. Compares current weight to hospital discharge weight.	4. Assesses for changes in sleep pattern.	4. Evaluates patient learning and provides reinforcement as needed.	4. Evaluates patient learning and provides reinforcement as needed.
4. Assesses sleep pattern.			
5. Performs lab tests as ordered.			

From Lasater M: The effect of a nurse-managed CHF clinic on patient readmission and length of stay. *Home Healthcare Nurs* 14(5):351-356, 1996.
H&P, history and physical.

TABLE 6-1	Critical Path for Follow-up Care of the Patient with CHF—cont'd			
Visit/Week #1	**Visit/Week #2**	**Visit/Week #3**	**Visit/Week #4**
Nutrition Patient: 1. States attempts to limit sodium intake. 2. Describes food and fluid intake. Nurse: 1. Assesses patient knowledge of low sodium diet. 2. Assesses appetite and signs/symptoms of abdominal bloating or constipation. 3. Assesses availability of proper food.	**Nutrition** Patient: 1. Maintains stable/appropriate body weight. 2. Demonstrates appropriate food selection. 3. Completes food diary for 3 days to 1 week. Nurse: 1. Assesses knowledge of diet and instructs in appropriate food choices as needed. 2. Consults dietitian as indicated.	**Nutrition** Patient: 1. Continues to maintain stable and appropriate body weight. 2. Demonstrates appropriate food selection. Nurse: 1. Reviews food diary for empty calories, high-sodium foods, fulfillment of U.S. dietary guidelines (food pyramid). 2. Continues nutrition counseling.	**Nutrition** Patient: 1. Continues to maintain stable and appropriate body weight. Nurse: 1. Continues to assess/intervene as needed.
Safety, Health Promotion & Prevention Patient: 1. States when to call MD, Nurse, 911 (chest pain, SOB, weight gain >3 lbs, falls, new onset edema). Nurse: 1. Begins home safety assessment. 2. Posts emergency numbers.	Patient: 1. Knows emergency phone numbers. 2. Decreases home safety risks. 3. Verbalizes fears/concerns related to illness. Nurse: 1. Listens and validates concerns.	Patient: 1. Demonstrates health promotion behaviors. 2. Verbalizes coping mechanisms. Nurse: 1. Continues home safety evaluation. 2. Assesses patient anxiety and coping.	Patient: 1. Performs activities that increase self-esteem (gardening, painting, sewing, etc.) Nurse: 1. Continues to assess and promote health maintenance and health promotion behavior.

SOB, shortness of breath.

Box 6-1	*Hypertension Questionnaire (True/False)*

1. Hypertension is usually caused by nerves.
2. Hypertension treatment does not prolong life but it does make you feel better.
3. Both hypertension and cigarette smoking greatly increase the risk of heart attacks and strokes.
4. Hypertension is uncommon in our community (less than 1 adult in 100).
5. Less salt in your diet can cause hypertension.
6. Hypertension makes you more likely to have a stroke later in life but not a heart attack.
7. A heavy alcohol intake can cause hypertension.
8. Most headaches are caused by hypertension.
9. Drug therapy for hypertension must cause bothersome side effects to be effective.
10. Proper control of hypertension can prolong life.
11. Most people with hypertension do not know they have it.
12. Hypertension can often be cured after a few courses of tablets.
13. Obesity (overweight) is a common cause of hypertension.

From Carney S and others: Hypertension education: patient knowledge and satisfaction, *J Hum Hypertens* 7:505-508, 1993.

TABLE 6-2	**Percentage of Respondents Answering True, False, and Not Sure on Each Item of the Nutrition Quiz ($N = 606$)**		
Quiz Item	True (%)	False (%)	Not Sure (%)
Ounce for ounce, chicken contains roughly the same amount of cholesterol as beef.	7.3*	78.6	14.1
Hydrogenated vegetable oil increases cholesterol levels more than nonhydrogenated vegetable oil.	38.9*	23.0	38.1
If a 100-calorie portion of food contains 4 g fat, more than 30% of its calories are from fat.	36.6*	17.7	45.7
No foods from animal sources contain dietary fiber.	36.6*	32.7	30.7
Two eggs over light contain more cholesterol than the daily limit recommended by the government.	55.6*	21.3	23.1
To reduce your cholesterol level, it is more important to reduce the amount of saturated fat you eat than the amount of dietary cholesterol.	65.6*	13.7	20.7
Plant foods contain no cholesterol.	43.6*	31.7	24.7
An ounce of Corn Flakes cereal contains more sodium than an ounce of potato chips.	14.7*	63.1	22.2
Two percent of the calories in 2% milk comes from milk fat.	49.7	22.7*	27.6
A 3-oz serving of lean ground beef contains fewer grams of fat than a 3-oz serving of chocolate ice cream.	48.8	26.0*	25.3

From Plous S, Chesne RB, McDowell AU: Nutrition knowledge and attitudes of cardiac patients, *J Am Diet Assoc* 95:442-446, 1995.
*Correct answer.

TABLE 6-3	Confidence Levels in Stair Climbing and Walking

Self-Efficacy for Stair Climbing					Walking Performance Scale					
	Definitely Cannot Do		Definitely Can Do					Did Not Try	Doing Regularly without Difficulty	
1. Climb 1 flight*	1	2	3	4	5	1. Walk 2 blocks†	1	2	3	4	5
2. Climb 2 flights	1	2	3	4	5	2. Walk 4 blocks†	1	2	3	4	5
3. Climb 3 flights	1	2	3	4	5	3. Walk 8 blocks (1 mile)†	1	2	3	4	5
4. Climb 4 flights	1	2	3	4	5	4. Walk 2 miles†	1	2	3	4	5
5. Climb 5 flights	1	2	3	4	5	5. Walk 4 miles†	1	2	3	4	5

From Gulanick M, Kim MJ, Holm K: Resumption of home activities following cardiac events, *Prog Cardiovasc Nurs* 6:21-27, 1991.
*1 flight = 12 stairs.
†Without stopping.

cholesterol levels by 10% through dietary modification, this is important information. Among people at high risk for coronary heart disease, modest reductions in serum cholesterol level are associated with an increase in life expectancy of up to 1 year. The responses in this study came from patients drawn from cardiology practices in New England, Southern California, and the Midwest.[51] The items on the questionnaire were designed to probe a variety of practical questions confronting persons who wish to follow a heart-healthy diet. All questions were pilot-tested for clarity and answers were independently confirmed by two registered dietitians. When these patients are taken as a group, their knowledge of nutrition is marginal; mean scores on the quiz did not exceed chance levels and were consistent with other surveys of nutrition knowledge.

Some cardiac patients fear resumption of physical activity until long after it is safe to do so, whereas others overestimate their capability. Providers have an important role in assisting patients in correct interpretation of their physical abilities and in providing instruction about home, social, and work activities. Gulanick, Kim, and Holm[30] developed a home activity assessment tool to guide discharge planning for these patients. Table 6-3 shows two scales that test confidence (self-efficacy) in stair climbing and walking performance. These and other scales can be used as a basis for teaching patients with low confidence to perform activities as their recovery allows.

Finally, identifying the needs of patients and spouses after an acute cardiac event is an important step in the development of nursing interventions to facilitate couples' psychosocial adaptation. A study of 49 such couples found that both patients and spouses identified the need for information as being the most important compared with all other needs.[47] Understandably, patients and spouses identified different needs as important; unfortunately, many of the needs that both patients and spouses ranked as being important or very important were perceived as unmet in 40% to 70% of the cases. Table 6-4 provides a listing of the needs and the percentage of patients and spouses who indicated that the need was not met either before or after discharge from the hospital. Apparently, information was not consistently delivered to the participating patients and spouses, or it was delivered at a time when patients and families were unable to absorb it. The findings show that patient and spouse need to be assessed both separately and as a dyad. The need to be prepared to deal with emergencies

TABLE 6-4 Patient and Spouse Needs Ratings and Percentage of Subjects Reporting Needs Not Met*		
Need Statement	**% Patient Needs Not Met**	**% Spouse Needs Not Met**
To know specific facts about my (the patient's) condition	26.1	20.8
To have honest explanations given in understandable terms	17.4	27.7
To talk to an M.D./R.N. about problems I or my family member may be facing	30.2	35.6
To know the expected course of the disease process	43.5	42.6
To receive specific instructions about care	25.5	25.5
To feel hope that I (my family member) will have a high quality of life	27.3	15.2
To receive information about what to do in an emergency	72.7	70.2
To receive information about expected physical course	26.7	31.9
To receive information about how to go about making life-style changes	42.2	47.6
To feel appreciated/valued by my family member	28.6	28.3
To receive information about life-style changes	46.5	38.3
To have my spouse assist me (be able to assist the patient) in making life-style changes	21.4	34.0
To feel as if others have my welfare in mind	5.0	39.0
To be able to talk with my family member about his/her concerns	35.7	26.7
To receive specific instructions about the return to sexual activity	46.2	48.8

Modified from Moser DK, Dracys KA, Marsden C: Needs of recovering cardiac patients and their spouses: compared views, *Int J Nurs Stud* 30:105-114, 1993.

*Wording in parentheses is that directed specifically to the spouse.

ranked highest among spouses and was most often unmet. For many family members the possibility of a future cardiac event can be a significant concern.

At present, few family members receive instruction in cardiopulmonary resuscitation (CPR), even though many of the attacks occur at home and the incidence of sudden death can reach as high as 50% in patients with advanced congestive heart failure. The concern of physicians that family members may feel burdened by this responsibility has been shown by some studies to be groundless.[19,42] Recent study has shown that CPR can be effectively taught through video-tape self-instruction in the home, with skills being practiced during the showing, like an exercise video. Cardboard manikins can be used both for the video and for practice. Training may be accomplished without an instructor, in one eighth the time of traditional CPR instruction.[6]

Other Topics

Self-management of chronic heart disease refers to those tasks individuals and families must undertake to maintain optimum health states and reduce the impact of disease on daily life, including handling clinical aspects of disease away from the hospital or physician's office. The "take

TABLE 6-4	Patient and Spouse Needs Ratings and Percentage of Subjects Reporting Needs Not Met*—cont'd		
Need Statement		% Patient Needs Not Met	% Spouse Needs Not Met
To be able to talk with my family member about my fears/ concerns		16.7	4.2
To receive information about expected psychological course		62.5	60.9
To talk to someone about my feelings		37.5	50.0
To have help with financial concerns		36.4	46.7
To receive information about feelings and emotions my spouse (I) may have during my (the patient's) recovery		19.3	69.3
To talk to someone about anger/frustration I may be experiencing		48.7	51.4
To talk to someone about my fears		52.5	52.6
To be told about other people or groups who can help with problems		59.0	59.5
To have time alone for myself		17.5	58.8
To be away from family member without worrying		36.8	41.0
To feel that others are going through the same things, that my experience is not unusual		25.0	35.7
To talk to others going through the same things		51.4	53.8
To have someone run errands or help with the house and/or cooking		11.1	50.0
To be able to offer meaningful assistance to the patient		n/a	28.3

PRIDE" program was organized around self-regulation processes: Problem selecting, Researching the daily routine, Identifying a heart self-management goal, Developing a plan to reach the goal, and Establishing a reward for reaching it.[11] The program's group-meeting format allows exchange of ideas and encourages role-modeling among the participants. The provider's role is to introduce accurate information, suggest strategies, and provide feedback to encourage new behavior, and enhance feelings of self-efficacy through praise and encouragement. A videotape is used, in which a model self-manager, who describes how she previously experienced fear and uncertainty, now demonstrates the PRIDE process. Participants use this process to establish a specific behavioral goal, write a contract, and gain skills in self-management.

Education for self-management of anticoagulation therapy with home testing and patient adjustment of medication dosage has been found to help patients achieve a degree of therapeutic effectiveness at least as good as traditional provider management.[1,54]

Educational materials for sickle cell disease, which predominantly affects African Americans, are not widely available.[4] Patients need education and support for managing disabling pain, and parents must be taught to recognize the danger signals that indicate need for immediate treatment.

PULMONARY PATIENT EDUCATION

General Approach

Almost all the work in pulmonary patient education focuses on asthma education, despite the fact that many people have other pulmonary diseases such as chronic obstructive pulmonary disease (COPD), which includes chronic bronchitis and emphysema. There are 14.2 million Americans with COPD, which is the fourth major cause of disability and fourth ranking cause of death.[17]

Morbidity and mortality from asthma have increased over the past decade despite improved understanding and advances in medical therapeutics. Thirteen million people in the United States have this disease, which is characterized by episodic symptoms, variable airflow obstruction and airway hyperresponsiveness, and inflammation. Asthma is the most common chronic disease of childhood, affecting 1 in 10 children. Among low-income families, many of whom have no health insurance, children with asthma have twice the odds of school failure as do those without the disease.[44]

Over the past decade several centers have developed effective, tested asthma self-management programs, although none has been demonstrated to have superiority. These programs, designed to help families learn how to become active partners in managing the disease, have been developed with patients and families of different social, educational, and economic backgrounds. It is important to note that no study evaluating these programs has shown an increase in morbidity as a result of patients or parents accepting more responsibility for their care. Those who have participated in such courses generally do not overtreat at home or delay seeking appropriate medical care.[34]

Educational Approaches and Research Base

A meta-analysis was completed of 11 randomized clinical trials that evaluated the impact of interactive self-management teaching programs on the morbidity of pediatric asthma.[3] The overall pooled effect size remained below 0.2—a small effect size—meaning that these programs seem to have little influence on morbidity outcomes. Generally, studies restricted to school-aged children showed a more significant reduction of morbidity during the year after the teaching intervention. It is suggested that studies need to be stratified according to severity of the disease and that control groups be limited to very brief instruction on medications and how to use them properly.[39] It is possible that these two changes in study design would result in raised effect sizes.

A summary of studies evaluating the cost of asthma education programs for children showed that savings resulted from fewer hospitalizations and emergency department visits.[53] There also seemed to be improvements in attitude and self-management skills and less school absenteeism. Two recent meta-analyses by Devine[16] and Devine and Pearcy[17] summarize studies in asthma and in COPD self-management education. Education provided to persons with asthma has shown benefits in reduced occurrence of asthma attacks, increased peak expiratory flow rate, improved functional status, better adherence to treatment regimen, improved utilization of health care and use of as-needed medications, improved psychological well-being, and increased psychomotor knowledge of inhaler use. Devine concludes that these educational services are well justified by the existing research. Educational interventions for COPD are usually packaged as pulmonary rehabilitation and include large muscle exercise and sometimes other psychosocial or behavioral interventions. Devine and Pearcy's review of 65 studies of such interventions covering the period from 1954 to 1994 demonstrated statistically significant beneficial effects on psychological well-being, endurance, functional status, dyspnea, and adherence to treatment regimens.

Adults with Asthma

When asthma is managed appropriately, hospitalization is rarely required. Yet 43% of its economic impact is related to use of emergency services and hospitals, presumably resulting from failure of patients to effectively use preventive treatment. Adherence to preventive regimens does not improve with the severity of asthma. Table 6-5 and Boxes 6-2 and 6-3 describe the structure of asthma education as delivered in an office setting and asthma self-management plans for adults and children.[59] A version of this plan should be carried in the patient's wallet. Note that the plans integrate changes in peak expiratory flow rate (PEFR) measurements (which can detect airway obstruction before symptoms occur) or symptoms with written directions to introduce or increase therapy. The highest level of lung function a patient is able to achieve after 1 to 2 weeks of aggressive therapy is the personal best for that patient and is used as a standard. This value should be reassessed annually in adults and periodically in children. Asthma episodes rarely occur without warning; the symptoms patients experience at different degrees of falling from the personal best vary widely from patient to patient, but generally are consistent for each patient.[25] Identification and avoidance of triggers are also part of the plan; grasses, dust, temperature change, smoke, pets, cockroaches, upper respiratory infections, and exercise are common ones. Directions for use of a peak flow meter are shown in Box 6-4.

Each asthma plan must be individualized, taking into account the patient's personal best peak flow number and asthma signs and symptoms. Behavioral goals of an asthma plan are early recognition of a change in the state of asthma stability that leads to early intervention for an exacerbation and sufficient confidence in the ability for self-management.

Because many classes of asthma medications are available in metered dose inhalers (MDI), learning the proper technique for self-administration is important. Only 20% to 40% of patients with asthma use the MDI correctly. Correct steps are the following: (1) take the cap off, (2) shake the MDI, (3) exhale to residual volume or functional residual capacity, (4) activate the inhaler with or slightly after the onset of inhalation, (5) take a steady deep inspiration, (6) hold

breath for 10 seconds or as long as possible, (7) wait at least a minute before the next puff.[56] Among a group of adults, problems included actuation of the canister before or at the end of inspiration, halt of inspiration after the release of the aerosol into the mouth, breathhold of less than 5 seconds, and actuation of the canister more than once during the same inspiration. Older adults have been found to have more difficulty; education and re-education are vital. Spacers, which cause a delay between activation of the device and inhalation by the patient, may be helpful.[15] There is some question about whether health care providers know what to teach. In one study, more than half of house staff members and 82% of nurses were judged to be poor in their ability to use the inhaler.[35]

Patients require frequent reinforcement of their self-management. The most common and important factor associated with a fatal outcome has been inability of the patient to recognize the severity of the attack. And it is patients who have the most severe asthma, with the greatest degree of bronchial hyperresponsiveness, who have the worst perception of the severity of airflow obstruction. These patients should be targeted for aggressive education and follow-up.[24] Indigent asthmatic patients who frequently use the emergency department as their primary source of care do respond well to repetitive education and follow-up, including removal of barriers to self-care, with significant decreases in the number of hospitalizations.[26,38]

The mortality from asthma is particularly high among racial and ethnic minorities compared with whites. In comparison with other patient groups, adults with asthma who have less education and lower income are likely to receive care that has less continuity and is less intensive after hospital discharge. These patients also have worse health and lower levels of physical and pulmonary function.[31] Asthma education programs frequently require multiple patient education sessions and extensive use of written materials, which may create impossible or difficult learning conditions for these patients. On the other hand, a nurse outreach worker assigned to

TABLE 6-5	Essentials of Office Education for Patients with Asthma		

Questions to Ask	Educational Information in Easy-to-Understand Format	Skills to Teach the Patient and Have Demonstrated to Prove Proficiency
First Office Visit		

What does having asthma mean to you?	Basic asthma facts
	  Chronic lung disease
	  Role of airways
	  Inflammation
	  Role of bronchoconstriction
	  Intermittent airway
	    narrowing
		Inhalers and spacers (see patient information handout)

What medicines have you taken for your asthma and did they help?		Introduce self-management plan (see Boxes 6-2 and 6-3)
What do you expect from asthma treatment?		Symptom monitoring Introduce use of peak flow monitoring if time permits (see patient information handout, Box 6-4)
What do you want to accomplish with this visit?		

Do you have any other questions for me today?	Asthma medications
	  Anti-inflammatory agents
	  Rescue medications: short-
	    acting bronchodilators to
	    relax smooth muscles
	Bring list of all medicines and frequency of use to all appointments
	Supply patient with office and hospital telephone numbers for advice	

Second Office Visit (2 to 4 Weeks after the First Visit or Sooner, as Needed)		
What medications are you taking and how often?	Use two types of medication Reminder to bring peak flow meter and inhalers to all visits	Self-management plan: incorporate symptoms and peak flow monitoring
What problems have you had using your medications?		Review goals

Show me how you use your inhalers	Role of environmental control
	  Allergens
	  Irritants
		Adjust peak flow monitoring as needed

Show me how you use your peak flow meter (if provided at first visit)		Instruct patient in use of peak flow daily record and the need to bring meter and records to all visits (see Box 6-4) Correct inhaler and spacer technique (patient should demonstrate proficiency at every visit)
All Subsequent Visits		

Ask all questions asked in previous visits	Review role of medications
	  Anti-inflammatory
	  Bronchodilators
		Patient demonstrates technique in using inhaler, spacer and peak flow meter

Ask if goals of therapy are being met	Review environmental control measures	Review and change self-management plan to meet goals of therapy
Ask patient, "What questions do you have about the self-management plan? Are you using it?"	Review peak flow meter results in daily record, as needed	
Ask patient, "Do you have any new concerns about the therapy or your medications?"		

From Stoloff SW, Janson S: Providing asthma education in primary care practice, *Am Fam Physician* 56:117-126, 1997.

Box 6-2	*Self-Management Plan for the Treatment of Asthma*

Asthma is a disease of the airways in the lungs. The disease causes them to become inflamed, and this results in swelling and blockage. This makes it more difficult for you to breathe. Some simple steps can help you improve the management of your asthma. First, it's helpful to identify factors that trigger asthma episodes. You can then try to avoid the asthma triggers you and your doctor have identified. Keeping a record of your asthma symptoms and medications, and tracking your peak expiratory flow rate (PEFR), will also help you and your doctor manage your asthma. Use your peak expiratory flow meter every morning, or more often if needed, to measure the amount of airway blockage you have. Keep a daily record of the rates to show your doctor. Always use your peak flow meter at least once or twice a week. The morning rate is the best indicator of airway blockage. Be sure to write down your results. Use your peak flow meter more often if you notice decreasing flow rates or if you have symptoms of asthma or an upper respiratory infection (cough, wheeze or chest tightness). When the PEFR results are falling, use the meter and write down the results at least twice a day, every day, so you can show them to your doctor.

First, you need to find out your "personal best" PEFR; your doctor will tell you how. The following explains how to manage your asthma according to your symptoms and your PEFR score:

A. If you don't have any symptoms that affect your work and play (no cough, no wheeze, no chest tightness) and your PEFR is greater than 80%-85% of your personal best:

   Continue your normal maintenance dose schedule of medications:

   —Inhaled steroids, leukotriene modifiers (Accolate, Zyflo), cromolyn (Intal) or nedocromil (Tilade)

   —Oral theophylline

B. If you have symptoms (such as coughing, wheezing, chest tightness, waking at night with cough) and/or your PEFR is less than 80% of your usual results:

   Use an inhaled bronchodilator. Take one puff and wait 1 to 2 minutes; then another puff. You may take a third or fourth puff after waiting an additional 1 to 2 minutes between each puff. To determine the need for additional puffs, use the peak flow meter to check your PEFR. Use the best of three PEFR measurements. You may take more albuterol every hour to every 4 to 6 hours, depending on your PEFR results.

Double the dose of inhaled corticosteroid medication and take it more often, up to four times a day. (The maximum dosage for cromolyn and nedocromil is two puffs four times a day, unless your doctor tells you otherwise.) Don't take more than the following dosages of inhaled corticosteroids:

   Beclomethasone (Beclovent, Vanceril), 20 puffs a day

   Triamcinolone (Azmacort), 16 puffs a day

   Flunisolide (AeroBid), 8 puffs a day

   Budesonide (Pulmicort), 4 puffs a day

   Fluticasone (Flovent), 800 to 1,600 µg a day

Keep taking the increased dose until your PEFR is 80% (or better) of your personal best PEFR. Keep taking the increased dose for the same number of days it took you to get back to this PEFR level.

   Reminder: Always be sure your technique of using the metered-dose inhaler is correct; if you aren't sure, call or visit your doctor.

C. If your symptoms are still getting worse even though you are following the above recommendations and/or if your PEFR is 60% or less of your personal best, start taking oral prednisone in the dosage prescribed by your doctor and call your doctor's office.

D. If your PEFR is 50% or less of your personal best, or if your PEFR is less than 150 to 200 liters per minute:

   Call your doctor's office right away and go directly to the office or to the hospital emergency department, as directed.

Doctor's office telephone: _____

Hospital emergency department telephone: _____

If you have any questions about this information or if you are having difficulty with your medicines or with the peak-flow meter, ask your doctor for information and help.

From Stoloff SW, Janson S: Providing asthma education in primary care practice, *Am Fam Physician* 56:117-126, 1997.

How Asthma Affects the Body

Your doctor has told you that your child has asthma. Your doctor has probably also told you that asthma is a disease of the airways. The disease causes inflammation that blocks the airways. This blockage makes it hard for your child to breathe.

How to Help Control Asthma

It's helpful to identify the triggers of your child's asthma. Your doctor will help you find out what they are and then help your child avoid them. Common asthma triggers are: house dust; mold; pets; pollen from trees, grasses and weeds; tobacco smoke; certain foods, and certain smells, like perfume, paint and household cleaners.

How to Keep an Asthma Record

In managing asthma, it's important to keep track of your child's symptoms, medicines and peak expiratory flow rate (PEFR).

The colors of a traffic light can help you learn your asthma medicine:

A. Green means Go—use preventive (anti-inflammatory) medicine.
B. Yellow means Caution—use quick-relief medicine (short-acting bronchodilator) in addition to preventive medicine.
C. Red means Stop—get help from a doctor.

How to Measure Flow Rates

Measure your child's PEFR once a day when he or she gets up in the morning, always before taking any medicine. Write down the best of three scores. The measurement tells you and your doctor how much airway blockage is present. If your child's PEFR results are going down, you should measure again several times during the day and write down these additional PEFR results.

A. Green—Go Zone

Breathing is good, with no cough, wheeze or problems during exercise or play. The PEFR is 80% to 100% of the personal best:

Continue giving your child the normal maintenance dose of medicine. This may be as follows:

Inhaled corticosteroids, cromolyn (Intal) or nedocromil (Tilade)
Oral theophylline

B. Yellow—Caution Zone

Symptoms are present (cough, wheeze, chest tightness or waking up in the night with symptoms) and/or the child's PEFR is less than 80% of personal best:

Have your child take one puff of bronchodilator medicine and wait 1 to 2 minutes; then take a second puff. Your child may take a third or fourth puff after waiting an additional 1 to 2 minutes between each puff.

To determine the need for additional puffs, check the child's PEFR; use the best of three PEFR measurements. Check the PEFR every hour and have your child use the bronchodilator every 1 to 6 hours, depending on the PEFR results.

Double the dose of inhaled corticosteroid medicine and give the medicine more often, four times a day. The maximum dosage for cromolyn and nedocromil is two puffs, four times a day, unless your doctor tells you otherwise. Don't give your child more than the following dosages of inhaled corticosteroids:

Beclomethasone (Beclovent or Vanceril), 16 puffs a day

Triamcinolone (Azmacort), 12 puffs a day

Flunisolide (AeroBid), 5 puffs a day

Budesonide (Pulmicort), 4 puffs a day

Fluticasone (Flovent), 440 µg per day

Keep giving the increased dose until your child's PEFR is about 80% (or better) of his or her personal best. Give the increased dose for the same number of days it took your child to get back to normal PEFR before you go back to the previous maintenance dose.

Be sure to watch your child's technique in using the inhaler and the spacer. Wash the spacer's mouthpiece every week.

C. Red—Stop—Danger Zone

You have followed the previous instructions but your child is having trouble breathing and talking, and/or your child's PEFR is 60% or less of his or her personal best:

Start giving your child oral prednisone in the dosage prescribed by your doctor; call your doctor to tell about this asthma flare.

D. If your child's PEFR is 50% or less of personal best:

Call your doctor's office right away and go directly to his or her office or to the hospital emergency department, as instructed.

Doctor's office telephone: _____

Hospital emergency department telephone: _____

Any Problems?

If you have any questions about this information or if you have trouble using the medicines or the peak flow meter, call your doctor and ask for more information and help.

_____

From Stoloff SW, Janson S: Providing asthma education in primary care practice, *Am Fam Physician* 56:117-126, 1997.

Box 6-4	*Correct Use of a Peak Flow Meter*

INSTRUCTIONS: *To ensure that your peak flow measurements are correct, you must use the peak flow meter correctly. If you have difficulty with these directions or if you have any questions about using a peak flow monitor, please be sure to talk with your doctor.*

1. Stand up.
2. Move the indicator on the peak flow meter to the the bottom of the numbered scale.
3. Breathe out all your air and then take as deep a breath as you can (fill your lungs with air)
4. Put the mouthpiece of the meter in your mouth and close your lips around it.
5. Blow out as hard and as fast as you can.
6. Repeat steps 2 to 5 two more times (for a total of three times).
7. Write down the highest of the three numbers in your asthma record book.

———
From Stoloff SW, Janson S: Providing asthma education in primary care practice, *Am Fam Physician* 56:117-126, 1997.

families from a health maintenance organization with a 70% black inner-city population achieved a marked reduction in the rate of hospitalization and emergency ward utilization for pediatric patients with asthma.[28] This method of delivering education may be better suited to the needs of this population.

It is extremely useful to understand, from the patient's perspective, the experience of having asthma.[2] Until recently psychological factors were thought to play a major role in asthma, a notion that served to discredit it as a "real illness." The medical notion that a chronic illness can be controlled is a common theme in American medical practice, yet the limits of control are not commonly discussed, placing the patient in the position of feeling responsible for control. This disease is characterized by stable periods punctuated by unpredictable flares. Health professionals may assume that persons with asthma who frequently use emergency services are not taking proper preventive measures and therefore are at fault for their asthma being out of control.

Many patients feel that they walk a "tightrope" between delaying formal medical intervention and seeking treatment too soon. In addition, they face uncertainty about the quality and speed of care they are likely to encounter in an emergency room, which affects their feelings of being able to control their illness. Experienced physicians have been found to underestimate the severity of symptoms. Thus these patients walk a fine line in attempting to fulfill practitioners' expectations about how they should manage their asthma and, given the nature of the disease, ascertain what seems actually to be possible.

Children with Asthma

Asthma education for children should alert parents to recognize the symptoms, which may be interpreted as a persistent cold or lack of physical stamina, and for those at high risk, to practice trigger avoidance. Evans and others[23] estimate that underdiagnosis and undertreatment may affect as many as half of the true population of children with asthma.

Although most asthma is manifest before 6 years of age, and about half before age 3, there are few programs available for children younger than 7 years and their families. A randomized controlled trial of the subjects in the Wee Wheezers Asthma Education Program showed increased symptom-free days, fewer nights of parental sleep interruption, and significantly better asthma management in comparison with control subjects. The program used very interactive and visual teaching methods, including films of real children and symptoms of varying severity in the emergency department so parents could recognize these symptoms in their own children, interviews of actual parents of children with asthma as discussion triggers for the way the disease affects the family, development of skills in determining their child's breathing rate, in-class practice and at-home assignments, behavioral contracts including prohibition of cigarette smoking in the house, and a group format which provides vicarious mastery experiences and social comparison.[64] A study of low-income African-American mothers of preschoolers with asthma usually diagnosed before 18 months showed children participating in their management by 20 months. A full description of participation by age may be found in Brown and others.[7] For example, a 3 year old should be able to identify asthma triggers with adult help and a 7 year old should be able to do it independently.

Asthma education for school-aged children is better developed. In addition to skill development as in adults, attention to disruption of peer and sibling relationships and loss of self-esteem due to limitations in physical activity is important. Asthmatic children experience emotional problems at twice the rate of well children.[33]

Teaching approaches can include camps for children that offer puppets, games, crafts, songs, and experiential learning. There are 125 asthma specialty camps nationwide, mostly of 1 to 2 weeks' duration. These environments offer opportunities for learning about triggers from horseback riding or jazz aerobics. These activities show that with proper planning, children with asthma can participate in physical activity, with counselors serving as coaches in asthma management.[43] In one such camp each child took corrugated tubing with a compressed sponge rolled up inside to simulate airway linings and then breathed through it. Dipped into water, the sponge swelled to take up most of the internal diameter of the tubing, and children breathing through it experienced the differences in resistance. Box 6-5 provides a script for Waldo the puppet. Such teaching-learning activities offer an excellent example of active teaching, well planned for the developmental levels of the children, and clearly focused on the important outcomes of skill in performing self-care and development of feelings of self-efficacy.[9]

A very helpful study found that families' cognitive beliefs and behavioral skills in managing asthma emerge in four successive phases as outlined in Table 6-6. Of the sample studied, 83% could be classified as being in phases one or two (precompliant). This work makes clear the point that self-regulation of asthma should be seen as a complex developmental process rather than a simple educational process. Moving to a higher stage involves changes in fundamental beliefs about the illness, in the home care environment, in relationships with health providers, in self-perception of vulnerability, and in perceived self-efficacy in coping with symptoms. The changes necessary to adopt a preventive asthma regimen instead of merely reacting to symptoms are more difficult for poorly educated populations because of limited knowledge about health, tight economic resources, and fewer environmental options.[66] A significant number of families are unresponsive to self-regulatory training in its present form, which is not designed around developmental phases. The higher the phase the more effective the self-management (Box 6-6).

Social skills involve interaction with health care providers, as well as interactions in school, home, and work environments. Poorly controlled asthma can have a significant negative impact on a child's self-image, activity level, fitness, and relationships. It is often helpful to send grandparents and other members of the extended family to an asthma education program.

COPD Self-Management Education

An example of a well-designed pulmonary rehabilitation program for persons with COPD has been reported by Scherer, Schmiedler, and Shimmel.[55] Patients had 1-hour classes 3 times a week for 12 weeks with education in self-care, nutrition, stress management, and anxiety control, retraining in breathing techniques and dyspnea control, and work simplification followed by training and workout sessions. Because these patients often lack confidence in their ability to avoid breathing difficulty, it is important to build in techniques to increase patient self-efficacy—performance accomplishments, vicarious experience in watching others, verbal persuasion, and teaching control of emotional and physical arousal states. Community outings and active practice of pacing and energy conservation techniques into activities of daily living enhance skills and self-efficacy.[61] Patients with higher self-efficacy showed a significant

Box 6-5	*Script for a Puppet Show*

Session 1

Waldo, a puppet with asthma, speaks with the children. He first introduces them to his lungs when they are symptom free. He shows them his trachea and then his airways as they gradually narrow to end in air sacs. He points out how the tubes are all wide open and how easily his lungs fill with air and then empty. Waldo gets exposed to a trigger and starts to wheeze. He then introduces them to his lungs during an asthma episode. He shows them how the muscles wrapping his lungs get tight and squeeze his airways and describes how the linings of his airways swell and take up too much space, making it really hard to move air. He uses an inhaler, carefully demonstrating good technique, and soon is breathing easier. His inhaler demonstration includes asking the audience to help him count while he holds his breath and while he waits between puffs.

Session 2

The Doc interacts first with the audience, asking if they know what triggers are and responds to the audience's answers. He discusses a bit about triggers and invites the audience to watch while his patient, Cleveland, encounters many triggers during his day. Cleveland starts his day sleeping. While he sleeps, Might Dust Mightious sneaks in and causes Cleveland to have an asthma attack. Dust Mightious talks about how Cleveland can keep him away if he finds out who causes his problems when he sleeps. Cleveland then wakes coughing and wheezing. His mother gives him his inhaler and, with the help of the audience, coaches him to use it correctly. She then sends him out to play.

A mouse comes on the scene and interacts with the kids. He compliments them on their great assistance so far and invites them to help Cleveland stay out of trouble. Cleveland goes for a walk in the neighborhood and walks past a smoking cigarette, which he knows could trigger a wheeze. He quickly gets away from it explaining that since he just used his inhaler, getting away will be enough. He then passes a truck and again has to get away quickly. He decides to go for a walk in the woods away from all those terrible triggers.

Mouse returns to chat with the children about how Cleveland did, what a great help they are and what problems they think Cleveland might encounter in the woods. The mouse again asks the children in the audience to help Cleveland avoid his triggers or do the right thing if he is exposed to triggers.

Cleveland walks in the woods and encounters a flock of birds, which drop feathers on him. This is another trigger and with the children's advice, he runs off again (still protected by his inhaler). He then sees flowers growing by the path, stops to sniff them, and gets a face full of pollen. With the audience's advice, Cleveland runs sneezing away from the flowers. He decides next to go to the pond where he thinks he will be safe from triggers. There he meets an alligator who scares him so badly that he wheezes until he can calm down. Cleveland decides to just go back home and on the way he gets rained on. He knows that wet weather often triggers his asthma so he hurries on home. He also knows that it has been hours since his inhaled reliever medicine and he knows with all those triggers he should not be out without his medicine.

Mouse comes back to tell the children what a super job they did helping Cleveland make good decisions. He also points out that most people don't have so many triggers and should do a better job of recognizing and avoiding them.

Session 3

Waldo and Jake have been playing soccer. Jake is wheezing and is short of breath. Waldo discerns that Jake didn't use his preventer medicine before soccer and encourages him to use his inhaler. Jake does so but with terrible technique. Waldo points this out and with the help of the audience, he coaches Jake through correct use. They go back out for the second half of their soccer game and when it is over, Jake is again having trouble breathing. Waldo encourages him to go see his mother.

The mouse comes in to ask the kids their opinions about Jake and Waldo's approaches to Jake's problems breathing. They discuss correct inhaler use.

Jake finds his mother in the garden and tells her he is having trouble breathing. She asks if he used his inhaler. He says yes, and she immediately gives him a nebulizer treatment. During this, she tells him what a good thing he did to use his inhaler first and come right to her when it didn't work. The nebulizer treatment doesn't help. They check Jake's peak flow and it is very low. Jake's mother calls the doctor, and they arrange to go to the office.

The mouse returns to chat with the audience about the decisions Jake and his mother made.

From Capen CL and others: The team approach to pediatric asthma education, *Pediatr Nurs* 20:231-237, 1994.

Continued

Box 6-5	*Script for a Puppet Show—cont'd*

Nurse Dawn talks to Jake and his mother about what a good job they did. She describes The Doc's plan to start Jake on a daily medication that he must take twice each day without fail. She helps him figure out a way to do this by keeping his medicine with his toothbrush. She describes the use of prednisone just for five days and why it is necessary. She also talks about using his inhaler before he exercises. She then tells him to keep using his peak flow meter and to always call if his number is too low.

Ideas for Props

Rain: A squirt gun can be fired from behind the theater.

Smoke/car exhaust: A nebulizer behind the scenes produces a nice mist.

Pollen: Yellow paper punches dropped into silk flowers can be shaken out to simulate pollen.

Lungs: Felt-covered cotton cording of different sizes is glued into the shape of airways with cotton balls, or small Styrofoam balls glued in clusters on the ends. Branches are wrapped with red ribbon (tightly on the wheezy set). Everything below the trachea is placed into clear plastic bags with one end of a piece of tubing inserted into each bag. Behind the scenes air can be blown in or sucked out of the bags.

Holding objects up without being seen can be accomplished by making mittens out of the leftover sheet (they are too long and need to be cut off) so the hand holding the object "disappears" into the background.

From Capen CL and others: The team approach to pediatric asthma education, *Pediatr Nurs* 20:231-237, 1994.

TABLE 6-6	Family Characteristics by Phase of Asthma Self-Regulation

Phase 1	*Asthma symptom avoidance.* The patient or family may perceive a periodic cough or wheeze, but they do not attribute these symptoms to an inherent physiological vulnerability with serious health-threatening outcomes if untreated. They try to avoid asthma symptoms nonmedically through activity restrictions and emotional calming.
Phase 2	*Asthma acceptance.* The patient or family accepts asthma as a serious health-threatening disease, but they respond to asthma only reactively (nonpreventively), primarily by using bronchodilators. Their main pharmacological efforts are toward a rescue from acute episodes, and they are resigned to the recurrence of exacerbations.
Phase 3	*Asthma compliance.* The patient or family seeks to prevent and control asthma symptoms by following the physician's treatment recommendations and is therefore less likely to need emergency treatment. However, they lack the confidence to self-regulate asthma because they are unskilled at preventively altering medications.
Phase 4	*Asthma self-regulation.* The patient or family develops an adaptable medical plan in consultation with the physician. They monitor lung functioning with peak flow meters or symptom recognition and can identify early warning signs of inflammation. They adjust their medical regimens on the basis of self-monitored signs, symptoms, or contact with triggers and are confident of their efficacy in implementing the plan and in contacting their doctor when modifications are needed.

From Zimmerman BJ and others: Self-regulating childhood asthma: a developmental model of family change, *Health Educ Behav* 26:55-71, 1999.

Box 6-6	*Asthma Self-Regulatory Phase Items and Scoring Criteria*

PHASE	ITEM
2	1. Do you ever worry that you may not be able to get to the doctor or hospital in time to get the care your child needs for an attack? Why or why not? *Responses that fail to indicate worry about asthma are not credited with passing; any mention of worry is scored as passing.*
2	2. How much do you feel that your child's asthma restricts daily activities or prevents him or her from being able to do the things he or she would like to do? *Responses that fail to indicate asthma restrictions are not credited with passing; any mention of restrictions is scored as passing.*
2	3. How serious can your child's asthma be? *Responses that fail to indicate that asthma is potentially life threatening for the child or that asthma has potential long-term consequences are not credited with passing; responses that mention limitation in lives or long-term consequences are scored as passing.*
2	4. Do you feel that your child's asthma could possibly be life threatening if nothing is done to treat it? Why or why not? *Disagreement that asthma can be life threatening is not credited with passing; agreement is scored as passing.*
3	5. How important is it for your child to have regularly scheduled appointments with the doctor for his or her asthma? Why? *Responses that fail to indicate that the child keeps regularly scheduled doctor visits for asthma are not credited with passing; responses that indicate that the child keeps regularly scheduled doctor visits are scored as passing.*
3	6. How important is it to take all the medicines at the exact dosage that the doctor has prescribed? Why? *Responses that fail to indicate adherence to the prescribed pharmacotherapy are not credited with passing; responses that indicate adherence are scored as passing.*
3	7. If the asthma medicine that the doctor prescribes doesn't seem to help your child, how important is it to continue giving it? Why? *Responses that fail to indicate consultation with the doctor before changing asthma medication are not credited with passing; responses that indicate consultation with the doctor for alterations of pharmacotherapy are scored as passing.*
4	8. Do you have any special method to check for early signs of an oncoming asthma attack? What is it? *Responses that fail to specify early symptoms of an attack are not credited with passing; responses that specify early symptoms are scored as passing.*
4	9. Do you have a special procedure that you follow starting at the first sign of an asthma attack? What is it? *Procedures that fail to specify the rescue medicines that must be administered at the first sign of an attack are not credited with passing; procedures that specify the rescue medicines are scored as passing.*
4	10. Do you have a systematic plan to adjust your child's medicine if his or her pattern of symptoms gets better or worse? What is it? *Responses that indicate the failure to work out a stepped pharmacological plan with the doctor are not credited with passing; stepped plans that have been worked out with the doctor are scored as passing.*
4	11. Do you have any special procedure for observing changes in your child's symptoms after you give him or her asthma medicine? What is it? *Responses that fail to indicate the necessity of personally monitoring specific symptoms are not credited with passing; responses that indicate the necessity of personally monitoring specific symptoms are scored as passing.*

From Zimmerman BJ and others: Self-regulating childhood asthma: a developmental model of family change, *Health Educ Behav* 26:55-71, 1999.

increase in activity. Pulmonary rehabilitation has also been reported as part of short-stay inpatient services.

National Standards and Tested Programs

Literature citations for evaluations of asthma self-management programs are included in Box 6-7.[49] Unfortunately, there are few carefully developed standardized measurement tools available to assess knowledge and skills for care management, levels of self-management behavior, psychological and physical functioning, and appropriateness of health care use.[12] In addition, few physicians have adopted proven asthma education programs as a regular part of care even though five-fold savings have been identified over the cost of using a program such as "Living with Asthma" and "Open Airways."[52]

SUMMARY

The most structured areas of cardiovascular patient education are reduction of risk factors, presentation for MI, cardiac rehabilitation and management of congestive heart failure. For pulmonary education, they comprise self-management programs for asthma. In the cardiovascular field investment has been for large-scale community trials and educational campaigns. Pulmonary patient education investment is primarily in tested programs of instruction for families of children with asthma, perhaps because approximately 10% of residents in the United States have asthma or wheezing at some time. Cardiovascular and pulmonary diseases are major health problems. Lack of standardized program development in the many other areas in which patient education could be helpful is unfortunate.

Box 6-7 | *Patient Education and Management of Asthma*

Patient education is a powerful tool for helping patients gain the motivation, skill, and confidence to control their asthma.[1,2] Patient education should begin at the time of diagnosis and be integrated with continuing care. All members of the health care team should participate in the process.

Building a Partnership

Much of the day-to-day responsibility for managing asthma falls on the patient and the patient's family. Active participation by the clinician, the patient, and the patient's family in a partnership can improve patient adherence to the treatment plan and stimulate improvements in asthma management.[3,4] The partnership concept includes open communication, joint development of a treatment plan by the clinician and patient, and encouragement of the family's efforts to improve prevention and treatment of the patient's symptoms. An important step in building

the partnership is to ask questions early in each patient visit to identify the patient's main concerns about and expectations for treatment. Patients can focus fully on the clinician's recommendations only after these have been addressed.[5]

The Content of Teaching

Patient education involves helping patients understand asthma, helping patients learn and practice the skills necessary to manage asthma, and supporting patients for adopting appropriate asthma management behaviors and adhering to the treatment plan. Providing information contributes to but is not enough by itself to accomplish these objectives. Developing the patient's asthma management skills as well as the patient's confidence that the patient can control asthma is also required.

From National Asthma Education Program: *Guidelines for the diagnosis and management of asthma,* Bethesda, MD, 1991, National Heart, Lung, and Blood Institute.
PEFR, peak expiratory flow rate.

| Box 6-7 | *Patient Education and Management of Asthma—cont'd* |

The full report, *Guidelines for the Diagnosis and Management of Asthma,* presents a complete discussion of suggested patient education programs and provides sample handouts. Areas and topics to be considered in patient education for asthma include:

- *Definition of asthma:* With an emphasis on the chronic nature of asthma and goals of therapy.
- *Key points about signs and symptoms of asthma:* The main symptoms of acute asthma episodes, the variability of symptoms among patients, the need to recognize and treat even mild symptoms, the importance of PEFR measurements in detecting early symptoms.
- *Characteristic changes in the airways of asthma patients and the role of medications:* Inflammation, bronchospasm, and excessive thick mucus; inhaled steroids, cromolyn, and bronchodilators.
- *Asthma triggers and how to avoid or control them:* Allergens and irritants, viral respiratory tract infections, and exercise.
- *Treatment:* The need for individualized continuing care, adverse effects and how to reduce them, the need for preventive treatment, the importance of early treatment of acute episodes.
- *Patient fears concerning medication:* Responses to common fears include the following: inhaled steroids are safe and efficacious; toxicity effects can be minimized by reducing the dosage; asthma medications are not addictive; continuous use does not reduce effectiveness.
- *Use of written guidelines:* Including medication plans for maintenance therapy and managing exacerbations as well as criteria for detecting onset of symptoms, initiating treatment for acute episodes, seeking emergency care, and recognizing when long-term treatment is less than optimal.
- *Use of written diaries:* To record asthma triggers, symptoms, actions taken, and PEFR in order to see patterns and report to the clinician.
- *Correct use of inhalers.*
- *Criteria for premedicating to prevent onset of symptoms:* Before exercise, before exposure to allergens, cold air, or irritants.
- *Optimal use of home peak expiratory flow rate monitoring:* To help decide when to initiate or terminate treatment, when to seek emergency

care, or when to consider additional chronic treatment because of, for example, high variability in PEFR readings or evening dips below morning PEFR levels.

- *Evaluation of results of treatment plan:* Review whether the goals of therapy are being achieved; identify any adherence problems in order to overcome barriers or to negotiate changes in the treatment plan. Adherence to the treatment plan is enhanced when the plan is simplified as much as possible and when the plan considers both the patient's ability to afford the medications and the payment method.
- *Fears and misconceptions:* Asthma is not caused by psychological factors; most deaths are related to undertreatment and are rare in children; people with asthma should live full and active lives; with proper treatment asthma does not lead to permanent lung disability.
- *Family understanding and support:* Need for family education about asthma, need for help in managing an acute exacerbation.
- *Communication with the child's school:* By parents and by the clinician.
- *Feelings about asthma:* Need for acknowledging negative feelings and their validity; possible need for obtaining referrals to self-management programs, counseling, and social services.

References

1. Feldman CH, Clark NM, Evans D: The role of health education in medical management in asthma. *Clin Rev Allergy* 1987; 5:197-205.
2. Mellins RB: Patient education is key to successful management of asthma. *J Rev Respir Dis* 1989; S47-S52 (Suppl).
3. Schulman BA: Active patient orientation and outcomes in hypertensive treatment. *Med Care* 1979; 17:267-280.
4. Clark NC: Asthma self-management education: research and implications for clinical practice. *Chest* 1989; 95:1110-1113.
5. Korsch BM, Gozzi EK, Francis V: Gaps in doctor-patient communication. I. Doctor-patient interaction and patient satisfaction. *Pediatrics* 1958; 42:855-871.

References

1. Ansell JE and others: Long-term patient self-management of oral anticoagulation, *Arch Intern Med* 155:2185-2189, 1995.
2. Becker G and others: The dilemma of seeking urgent care: asthma episodes and emergency service use, *Soc Sci Med* 37:305-313, 1993.
3. Bernard-Bonnin A-C and others: Self-management teaching programs and morbidity of pediatric asthma: a meta-analysis, *J Allergy Clin Immunol* 95:34-41, 1995.
4. Bird ST and others: Patient education for sickle cell disease: a national survey of health care professionals, *Health Educ Res* 9:235-242, 1994.
5. Blank FSJ and others: Development of an ED teaching program aimed at reducing prehospital delays for patients with chest pain, *J Emerg Nurs* 24:316-319, 1998.
6. Braslow A and others: CPR training without an instructor: development and evaluation of a video self-instructional system for effective performance of cardiopulmonary resuscitation, *Resuscitation* 34:207-220, 1997.
7. Brown JV and others: Asthma management by preschool children and their families: a developmental framework, *J Asthma* 33:299-311, 1996.
8. Burke LE, Dunbar-Jacob JM, Hill MN: Compliance with cardiovascular disease prevention strategies: a review of the research, *Ann Behav Med* 19:239-263, 1997.
9. Capen CL and others: The team approach to pediatric asthma education, *Pediatr Nurs* 20:231-237, 1994.
10. Carney S and others: Hypertension education: patient knowledge and satisfaction, *J Hum Hypertens* 7:505-508, 1993.
11. Clark NM and others: Self-regulation of health behavior: the "take PRIDE" program, *Health Educ Q* 19:341-354, 1992.
12. Clark NM, Nothwehr F: Self-management of asthma by adult patients, *Patient Educ Couns* 32: S5-S20, 1997.
13. Cleeman JI, L'enfant C: The National Cholesterol Education Program, *JAMA* 280:2099-2104, 1998.
14. Daley S and others: Education to improve stroke awareness and emergent response, *J Neurosci Nurs* 29:393-396, 1997.
15. Daniels S, Meuleman J: Importance of assessment of metered-dose inhaler technique in the elderly, *J Am Geriatr Soc* 42:82-84, 1994.
16. Devine EC: Meta-analysis of the effects of psycho-educational care in adults with asthma, *Res Nurs Health* 19:367-376, 1996.
17. Devine EC, Pearcy J: Meta-analysis of the effects of psychoeducational care in adults with chronic obstructive pulmonary disease, *Patient Educ Couns* 29:167-178, 1996.
18. Devine EC, Reifschneider E: A meta-analysis of the effects of psychoeducational care in adults with hypertension, *Nurs Res* 44:237-245, 1995.
19. Dracup K and others: Is cardiopulmonary resuscitation training deleterious for family members of cardiac patients? *Am J Public Health* 84:116-118, 1994.
20. Dracup K and others: Causes of delay in seeking treatment for heart attack symptoms, *Soc Sci Med* 40:379-392, 1995.
21. Dracup K and others: The physician's role in minimizing prehospital delay in patients at high risk for acute myocardial infarction: recommendations from the National Heart Attack Alert Program, *Ann Intern Med* 12:45-51, 1997.
22. Dusseldorf E and others: A meta-analysis of psychoeducational programs for coronary heart disease patients, *Health Psychol* 18:506-519, 1999.
23. Evans D and others: Improving care for minority children with asthma: professional education in public health clinics, *Pediatrics* 99:157-164, 1997.
24. Fishwick D, D'Souza WD, Beasley R: The asthma self-management plan system of care: what does it mean, how is it done, does it work, what models are available, what do patients want and who needs it? *Patient Educ Couns* 32:S21-S33, 1997.
25. Flaum M, Lang CL, Tinkelman D: Take control of high-cost asthma, *J Asthma* 34:5-14, 1997.
26. George MR and others: A comprehensive educational program improves clinical outcome measures in inner-city patients with asthma, *Arch Intern Med* 159:1710-1716, 1999.
27. Goff DC and others: Knowledge of heart attack symptoms in a population survey in the United States, *Arch Intern Med* 158:2329-2338, 1998.
28. Greineder DK, Loane KC, Parks P: Reduction in resource utilization by an asthma outreach program, *Arch Pediatr Adolesc Med* 149:415-420, 1995.
29. Gruesser M and others: Structured patient education for outpatients with hypertension in general practice: a model project in Germany, *J Hum Hypertens* 11:501-506, 1997.
30. Gulanick M, Kim MJ, Holm K: Resumption of home activities following cardiac events, *Prog Cardiovasc Nurs* 6:21-27, 1991.

31. Haas JS and others: The impact of socioeconomic status on the intensity of ambulatory treatment and health outcomes after hospital discharge for adults with asthma, *J Gen Intern Med* 9:121-126, 1994.

32. Heidenrich PA, Ruggerio CM, Massio BM: Effect of a home monitoring system on hospitalization resource use for patients with heart failure, *Am Heart J* 138:633-640, 1999.

33. Hendricson WD and others: Implementation of individualized patient education for Hispanic children and their families, *Patient Educ Couns* 29:155-165, 1996.

34. Howell JH, Flaim T, Lung CL: Patient education, *Pediatr Clin North Am* 39:1343-1361, 1992.

35. Interiano B, Kalpalatha K, Guntupalli K: Metered-dose inhalers; do health care providers know what to teach? *Arch Intern Med* 153:81-85, 1993.

36. Iso H and others: Community-based education classes for hypertension control, *Hypertension* 27:968-974, 1996.

37. Johnson JA, King KB: Influence of expectations about symptoms on delay in seeking treatment during a myocardial infarction, *Am J Crit Care* 4:29-35, 1995.

38. Kelso TM and others: Educational and long-term therapeutic intervention in the ED: effect on outcomes in adult indigent minority asthmatics, *Am J Emerg Med* 13:632-637, 1995.

39. Kesten S: Asthma education: a time for reappraisal, *Chest* 107:893-894, 1995.

40. Linden W, Stossel C, Maurice J: Psychosocial interventions for patients with coronary artery disease, *Arch Intern Med* 156:745-752, 1996.

41. Man-Son-Hing M and others: A patient decision aid regarding antibiotic therapy for stroke prevention in atrial thrombotic therapy for stroke prevention in atrial fibrillation, *JAMA* 282:737-743, 1999.

42. McLauchlan CAJ and others: Resuscitation training for cardiac patients and their relatives—its effect on anxiety, *Resuscitation* 24:7-11, 1992.

43. Meng A: An asthma day camp, *MCN Am J Matern Child Nurs* 22:135-141, 1997.

44. Meurer JR and others: The Awesome Asthma School Days program: educating children, inspiring a community, *J Sch Health* 69(2):63-68, 1999.

45. Missed opportunities in preventive counseling for cardiovascular disease—U.S. 1995, *MMWR Morb Mortal Wkly Rep* 47:91-95, 1998.

46. Morrison VL and others: Improving emotional outcomes following acute stroke: a preliminary evaluation of a workbook-based intervention, *Scot Med J* 43:52-53, 1998.

47. Moser DK, Dracup KA, Marsden C: Needs of recovering cardiac patients and their spouses: compared views, *Int J Nurs Stud* 30:105-114, 1993.

48. Mullen PD, Mains DA, Velez R: A meta-analysis of controlled trials of cardiac patient education, *Patient Educ Couns* 19:143-162, 1992.

49. National Asthma Education Program: *Guidelines for the diagnosis and management of asthma*, Bethesda, MD, 1991, National Heart, Lung and Blood Institute.

50. Pancioli AM and others: Public perception of stroke warning signs and knowledge of potential risk factors, *JAMA* 279:1288-1292, 1998.

51. Plous S, Chesne RB, McDowell AV: Nutrition knowledge and attitudes of cardiac patients, *J Am Diet Assoc* 95:442-446, 1995.

52. Ronchetti R and others: Asthma self-management programmes in a population of Italian children: a multicentric study, *Eur Respir J* 10:1248-1253, 1997.

53. Rutten-Van Molken MPMH, VanDoorslaer EKA, Rutten FFH: Economic appraisal of asthma and COPD care: a literature review 1980-1991, *Soc Sci Med* 35:161-175, 1992.

54. Sawicki PT: A structured teaching and self-management program for patients receiving oral anticoagulation, *JAMA* 281:145-150, 1999.

55. Scherer YK, Schmiedler LE, Shimmel S: The effects of education alone and in combination with pulmonary rehabilitation on self-efficacy in patients with COPD, *Rehab Nurs* 23(2):71-77, 1998.

56. Shresta M and others: Metered-dose inhaler technique of patients in an urban ED: prevalence of incorrect technique and attempt at education, *Am J Emerg Med* 14:380-384, 1996.

57. Simons-Morton DG, Cutler JA: Cardiovascular disease prevention research at the National Heart, Lung and Blood Institute, *Am J Prev Med* 14:317-330, 1998.

58. Soghikian K and others: Home blood pressure monitoring; effect on use of medical services and medical care costs, *Med Care* 30:855-865, 1992.

59. Stoloff SW, Janson S: Providing asthma education in primary care practice, *Am Fam Physician* 56:117-126, 1997.

60. Study: CHF education more than pays for itself, *Health Benchmarks* 4:144-146, 1997.

61. Votto J and others: Short-stay comprehensive inpatient pulmonary rehabilitation for advanced chronic obstructive pulmonary disease, *Arch Phys Med Rehabil* 77:1115-1118, 1996.

62. Wiles R and others: Providing appropriate information to patients and carers following stroke, *J Adv Nurs* 28:794-801, 1998.

63. Williams LS and others: Stroke patients' knowledge of stroke, *Stroke* 28:912-915, 1997.

64. Wilson SR and others: Education of parents of infants and very young children with asthma: a developmental evaluation of the Wee Wheezers program, *J Asthma* 33:239-254, 1996.

65. Zapka J and others: Health providers' perspectives on patient delay for seeking care for symptoms of acute myocardial infarction, *Health Educ Behav* 26:714-733, 1999.

66. Zimmerman BJ, Bonner S, Evans D, Mellins RB: Self-regulating childhood asthma: a developmental model of family change, *Health Educ Behav* 26:55-71, 1999.

Diabetes Self-Management Education

GENERAL APPROACH

Diabetes education is the most fully developed of all the fields of patient education practice and among the oldest, having begun in the 1930s. Nationally accepted standards have been adopted for accrediting programs of diabetes education and for certification for an interdisciplinary advanced-practice role of certified diabetes educator (CDE). In addition, randomized clinical trials have shown that stringent blood glucose control is associated with decreased risk of complications.[1] Intensive treatment is attempted to achieve glycemic control as close to the nondiabetic range as possible. Flexible adjustment of insulin dose, frequent monitoring of glucose levels (a minimum of four times a day), diet and exercise instruction, as well as frequent counseling and dietary adjustments are important. The National Diabetes Education Program, much like cardiovascular education programs, is in effect. Its goals include (1) increasing public awareness of the seriousness of diabetes, risk factors, and prevention; (2) promoting effective self-management; (3) improving knowledge of diabetes among health professionals; and (4) promoting policies that improve quality of and access to diabetes care.[17]

Approximately 8% of all adults in the United States have diabetes, and the percentage is proportionally higher in Hispanic, Native American, and African-American populations. Severe deficits in self-management skills such as glucose testing, diet, sick-day guidelines and foot care have been identified in 50% to 80% of adults and children with diabetes. More than half of persons with diabetes receive limited or no diabetes self-management education.[8] In addition, significant shortfalls in the quality of care for diabetes leave a great deal of room for improvement.[14]

EDUCATIONAL APPROACHES AND RESEARCH BASE

Several meta-analyses of studies on the effectiveness of diabetes education have been completed. A summary of 82 such studies showed a high effect for increase in patient knowledge, medium-sized effects for dietary compliance and urine-testing skill, and lesser-sized effects for glycosylated hemoglobin and blood sugar.[3] Most of the studies did not provide in-depth descriptions of the interventions that were used. A reanalysis of 73 of these studies found that patient education appeared to be more effective in younger patients.[4] For all patients, glycosylated hemoglobin levels improved between 1 and 6 months postintervention but decreased to 1-month levels after 6 months. Length of the educational intervention did not appear to influence outcomes. An independent meta-analysis found an effect size of 0.68 for diet instruction, with positive effects decreased but retained at 6- and 12-month follow-up examinations, excepting weight loss.[21]

Modern diabetes self-management programs reflect a movement away from a goal of regimen compliance to a goal of patient empowerment. Such programs include a strong emphasis on self-efficacy, as well as on the impact of diabetes on the totality of a person's life. Goals include enhancing the ability of patients to identify and set realistic goals, to apply a systematic problem-solving process, to manage the stress caused by living with diabetes, and to identify and obtain appropriate social support. The view that patients should define their blood glucose target, weighing the risk they are prepared to take and the efforts they are prepared to make, is still not the norm.

One study of patients' explanatory models of diabetes focused on difficulties in patients' life-styles and relationships; however, staff members viewed diabetes primarily as a pathophysiological problem.[9] Among the highly educated patients, the restrictions required to manage diabetes were seen as major obstacles to social relationships, causing things such as divorce, loss of jobs, sexual problems, the death of newborn children, and difficulty traveling. What patients viewed as fears, professionals discussed as difficulties, without the same depth of turmoil that patients felt. Staff members did not elicit patients' perspectives on their illness, and major difficulties for patients were unknown to the staff.

One experiential model of learning how to manage diabetes reflects a rich series of sequential stages, including the following[22]:

- Trying out the regimen with rigid adherence
- Making regimen modifications that are more compatible with daily schedules or that ameliorate untoward and often frightening body responses
- Experimenting with effects of foods, activities, and circumstances, such as stressful

situations, on blood glucose levels in an effort to find a regimen that would work for the patients
- Settling into a basic routine if the patient could recognize a predictable response pattern

Eventually, patients were able to apply their basic routines to new situations such as travel, illness, or change in work schedule; this adaptation sometimes required them to return briefly to trial-and-error activities. This approach allowed patients to tailor the regimen to their preferred lifestyles and perceived selves.

In this experiential model, body listening was interpreted as a crucial source of information and became more important to these patients than did monitoring from health providers and significant others.[22] In fact, a special form of training, called blood-glucose awareness training (BGAT), has been effective in teaching individuals with insulin-requiring diabetes to improve their ability to recognize blood glucose fluctuations, although it is still less accurate than actual measures—self-monitoring of blood glucose— and quite variable across patients. Patients use both internal cues (body feelings) and external cues (timing, type and amount of insulin, food, and exercise). Blood glucose estimates made by adults in this way have been found to be accurate about 50% of the time but dangerously inaccurate 15% of the time, failing to detect hypoglycemia and hyperglycemia.

The data suggest there are no symptoms consistently associated with hypoglycemia or hyperglycemia for all patients. Most patients appear to have one or more symptoms that are highly idiosyncratic, varying from patient to patient, and they are unaware of which symptoms are actually predictive in their own case. BGAT involves teaching patients how to identify symptoms sensitive and specific to their hypoglycemia and hyperglycemia. At an average of 4.9 years after training, these patients had improved glycosylated hemoglobin levels and fewer automobile accidents than did control subjects who received routine diabetes education. Booster training (periodic brief retraining) was important. This work suggests that teaching classic signs or symptoms of hypoglycemia or hyperglycemia may be seriously misleading. Only one symptom (feeling shaky) was predictive of hypoglycemia for more than half of those studied, and in some cases a single symptom predicted hyperglycemia for one patient and hypoglycemia for another. Postintervention levels were still far from ideal.[10]

Studies of learning conditions for persons with diabetes show that poor glycemic control in older persons with non-insulin-dependent diabetes mellitus is associated with decreased cognitive functioning, including verbal learning and memory, and the worse the control, the greater the impairment.[12] Depression is more prevalent in persons with diabetes than it is in the general population and is associated with poor glycemic control and decreased compliance with therapy. Pharmacotherapy for depression may be poorly tolerated or insufficient to produce full remission in as many as half of persons with diabetes with major depression or may not be prescribed.[19] As you know, depression makes learning and self-management difficult.

Teaching materials and approaches must reflect the fact that diabetes involves a complex regimen and often necessitates lifestyle changes on the part of a patient and family. Approaches must also be culturally sensitive. Brown and others[6] have carried out a series of studies in Starr County, Texas, a bicultural community on the Mexican border. The intervention is community-based, employs bilingual Mexican-American nurses from the community, uses videotapes filmed in Starr County showing community leaders describing their experiences with diabetes, and focuses on dietary choices consistent with Mexican American preferences. Preliminary data from the study show a decrease in glycosylated hemoglobin levels. Other studies of a similar but low-income population found that patients commonly relied on medication as a safety valve to compensate for not following their diet. They ate "normal" foods until a crisis in glucose levels and then ate more carefully until control was regained. Patients feared low rather than high

blood glucose because of its distressing symptoms. Even though patients knew what to do and were committed to taking care of themselves, many pushed the bounds of acceptable practice.[16] The community-based and community-involving approaches to attaining the tighter glucose control essential to the new standards of diabetes care of Brown and others[6] offer a different model of diabetes education—especially in high-incidence populations.

Games and active learning are excellent ways to teach both motor and cognitive skills to children. They provide learning conditions that are motivating and highly repetitive so that the knowledge is retained. Table 7-1 summarizes games used to teach children ages 7 to 12 years at the International Diabetes Center.[2] Assessment and evaluation tools are also important. Readers will recall that in Chapter 2 the transtheoretic model was described as useful for assessing whether patients were ready for behavior change. Boxes 7-1, 7-2, and 7-3 present sample questions for such an assessment of persons with diabetes; similar tools should be used for each important self-care behavior such as glucose testing or weight loss.[24] The outcomes of such an assessment allow an educator to match much more specifically the education to a patient's stage of readiness and to prioritize which of multiple target behaviors are most amenable to change. It should be remembered that some patients experience something like a religious conversion, when after many years of diabetes they finally realize its threat to their health and make a conscious decision to take better care of themselves. Most often the conversion occurs around major events in the lives of relatives or friends.[20]

A number of instruments are available to measure quality of life, attitudes, disease-relevant behaviors, and knowledge among children and adults with diabetes. These instruments may be found in the literature—four are reproduced and critiqued in Redman.[23]

Diabetes education is the area of practice most likely to have formal programs, especially in hospitals. Lowe, Hogue, and Delcher[18] write of the

Text continued on p. 166

TABLE 7-1 Games from the Children's Classweek Curriculum

Game	Objectives	Equipment	Instruction
What is Diabetes?	To identify body parts, to define diabetes and discuss possible causes, to demonstrate how food is digested	Brown wrapping paper (large roll, 3 ft wide, cut into pieces corresponding to children's height), paper cutouts of body parts (pancreas, heart, lungs, stomach, heart, brain), "What causes diabetes?" flashcards, models of stomach, sample breakfast foods (juice, milk, cereal, etc.)	Children trace an outline of each other on brown paper and then paste body parts to the corresponding area. Discussion involves defining each body part and its function. Using the diabetes flashcards, children work in small groups to decide which do/do not cause diabetes. Then the entire group reconvenes and discusses causes of diabetes. Each child is given a model stomach to fill with breakfast foods. Children's hands are used to simulate "digesting" food and the group discusses how food turns into blood sugar.
A Hanging Drop and Other Blood Sugar Mysteries	To state reasons for self blood glucose monitoring (SBGM), to describe/explain hemoglobin A_{1c}, to discuss steps necessary to get an accurate blood test using a meter, to describe pattern control, to describe ketone testing and its purpose	HbA_{1c} puppets, one apple, toothpicks, marshmallows, SBGM concentration gameboard and cards, various meters and equipment for demonstration, four colored pens, diabetes record book, Ketostix, life-size duplicate of a Ketostix, and color-code chart	Children act out the way hemoglobin and glucose function. Instructor demonstrates by placing marshmallows on toothpicks and sticking them into an apple (higher A_{1c} = more marshmallows). The class is divided into two or more teams for a concentration game. Each team member takes a turn to get a match on the board and after each match the team member must say whether the step is required for an accurate blood test. For the four-colored pen game each child is given a pen and record book. Children are told to circle morning regular insulin and lunch blood sugar in red, morning NPH and evening meal blood glucose in green, evening meal regular and bedtime blood glucose in blue, and evening meal NPH and morning blood glucose in black. Discussion is then held regarding the relationship between these insulins and tests and how adjustments might be made. In the Ketostix game children pick a Ketostix and match it to the area/color on the color-code chart.

Eating Right = Feeling Great and In Control	To understand the importance of consistency for blood sugar control and good nutrition for growth and development, to understand carbohydrate choices at meals and snacks, to learn what is included in each exchange list and what constitutes a portion	Writing board, erasable markers, examples of each type of macronutrient (eg, sugar and starch for carbohydrate, egg white for protein, margarine or oil for fat), Exchange Lists handout, large picture of Food Pyramid, supplies for Guess the Exchanges game	The class begins with a description of the macronutrients and micronutrients in foods. The food pyramid then is discussed and the components of each group are described. The exchange lists are compared with the food pyramid by listing similarities and differences. Discussion is held about carbohydrate, protein, and fat, and their effects on blood sugar, emphasizing that CHO has the greatest impact. The concept of starch, fruit, and milk affecting blood sugar the most also is discussed. Examples of each nutrient can be demonstrated. To help visualize portions, children play the Guess the Exchanges game. They go to different stations where a food is shown in two portions (one correct/one incorrect) and they are told to pick which portion is correct. The class then discusses the answers as a group.
Exchange Relay	To learn what foods are in each exchange group	Pictures of foods	The class is divided into two or more teams. Each person on the team is assigned one of the six exchange groups and must retrieve a food from that group from a large pile of pictures at the other side of the room. The first team to get all of the required foods wins the game. To reinforce learning, the foods chosen then are reviewed at the end of each race.
Weak and Wobblies, Trick or Treat 'Em	To define hypoglycemia, to describe how it feels to be hypoglycemic, to name at least three treatments for hypoglycemia and what supplies should be carried, to identify causes of hypoglycemia, to determine one's individual blood glucose target range	Targeting Blood Glucose game contents (board, markers, Nerf brand dart gun, hypoglycemia treatment center)	A general discussion of hypoglycemia is conducted in a group setting and each of the objectives is addressed. The game, Targeting Blood Glucose, then is played to reinforce proper treatment of hypoglycemia.

Continued

From Barry B: Games and activities to teach children about diabetes and nutrition, *Diabetes Educ* 21:27-30, 1995. *NPH*, neutral protamine Hagedorn; *CHO*, carbohydrate.

TABLE 7-1   Games from the Children's Classweek Curriculum—cont'd

Game	Objectives	Equipment	Instruction
Shop 'N Bop	To identify the main components of the new nutrition label, to identify guidelines for fat and sugar content when choosing foods, to demonstrate how to use the nutrition labels for doing carbohydrate counting	Nutrition Facts Label handout, grocery store	The Nutrition Facts Label handout is discussed in class, and children are told to highlight/circle serving size, total fat, and total carbohydrates. The class discusses how much fat to eat in one serving of food (<3 to 5 grams).
Sick Days Rummy	To identify the steps necessary to prevent diabetic ketoacidosis (DKA) when ill	Sick Days Rummy cards	The class discusses the proper steps to take for sick-day management and each step is listed on the board and reviewed. Sick Days Rummy is played by dividing the class into groups, each receiving a deck of cards. The object of the game is to collect the cards that contain all of the proper steps to follow for sick-day management.
Be the Teacher	To demonstrate to the class and instructors a topic learned during the children's classweek	Various diabetes teaching aids used during the week or a container filled with papers on which various diabetes topics are written	The class is divided into groups and each group is given a topic to present. They are allowed to use any prop or tool they have seen used for teaching in the past week. Each group has at least 1 hour to prepare and must present for at least 10 minutes. This game can also be played by placing in a container papers on which topics are written and having each child draw a topic. The child then has 1 minute to describe the topic, give examples, etc. The "teaching" by children can be videotaped to show to parents later.
Diabetes Hangman	To help teach concepts related to diabetes and management	Chalkboard or dry erase board, markers	This game is played just like regular hangman, except that diabetes-related words are used and the person who guesses the word must also give a definition of that word.
Exchange Bingo	To help teach about foods and portions from the exchange lists	Exchange Bingo cards, cover chips	This game is played just like regular bingo, except that the names of the six exchange groups are printed across the top of each card and below each name is a food and one serving/portion size. The object of the game is to cover six squares in a row, horizontally, vertically, or diagonally. Other options include covering the four corners or a coverall.

From Barry B: Games and activities to teach children about diabetes and nutrition, *Diabetes Educ* 21:27-30, 1995.

Box 7-1	*Sample Staging Questions*

Glucose self-monitoring: *Do you always check your blood sugar (glucose) in the way you were instructed to?*

_____ Yes, I have been doing so for more than 6 months (maintenance)

_____ Yes, I have been doing so but for less than 6 months (action)

_____ No, but I plan to in the next month (preparation)

_____ No, but I plan to in the next 6 months (contemplation)

_____ No, and I do not intend to in the next 6 months (precontemplation)

If you answered no above, how often do you check your blood glucose?

_____ Never

_____ Rarely

_____ Sometimes

_____ Often

_____ Usually

Diet: *Do you always follow your special diet in the way you were instructed?*

_____ Yes, I have been doing so for more than 6 months (maintenance)

_____ Yes, I have been doing so but for less than 6 months (action)

_____ No, but I plan to in the next month (preparation)

_____ No, but I plan to in the next 6 months (contemplation)

_____ No, and I do not intend to in the next 6 months (precontemplation)

If you answered no above, how often do you follow your diet?

_____ Never

_____ Rarely

_____ Sometimes

_____ Often

_____ Usually

From Ruggerio L, Prochaska JO: Introduction: sample staging, decisional balance, and self-efficacy questions. *Diabetes Spectrum* 6:22-24, 1993.

Box 7-2	*Sample Decisional Balance Questions*

How important is each of the following in deciding whether to take care of your diabetes as recommended?

Pros

When I follow my diet, there is less chance that I will have serious health problems.

When I test my glucose, I feel more in control of my life.

When I exercise, I see myself as a "healthy person."

When I take my insulin as recommended, I feel more responsible.

Cons

Following my diabetes diet gets in the way of other people's plans.

Testing my blood glucose makes me feel different.

My exercise routine interferes with other activities.

Injecting myself with insulin is painful.

From Ruggerio L, Prochaska JO: Introduction: sample staging, decisional balance, and self-efficacy questions. *Diabetes Spectrum* 6:22-24, 1993.

Box 7-3	*Sample Self-Efficacy Questions*

How confident (sure) are you that you would continue to follow the . . . aspect of your diabetes regimen in each of the following situations?

Diet: When I am on vacation.

Self-monitoring of blood glucose: When my fingers hurt from the last monitoring.

Exercise: When I am tired.

Insulin use: When I am with other people.

From Ruggerio L, Prochaska JO: Introduction: sample staging, decisional balance, and self-efficacy questions. *Diabetes Spectrum* 6:22-24, 1993.

TABLE 7-2	Diabetes Patient Educational Opportunities at Georgia Baptist Medical Center

Source	Service
Literature	Diabetes starter kits with educational materials on diabetes, insulin, diet, and exercise
Video learning series or closed circuit TV	Presentation of: 1. Diabetes information and essential components of treatment 2. "A Positive Approach to Diabetes" (video)
Bedside teaching by nurse	1. Insulin injection 2. Emphasis on signs/symptoms of hypo/hyperglycemia 3. Other survival skills as appropriate
Patient care assistant	Demonstration of fingerstick technique for blood glucose monitoring
Inhouse classes	Multidisciplinary teaching each Thursday, 2 to 3 PM; subject and location announced prior to presentation
Diabetes nurse consultant	Consultation by request (provide appropriate extension)
Diabetes resource nurse	Unit nurse liaison
Pharmaceutical services	Bedside teaching on therapeutic effect of insulin and oral agents for all new prescriptions
Nutritional services	Bedside assessment and teaching of appropriate diet prescriptions
Blood glucose monitoring	Delivery and instructional use of blood glucose monitor (optional service offered to GBMC patients)
Home health follow-up	Provided as appropriate (per physician order) for a minimum of two visits regarding compliance, safety, or other self-care deficits
Skin consultation	Skin and foot assessment with review of skin care
Chaplain	Assessment of psychosocial/spiritual needs
Preventive medicine	Supplemental literature on exercise

From Lowe DH, Hogue JK, Delcher HK: Evolution of a progressive self-directed diabetes education model. *Diabetes Educator* 20:199-203, 1994.

program of diabetes education at Georgia Baptist Medical Center that has broad-based and many educational opportunities and includes continuous staff development (Table 7-2). The role of diabetes nurse coordinator is described in Box 7-4 and includes clinical practice, case management, consultation, and staff education and extends into home care. The critical path for patients with newly diagnosed insulin-dependent diabetes mellitus could be strengthened by adding patient outcomes (Box 7-5).

Because managed care is changing patterns of service provision and because of the recognition that all persons with diabetes should have easy access to self-care management education in-cluding regular follow-up, new delivery modes are springing up. Work site-based programs have been shown to significantly improve control of the disease, which is very costly to employers if it is not well controlled.[7] For the same reason, health maintenance organizations may provide close follow-up of these patients through a nurse case manager and pay for their enrollees to attend a self-management educational program.[1] Hendricks and Hendricks[15] describe a freestanding outpatient diabetes disease management center to which managed care organizations could send patients.

Lack of payment for diabetes self-management education services has traditionally been a

Box 7-4	*Diabetes Nurse Coordinator Advanced Practice Role Delineation*

- Assesses physical, psychosocial, economic, and spiritual responses of patients, families, and significant others to actual/potential diabetes health-related problems.
- Determines with healthcare team the appropriate interventions for clinical problems and case-management issues based on needs assessment.
- Develops and coordinates continuous quality improvement systems based on patient outcome criteria.
- Develops practice standards for diabetes patient education.
- Functions as a liaison between patients, families, physicians, healthcare team members, and the Diabetes Advisory Committee (DAC), facilitating communication and quality patient care with regard to the diabetes patient population.
- Develops, plans, and implements diabetes programs based on assessment of patient/physician population.
- Serves as a consultant to healthcare professionals who request information, assistance, etc in diabetes and diabetes-related healthcare issues.
- Maintains a level of clinical and theoretical expertise necessary to provide consultation to the healthcare team members.
- Develops and evaluates critical pathways for diabetes management.
- Utilizes knowledge base concerning reimbursement issues whereby cost-effective diabetes patient care is identified.
- Supports, initiates, participates, and/or facilitates formal and informal research and relates findings to clinical practice and home health services.

From Lowe DH, Hogue JK, Delcher HK: Evolution of a progressive self-directed diabetes education model. *Diabetes Educator* 20:199-203, 1994.

Box 7-5	*Critical Teaching/Learning Path for Patients with Newly Diagnosed Insulin Dependent Diabetes*

Day 1

1. Review contents of diabetes kit, emphasize diary.
2. Patient acknowledges he/she is challenged with diabetes.
3. Patient views video learning programs.
4. Patient observes fingerstick.
5. Patient observes nurse administering insulin.

Day 2

1. Patient does fingerstick.
2. Patient demonstrates eye estimation of blood glucose.
3. Patient documents in blood glucose diary.
4. Patient is assisted with insulin administration.
5. Nutrition Service visits with patient.

Day 3

1. Patient assesses and identifies trends in blood glucose (see diary).
2. Patient demonstrates insulin administration and verbalizes rationale for insulin.
3. Review with patient the signs and symptoms of hypo/hyperglycemia.
4. Pharmacist consultation.
5. Diabetes nurse consultant visits with patient (optional).

Day 4

1. Blood glucose monitoring instruction.
2. Patient identifies trends in blood glucose (see diary).
3. Nurse explains glycosylate hemoglobin assay.
4. Patient verbalizes actions needed for high and low blood glucose.
5. Patient verbalizes diabetes education resources (e.g., ADA).

From Lowe DH, Hogue JK, Delcher HK: Evolution of a progressive self-directed diabetes education model. *Diabetes Educator* 20:199-203, 1994.
ADA, American Diabetes Association.

problem. More than 30 states have now passed legislation that mandates coverage of diabetes education and supplies. Medicare also reimburses for some supplies and for non-hospital-based education and training services furnished by a certified provider, with referral by a patient's physician.[15]

NATIONAL STANDARDS AND TESTED PROGRAMS

The first diabetes education programs accredited by the American Diabetes Association were recognized in 1987, with more than 375 programs approved since then. The standards against which programs are judged (see Appendix D) are primarily process standards; the usual expected content to be taught may be found in standard 12. In addition, several states have developed mechanisms to approve programs that meet the National Standards for Diabetes Patient Education Programs. Inasmuch as there are no reported studies that compare programs that meet the standards with those that do not, the impact of the standards on the quality of diabetes education remains undocumented. There is a trend toward referring to diabetes education programs as self-management education training programs.[11]

In addition to accreditation or recognition of diabetes education programs, certification is available to diabetes educators. The scope and standards of practice for CDEs are shown in Appendix D. National standards for diabetes self-management programs may also be found in Appendix D.

SUMMARY

Perhaps more than in any other area of practice, the success in patients with diabetes has demonstrated what can be accomplished with research, policies, standards, and services in support of self-management education. Yet large numbers of persons with this disorder are still not reached.

Study Questions

1. Read the article by Hardway, Weatherly, and Bonheur,[13] which provides an excellent example of one institution's evaluating its diabetes education practice and revising it. Make a list of the learning principles that strengthen the process undertaken by this institution.

References

1. Aubert RE and others: Nurse case management to improve glycemic control in diabetic patients in a health maintenance organization, *Ann Intern Med* 129:605-612, 1998.
2. Barry B: Games and activities to teach children about diabetes and nutrition, *Diabetes Educ* 21:27-30, 1995.
3. Brown SA: Studies of educational interventions and outcomes in diabetic adults: a meta-analysis revisited, *Patient Educ Couns* 16:189-215, 1990.
4. Brown SA: Meta-analysis of diabetes patient education research: variations in intervention effects across studies, *Res Nurs Health* 15:409-419, 1992.
5. Brown SA, Hanis CL: A community-based, culturally sensitive education and group-support intervention for Mexican Americans with NIDDM: a pilot study of efficacy, *Diabetes Educ* 21:203-210, 1995.
6. Brown SA and others: Symptom-related self care of Mexican Americans with type 2 diabetes: preliminary findings from the Starr County diabetes education study, *Diabetes Educ* 24:331-339, 1998.
7. Burton WN, Connerty CM: Evaluation of a worksite-based patient education intervention targeted at employees with diabetes mellitus, *J Occup Environ Med* 40:702-706, 1998.
8. Clement S: Diabetes self-management education, *Diabetes Care* 18:1204-1214, 1995.
9. Cohen MZ and others: Explanatory models of diabetes: patient practitioner variation, *Soc Sci Med* 38:59-66, 1994.
10. Cox DJ and others: Long-term follow-up evaluation of blood glucose awareness training, *Diabetes Care* 17:1-5, 1994.
11. Funnell MM, Haas LB: National standards for diabetes self-management education programs, *Diabetes Care* 18:100-116, 1995.

12. Gradman TJ and others: Verbal learning and/or memory improves with glycemic control in older subjects with non-insulin-dependent diabetes mellitus, *J Am Geriatr Soc* 41:1305-1312, 1993.

13. Hardway D, Weatherly KS, Bonheur B: Diabetes education on wheels, *J Nurs Staff Dev* 9:122-126, 1993.

14. Helseth LD, Susman JL, Crabtree PJ: Primary care physicians' perceptions of diabetes management, *J Fam Pract* 48:37-42, 1999.

15. Hendricks LE, Hendricks RG: Making a case for the CDE's role in outsourcing diabetes services to a freestanding outpatient diabetes disease state management center, *Diabetes Educ* 25:765-773, 1999.

16. Hunt LM, Pugh J, Valenzuela M: How patients adapt diabetes self-care recommendations in everyday life, *J Fam Pract* 46:207-215, 1998.

17. Leontos C, Wong F, Gallivan J, Lising M: National Diabetes Education Program: opportunities and challenges, *J Am Dietet Assoc* 98:73-75, 1998.

18. Lowe DH, Hogue JK, Delcher HK: Evolution of a progressive self-directed diabetes education model, *Diabetes Educ* 20:199-203, 1994.

19. Lustman PJ and others: Cognitive behavior for depression in type 2 diabetes mellitus, *Ann Intern Med* 129:613-621, 1998.

20. O'Connor PJ, Crabtree BF, Yanoshik K: Differences between diabetic patients who do and do not respond to a diabetes care intervention: a qualitative analysis, *Fam Med* 29:424-428, 1997.

21. Padgett D and others: Meta-analysis of the effects of educational and psycho-social interventions of management of diabetes mellitus, *J Clin Epidemiol* 41:1007-1030, 1988.

22. Price MJ: An experiential model of learning diabetes self-management, *Qual Health Res* 3:29-54, 1993.

23. Redman BK: *Measurement tools in patient education*, New York, 1997, Springer.

24. Ruggiero L, Prochaska JO: Introduction, *Diabetes Spectrum* 6:22-59, 1993.

Chapter 8

Education for Pregnancy and Parenting, and Educating Children

EDUCATION FOR PREGNANCY AND PARENTING

General Approach

Education for pregnancy, parenting, and educating children are established fields of practice in patient education. Although many of the goals remain the same, prenatal education has become more varied philosophically. All three fields reflect dramatic shifts in the way health is delivered and in the tremendous increase in self-management currently expected of patients and families.

Educational Approaches and Research Base

Ideally, prenatal education should begin before pregnancy, with formal classes starting before conception or early in pregnancy and extending across the childbearing year to 3 months after delivery. In actuality, formal early-pregnancy education has been neglected, formal midpregnancy education classes are not widely available, and most prenatal teaching that takes place during the third trimester prepares for birth. A fre-

quently used format is weekly classes in a community setting, in which the following topics are addressed[38]:

- Health maintenance: Prevention of urinary tract infections, Kegel exercises and exercise in general, smoking and alcohol ingestion, medication use, and nutritional intake
- Management of pregnancy and birth: Signs of complications, discomforts of pregnancy, potential complications of pregnancy, the birth plan, recognition of labor and preterm labor and preparation for it
- Parenting, as well as postpartum and infant care: Prebirth preparation for parenting, preparation for infant feeding, including breastfeeding, circumcision and cord care, and other topics

Box 8-1 provides an outline for prenatal education that includes both preconception and the trimesters. In addition, special classes may be held for pregnant adolescents, for first-time mothers older than 35 years of age, for adoptive parents, for those who have a scheduled cesarean

Box 8-1	*Outline for Prenatal Education*

At the earliest contact between client and nurse, a teaching plan is developed. This reflects the unique learning needs of each client and incorporates information that health care providers identify as essential for all pregnant women to know and information that clients identify as learning priorities. The outline is reviewed with the client and updated whenever necessary. Client referral to individuals or organizations sponsoring childbirth education can also be appropriate for meeting overall learning objectives.

Preconception

How pregnancy occurs (menstrual cycle)
Lifestyle factors with potential impact on becoming pregnant and on early pregnancy: drugs such as alcohol, nutritional status, general health, occupational and environmental considerations
Alternatives in childbirth settings and in obstetric caregivers
Pregnancy tests
Myths about conception and pregnancy

First Trimester

Feelings about pregnancy, ambivalence, developmental tasks of early pregnancy, age-related issues
Family reactions to pregnancy, first-trimester emotional responses of expectant fathers
Early-pregnancy physical changes
Sexuality during the first trimester
Lifestyle factors with potential impact on early pregnancy: drugs such as alcohol, nutrition (including prescribed vitamin and iron supplements), general health, exercise, rest, occupational and environmental considerations
Warning signs of early pregnancy

Fear of miscarriage (suggested presentation as a topic in a group setting)
First-trimester diagnostic tests for maternal/fetal well-being (as appropriate)
Client expectations for pregnancy and childbirth
Options available to client within the selected prenatal and delivery setting, tour of birthing facility
Anticipatory guidance regarding what to expect at prenatal visits
Sibling concerns, telling other children about pregnancy
Resources within the caregiving agency or private practice and within the community (including relevant literature)

Second Trimester

Feelings about pregnancy, acceptance of pregnancy, developmental tasks of midpregnancy, age-related issues
Family responses to progressing pregnancy, second-trimester responses of expectant fathers
Fetal growth and development
Midtrimester physical changes, relief of discomforts associated with enlarging fetus and physical changes
Sexuality during the second trimester
Lifestyle factors with potential impact on midpregnancy: drugs such as alcohol, smoking, nutrition (including prescribed vitamin and iron supplements), general health, exercise, body mechanics, rest, occupational and environmental considerations, stress
Changes in activities of daily living related to midtrimester
Warning signs of midpregnancy
Diagnostic tests for assessment of maternal/fetal well-being (as necessary)

From Sherwen LN, Scoloveno MA, Weingarten CT: *Nursing care of the childbearing family,* ed 2, Norwalk, CT, 1995, Appleton & Lange.

section or a vaginal birth after cesarean, for siblings, for grandparents, and for others.[38]

Some educational efforts have focused in detail on particular topics. For example, the benefits of adequate levels of folic acid in decreasing the risk of neural tube defects were promoted by a mass media campaign particularly targeted at low socioeconomic status women in the Netherlands. Although low-income women benefited from the campaign, those of higher income benefited more.[10] Special programs have been established to educate women who test positive for the hepatitis B virus during the prenatal period.[8]

Box 8-1	*Outline for Prenatal Education—cont'd*

Second Trimester—cont'd

Client's expectations for pregnancy and birth

Client's fears and anxieties related to second trimester

Sibling concerns

Client expectations for pregnancy and childbirth, confirmation of registration for third-trimester prenatal classes

Third Trimester

Feelings about pregnancy, developmental tasks of third trimester

Preparation for labor, delivery, and parenting (Content may be given by health care providers during prenatal visits or can be offered in greater depth during a series of prepared childbirth classes.)

Client expectations for labor and birth, progress of prepared childbirth classes

Family reactions to advanced pregnancy; third-trimester emotional responses of expectant fathers; sibling preparation

Late-pregnancy physical changes, management of discomforts related to late pregnancy

Sexuality during the third trimester

Lifestyle factors with potential impact on late pregnancy: drugs such as alcohol, nutrition (including prescribed vitamin and iron supplements), smoking, general health, exercise, body mechanics, rest, occupational and environmental considerations

Signs of labor, "true" labor versus "false" labor, physiology of labor and delivery, passenger, passage, powers, and psyche in labor

Positioning in labor

Techniques useful during labor and delivery (e.g., psychoprophylactic method, Bradley method)

Analgesia and anesthesia during labor and delivery, medications used during labor and delivery

Technology and childbirth, assessment of fetal maturity, potential for induction or augmentation of labor, potential use of electronic fetal monitoring, intravenous infusions, and so on

Variations in labor

The high-risk experience: potential for operative obstetrics (e.g., forceps, episiotomy, cesarean childbirth); potential for transfer from birthing center, home, or birthing room because of obstetric complications; potential for family-centered birth despite operative obstetrics

Warning signs of late pregnancy, signs and symptoms of premature labor

Review of birth plan, anticipatory guidance regarding what can be expected within the selected labor and delivery setting

Discussion of fears and concerns related to late pregnancy, labor and delivery, or postpartum

Tour of labor and delivery setting

Preparations for client's stay in hospital or birth center, preparations for a home birth

Preparations for other family members during client's birthing experience and immediate recovery (e.g., child care for siblings)

Preparations for the newborn, selection of a pediatric caregiver (may include a prenatal introductory meeting)

Infant nutrition, preparation for breastfeeding or bottle feeding

Early parenting

What to expect from caregivers and the health care system during labor, delivery, and postpartum

Anticipatory guidance for postpartum (includes physical and emotional changes, family changes, and strategies for coping)

Resources available during third trimester and postpartum

The Resource Mothers program for women with maternal phenylketonuria (PKU) aims to increase positive outcomes for their babies by improving metabolic control. The majority of young women with PKU discontinue the restrictive diet during middle childhood and have difficulty resuming it, sometimes complicated by limited intellectual abilities and low socioeconomic status. In one population studied, more than 80% of pregnancies involved inadequate metabolic control. The Resource Mothers program includes 40 hours of instruction and home visitation to develop skills in cooking, shopping, meal planning, and preparation for the baby. The mean number of weeks it took to reach metabolic control was shorter in the studied intervention group than in the control group, and their babies were better developed.[35]

Infant communication education, focusing on infant behaviors, states, and communication cues, has also been presented prenatally to first-time mothers, taught in part by videotape. This randomized controlled trial found significant differences in early mother-infant interaction, which is known to facilitate bonding and infant development.[24]

There is some evidence that women have transient deficits in cognitive function postpartum, particularly in memory function and attention. This finding has major implications for informed consent, discharge planning, and instructions for subsequent care of the newborn infant. There is strong support for the conclusion that this is not a side effect of intrapartum narcotic medication but rather is caused by the stress of labor and delivery. In one study the women's scores on cognitive tests had returned to normal by the second postpartum day, although other studies have found them to be altered for a longer duration.[12] Equally interesting is the finding that maternal self-efficacy in coping with labor, which can be a goal of pregnancy education programs, significantly contributes to a lessened perception of pain during labor. Recall from Chapter 2 that development of self-efficacy may occur through previous experience with significant pain, watching others perform successfully, verbal persuasion, and knowledge that develops during childbirth-preparation classes.[26]

Several excellent meta-analyses of studies of prenatal education have been completed, although two were published long enough ago to need updating. Jones'[22] summary of 27 studies completed through the early 1980s found a moderate effect size as a result of childbirth education: parents were more attentive and responsive to their infants, were more satisfied with the behavior of the infants, and spent more time playing with and cuddling their infants. Few negative effects were found. Larger effect sizes were obtained for middle-income parents (0.40)

compared with parents of low income (0.16). A research summary of adolescent pregnancy education programs found average effect sizes of 0.35.[25] It is important to remember that potential adverse effects of prenatal education include fear created by the classes, pressure to conform, and anger or guilt when expectations raised by the classes are not met.[13]

An analysis of 11 randomized trials of prenatal smoking cessation interventions found a 50% increase in smoking cessation.[31] Although there was a high rate of return to smoking among women who were abstinent during pregnancy, approximately one third stopped smoking permanently. Interventions that were more intensive, with multiple contacts, multiple formats, and some form of follow-up, were more effective. The outcomes these programs can effect are important because maternal smoking causes an estimated 20% to 30% of the low birth weight rate and 10% of infant mortality in the United States.

Finally, a meta-analysis of 13 studies of parenting interventions based on the Neonatal Behavior Assessment (NBA) Scale showed an effect size of 0.4—a small to moderate beneficial effect—on quality of later parenting. The NBA assesses an infant's alertness to auditory and visual stimuli, ability to tune out distraction, responses to stress, soothability, motor functioning, and reflexive behaviors.[17] It is administered by a trained examiner in the parent's presence or the parents are trained to administer the instrument to their infants. In either case, the effect should be to educate the parent about the infant's capabilities.[9] Studies using the NBA as a teaching tool have also shown strong results with groups such as depressed mothers.[17]

A special area of concern currently is patient education to aid in the early detection and treatment of preterm labor, which is part of a larger program of management. Of all preterm births, about 80% are the direct result of preterm labor, defined as the presence of uterine contractions with progressive cervical dilation or effacement, or both, occurring before 37 weeks' gestation. Programs for prevention have had inconsistent results in decreasing overall preterm birth rates, in part because risk-scoring systems still fall short of identifying most patients who experience the problem. Goldenberg and Rouse[15] conclude that most medical interventions designed to prevent preterm birth, including patient education, do not work. Despite this view, professional opinion still supports teaching patients to monitor for and promptly report symptoms of preterm labor (uterine contractions every 10 minutes or less, menstrual-like cramps, low dull backache, pelvic pressure, changes in vaginal discharge, urinary frequency, or intestinal cramping).[28] Women have found the symptoms ambiguous in that they were subtle, lacked a pattern, and unpredictably waxed and waned and thus were confused with the expected discomforts of pregnancy.

A developmentally oriented framework to understand what parents need to know flows from what is known about sensitive caregiving being critical in the development of a secure attachment relationship. Knowing the behav-ioral characteristics, strengths, and preferences of one's baby provides this foundation as does understanding infant state and its modulation and infant behaviors and cues. Infant state refers to the six levels of consciousness associated with coherent patterns of behavior. The full alert state is perfect for feeding, teaching, playing, and interacting. Over time infants maintain this state for longer periods. Parents may benefit from a review of a range of interventions to arouse and soothe their infant as they learn what works best for their child. The pleasure and feeling of efficacy that comes from synchronous interaction with their infant is highly reinforcing to parents.[16]

After birth some parents of gravely ill infants face difficult decisions about withdrawal of the neonate's life supports and limiting resuscitation efforts in the neonatal intensive care unit (NICU). Education is almost always necessary to help them cope and be full participants. Box 8-2 presents questions for physician and parents; these

---

| **Box 8-2** | *Questions for the Physician and Parents in the Neonatal Intensive Care Unit Setting* |

1. How do you understand Billy's medical problems?
2. Has anything like this ever happened to you before?
3. What do you feel may have contributed to Billy's illness?
4. Is there anything that we are doing or not doing to Billy that is worrying you?
5. Do both of you see Billy's medical problems and the decision that we are facing in the same way? Do either of you see anything differently?
6a. Have you been able even to consider that Billy, being this ill, is in danger of not getting better or actually dying?
6b. Just as we fear not being able to save every child, we also fear going too far, even worsening their suffering, when our efforts are futile. Do you think that this could happen to Billy?
6c. If I am sure that certain treatments will cause suffering for Billy without really helping him then I won't be able to do those things. We always tell parents when we think this time is approaching. [Initially] For Billy things have not reached this point and we hope they do not. [Later] For Billy we could be there in a matter of hours. (A brief period of silence will allow parents to respond.)
7. Do you feel I'm helping or guiding you too much or too little?
8. How do your religious or cultural values influence this decision?
9. What was your main reason for deciding the way you did?
10. How do you feel about holding the baby when the machines are removed?

From Jellinek M and others: Facing tragic decisions with parents in the neonatal intensive care unit: clinical perspectives, *Pediatrics* 89:119-122, 1992.

Box 8-3   *Positioning and Handling Techniques*

Positioning

- Horseshoe rolls (blankets made into a roll, shaped as a horseshoe, and placed around infant as boundaries)
- Head roll (blanket roll placed at top of bed so that, if infant pushes with legs, there is a boundary)
- Swaddling (with either blanket or T shirt if infant is small)
- Sheepskin
- Hands to face

Handling

- Try to wake infant slowly (with soft touch or voice) before performing care.
- When performing caregiving activities, make sure infant remains in flexed position.
- Offer infant finger for grasping.
- Offer infant pacifier for nonnutritive sucking.
- If infant demonstrates various disengagement cues, give infant a break from the activity.

From Krebs TL: Clinical pathway for enhanced parent and preterm infant interaction through parent education, *J Perinat Neonatal Nurs* 12(2):38-49, 1998.

---

same questions and their answers are also highly relevant for caregiving by other staff members. They are meant to assess parent understanding, as well as guilt they may be feeling, their worries about painful procedures, and ways to deal with the ambiguity that is frequently a part of these situations.[19]

Likewise, the transition from NICU to home is stressful for parents and requires concentrated instruction for them to become competent and confident in the care of the infant. Prematurity may have been the reason for NICU treatment; premature infants are often less responsive and more difficult to care for than are healthy full-term infants. Because of the immaturity of the central nervous system, these infants' behavior is more disorganized and unpredictable. They show less effective care-eliciting behavior and may not cry to signal the need for care, causing asynchrony in the parent-infant dyad; feeding is often characterized by slow food intake and excessive body movements or frequent spitting up; and they are more likely to have residual medical problems that require treatment at home.

Parents need to be taught basic caregiving, regulation of temperature, growth and development, and infant stimulation, and they must learn to recognize the signs and symptoms of illness, including abnormal breathing patterns.

Box 8-4   *Infant Cues*

Disengagement Cues	**Engagement Cues**
• Hiccoughs	• Hands to midline
• Apnea	• Sucking
• Bradycardia	• Lip pucker
• Color changes	• Gazing
• Finger splaying	• Flexion
• Arching	• Smiling
• Extensions	• Grasping
• Grimacing	

From Krebs TL: Clinical pathway for enhanced parent and preterm infant interaction through parent education, *J Perinat Neonatal Nurs* 12(2):38-49, 1998.

Despite agreement on discharge preparation needs, there is little evidence to indicate whether parents are currently being well prepared for their infant's discharge. Boxes 8-3, 8-4, and 8-5 describe specific skills for positioning and handling, environmental enhancements, and reading of infant cues that these parents need to learn.[23] Interventions to facilitate parent-infant interactions include guiding parents to maximize periods of infant attentiveness and educating parents in specific interacting behaviors. Developmental delays are more likely in interaction mismatch—for example, when the parent contin-

Box 8-5	*Environmental Enhancements*

Dim lights during day, provide dark environment at night

Use isolette cover to help modify lighting

Institute quiet time around bedside when infant is sleeping

Introduce music or parent tapes when infant is developmentally ready (~ 33 to 35 weeks)

Place pictures of family at bedside for infant to look at when developmentally ready (~ 33 to 35 weeks)

Cluster caregiving times

From Krebs TL: Clinical pathway for enhanced parent and preterm infant interaction through parent education, *J Perinat Neonatal Nurs* 12(2):38-49, 1998.

ues to play despite the infant's overt behavioral signs of overstimulation. Outcome goals are for parents to (1) recognize their infants' engagement and disengagement cues, (2) respond appropriately to their infants' cues, and (3) perform caregiving activities according to their infants' cues.[23] Support groups for parents of preterm infants can help to normalize parental experiences and provide much needed information and family support.

Table 8-1 provides a list of topics thought to be important to learn, the staff and parents' perception of importance (on a scale of 1 as very unimportant to 5 as very important), and whether the topic was discussed.[37] Note the significant discrepancies between parents and staff members on some items. Parents who receive inadequate discharge preparation may not feel competent or confident of their ability to care for their newborn. If you were working in this NICU, what would you do with the results of this survey?

Policies of most NICUs include teaching caretakers cardiopulmonary resuscitation (CPR) before discharge of the infant. These caretakers report decreased anxiety and increased feelings of control without an increased sense of responsibility and burden. It is important to remember that research has shown that within 6 months only one third of those educated at hospital discharge were able to perform CPR satisfactorily.[11,29] Thus reassessment and reinstruction periodically are important. Box 8-6 provides a description of emergency skills education for parents, of which CPR instruction is a part.[30] In addition to the class content outline, it would have been extremely useful to see outcome objectives and measures to determine how well they were being met. Construct objectives you think would be required.

Traditional pediatric care is based on the assumption that parents have the basic knowledge and resources to provide a nurturing, safe environment. Free home visitation is a widespread early intervention strategy in most industrialized nations other than the United States. In England every prospective mother is visited at home at least once before birth with six more visits before the child is 5 years of age. Special attention is focused on those in greater need of service, including mothers of low-birth-weight and premature children with chronic illness and disabilities, low-income unmarried teenage mothers, families with a history of substance abuse, and parents with a low intelligence quotient. The purpose of the visits is active promotion of positive health and infant caregiving and a decrease in family stress.[2] Parenting education programs for low-income parents of young children produce a significant decrease in verbal and corporal punishment and a significant increase in nurturing behaviors, with children's behavior improving significantly. The abusive parent has been characterized as having low tolerance for frustration, impaired parenting skills, a sense of incompetence in parenting, unrealistic expectations of children, inappropriate expression of anger and social isolation.[14]

It has been shown that child abuse is more prevalent among parents of children with a subtle handicap, and preterm infants are highly represented in this group of abused children. Although abuse has many causes, a teaching approach to help parents recognize their preterm infant's behavioral cues and to develop confi-

TABLE 8-1	Results of Staff Discharge Teaching Survey and Comparable Items from the Parent Retrospective Transition Interview			
		Importance		**Was Topic Discussed?**
Questionnaire Item		**Staff**	**Parents**	**Staff (%)**	**Parents* (%)**
Feeding					
1. How much and how often to feed baby		4.9	4.7	100	96
2. What to do if baby isn't eating enough		4.9	4.3	94	24
3. Help if I wanted to breastfeed		4.8	3.4	97	56
4. What to do if baby sleeps through feedings		4.4	4.1	91	64
Bathing					
5. How to bathe and how often		4.3	4.4	97	93
6. How to keep baby's hair clean		4.1	4.1	100	73
Sleeping					
7. How long baby should sleep at one time		3.8	3.7	68	20
8. How often baby should nap		3.5	3.6	56	14
9. How to tell if baby is sleepy		3.1	3.3	44	14
10. What to do when baby won't sleep		3.9	4.0	67	22
Crying					
11. How much baby might cry		3.5	3.8	47	13
12. What to do when baby cries		4.2	4.4	88	38
13. What to do if baby cries too much or not enough		3.9	4.0	67	9
Playing					
14. How to encourage baby to interact with mom		4.3	4.2	88	38
15. How to tell when baby is ready to play		3.4	3.8	44	9
16. Tricks to keep baby involved in play		3.2	3.6	32	2
17. How to make or find interesting things to put in baby's crib		3.7	4.0	74	47
Baby's Unique Characteristics					
18. Baby's personality/temperament		4.0	4.2	85	53
19. How baby lets his/her needs be known		4.2	4.3	94	59
20. Baby's response to handling		4.1	4.4	82	47
Monitoring Baby's Health					
21. How to recognize differences between normal breathing patterns and those that indicate illness		4.8	4.4	91	38
22. How to recognize the difference between spitting up and vomiting		4.4	4.4	77	38
23. How to recognize the difference between regular stools, diarrhea, and constipation		4.6	4.6	82	58
24. How to get in touch with the NICU staff		4.6	4.8	100	100

From Sheikh L, O'Brian M, McCheskey-Fawcett K: Parent preparation for the NICU-to-home transition: staff and parent perceptions, *Children's Health Care* 22:227-239, 1993.
*Parent data represent percentage of those who responded to the question; when a topic was not relevant for a particular mother and infant, it was recorded as not applicable.

TABLE 8-1	Results of Staff Discharge Teaching Survey and Comparable Items from the Parent Retrospective Transition Interview—cont'd			
	Importance		**Was Topic Discussed?**	
Questionnaire Item	**Staff**	**Parents**	**Staff (%)**	**Parents* (%)**
Taking Care of Baby's Health				
25. How to give medications	5.0	4.8	100	100
26. How to take baby's temperature	4.9	4.6	100	98
27. How to use a bulb syringe	4.9	4.4	100	84
28. What to do if someone living at home gets sick	3.9	4.3	42	27
29. How to give CPR	4.9	4.8	100	64
Medical Care				
30. How soon to schedule a visit with baby's primary care physician	4.8	4.8	100	93
31. How baby's medical records are transferred	3.3	4.1	38	27
32. How to get help in an emergency	4.9	4.7	94	64
33. How to pay for the hospital stay	3.8	4.1	71	42
Learning More about Prematurity				
34. How to get in touch with other parents of preemies	3.4	3.6	47	5
35. Books or pamphlets about prematurity	4.1	4.5	97	46
36. Where to get preemie diapers and clothing	3.6	3.9	82	47
37. Awareness of normal and delayed growth and development	4.2	4.5	67	38
38. Suggestions on ways to encourage baby's growth and development	4.1	4.4	68	22
39. When to schedule baby for developmental follow-up	4.2	4.6	85	73
With Family and Friends				
40. Who should hold and handle baby	3.4	3.5	68	33
41. How relatives and friends might react to the baby	3.3	3.3	32	7
42. Whether it is okay to leave the baby with another caretaker	3.6	3.6	53	38
43. How much clothing baby needs indoors and outdoors	4.1	4.1	82	47

Box 8-6	*Emergency Skills Education Parent Class Content Outline*

Introduction: Purpose and organization of the class

Emergency Medical Services System: Access and use
  a. "911"
  b. Other

Causes and prevention of injury

ABC's of lifesaving

Management of foreign body airway obstruction
  Conscious victim
  a. Lecture: Assessment of airway obstruction in the conscious victim and actions to relieve the obstruction
  b. Demonstration of skills needed to relieve the obstructed airway
  c. Mannequin practice and skills demonstration by participants
  Unconscious victim
  a. Lecture: Assessment of airway obstruction in the unconscious victim and actions to relieve the obstruction

  b. Demonstration of skills needed to relieve the obstructed airway
  c. Mannequin practice and skills demonstration by participants

Rescue breathing
  a. Lecture: Assessment of the need for rescue breathing
  b. Demonstration of rescue breathing techniques

Cardiopulmonary resuscitation
  a. Lecture: Assessment of pulselessness to determine the need for CPR and determination of the effectiveness of CPR when given
  b. Demonstration of CPR skills
  c. Mannequin practice and skills demonstration by participants

Closing
  a. Questions and answers
  b. Refer participant to CPR courses in their communities for further information and reinforcement of skills

From Moynihan P, Naclerio L, Kiley K: Parent participation, *Nurs Clin North Am* 30:231-241, 1995.

dence in the infant's competence is a way of building self-efficacy.

In a study of interventions provided by clinical nurse specialists who followed very low-birth-weight infants from hospital to home, 68% were teaching interventions.[5] Before discharge, parents were required to demonstrate satisfactorily the basic caretaking skills (such as bathing, handling, feeding, soothing, taking the infant's temperature, providing skin care, and preventing infection) and a basic knowledge of any medications or special procedures required in the infant's care. It was important to teach adaptations of basic care because of prematurity of the infant, including use of "preemie" nipples, problems of reflux, and frequent feeding problems caused by diminished or weaker sucking and reduced gastric capacity. The need to maintain warmth because of less advanced neurological development, less adipose tissue, and thinner, more fragile skin was taught. Infant stimulation and how to gauge developmental milestones were also addressed.

Management of chronic illness in children requires a special approach to education frequently difficult to deliver in acute care settings. For example, McCrindle and others[27] provide data on an old problem that could be solved with appropriate education. Most children with heart murmurs are found to have no significant heart disease; yet many parents believe a heart murmur to be an actual heart lesion. Restrictions and emotional distress may therefore be imposed on the child despite the absence of significant heart disease. The data in this study show that 1 month after assessment, 10% of parents continued to believe that their child had a heart problem, although none could describe or specify a lesion.

Advances in the treatment of childhood diseases have created a population of technology-dependent and medically fragile children whose life expectancy is unknown and whose future quality of life is unpredictable. The family, of course, has to cope with the uncertainty. As much as the family may understand what can be known about their child's condition, certain triggers heighten awareness of the uncertainty concerning the child's survival. Triggers are routine medical appointments; body variability, inasmuch as the initial presenting symptoms frequently were not seen as harbingers of a serious illness; key words and provocative questions such as "remission"; changes in therapeutic regimen, including a therapeutic success; evidence of negative outcomes; new developmental demands; and nighttime. The responsibility for management of this chronic uncertainty has been largely left to the parents and their ingenuity, without much deliberate assistance from health care providers. Cohen[7] reports that parents who are trying to attain some degree of family normality by consciously controlling the awareness of the seriousness of their child's illness are thwarted by health professionals who mistakenly assess their behavior as denial.

Although there will always be triggers, attending to them has the potential to reduce some of the stressful events experienced by these families. For example, when a child is seen for a routine medical appointment, there should be no time lag between the physical examination and the explanation of the findings to the parents. Anticipatory guidance that will enable parents to recognize normal or common behavioral and physiological alterations has the potential to reduce uncertainty for parents who may lack plausible alternative explanations for the variation in their child's usual behavior or who may be unsure of how to change their own behavior in relation to the child's changing needs. The simple act of teaching parents to use a stethoscope to recognize abnormal breath sounds has been shown to be a significant factor in reducing uncertainty about the status of a child who has cystic fibrosis.[7] It gives the parents immediate feedback and some sense of control to be able to distinguish an actual problem from a false alarm.

National Standards and Tested Programs

Both childbirth educators and lactation consultants can be certified through international associations.

EDUCATING CHILDREN

General Approach

Theory and research about how children learn are presented in Chapter 2. In addition, several earlier chapters include examples of education for health problems, such as asthma, that commonly affect children. Some earlier sections of this chapter that focus on education for parenting also include an educational component for children. This section provides examples of how patient education services primarily focused on children are being offered in communities and health care institutions.

A distinct philosophy guides educational programs for children. It is articulated in a statement by the American Academy of Pediatrics on child life programs.[1] The statement notes that these programs have become the standard in pediatric settings to address the psychosocial concerns that accompany hospitalization and medical care. Child life specialists facilitate coping and adjustment of children and families by providing play experiences, presenting information about events and procedures, and establishing supportive relationships to encourage family involvement in each child's care. These activities are shared by members of the health care team and the child life specialist.

Play is a central part of child life programs because it sustains normal development and because play episodes allow children to process their concerns and cope with health treatments. Clinical data support the value of play in reducing the emotional disturbance of children in hospitals and clinics. Preparation programs that introduce children and their families to the circumstances and procedures they will encounter also reduce emotional disturbance. Family resource centers that make educational materials available can assist in the goal of helping to reduce parental anxiety, which can be transmitted to children.[1]

Educational Approaches and Research Base

Although not all education of children takes place as part of a formal child life program, there is general acceptance of the need to design education according to the developmental levels of recipients and with the essential involvement of families.

Of the four summaries of research on patient education for children shown in Appendix C, none is recent. Those that use techniques of meta-analysis generally provide a more reliable summary of the research available a few years before the time they are published. Broome, Lillis, and Smith[4] found that pain-management programs for children resulted in at least a 30% reduction in their distress responses.

Because an understanding of internal anatomy is useful to much health teaching, it is helpful to have available a summary of research about children's knowledge of internal body parts. Preschool-aged children, who may be in the preoperational stage of cognitive development, have only a vague idea that something is going on inside their bodies. Internal body image is not a significant part of children's body image until age 5 to 6 years. They seem to make the most dramatic gains in this knowledge at about age 8 years, corresponding to expected entry into the concrete operational stage of cognitive development. From that age forward, children usually have rudimentary information about the brain, heart, bones, and stomach but only minimal knowledge of the nervous system, parts of the gastrointestinal system besides the stomach, the circulatory system, or the immune system.[21]

Little information is available about possible cross-cultural differences in children's knowledge of internal anatomy or about the mediating effects of altered health status. It is believed that it is not until close to the midteenage years that individuals achieve the conceptual-integrative capacity to simultaneously relate the multiple factors involved in understanding diabetes and its control.[21]

Much education for children in medical settings focuses on helping them through procedures; misunderstandings, fears, and fantasies often manifest as overt upset behavior during procedures. Figure 8-1 shows portions of a coloring book about intravenous (IV) therapy for children between the ages of 3 and 11 years. It is expected that after the teaching session, children will be able (1) to explain at least one reason why IV therapy is used, (2) to verbalize two sensations they will see, feel, or smell during IV insertion, (3) to demonstrate their role during the IV insertion, and (4) to describe what they will feel when the IV line is removed.[39]

Because children at the preoperational stage are egocentric, the first frame of Figure 8-1 is blank for them to draw a self-portrait. The booklet is designed to be used in conjunction with an IV pump, dolls, syringes, a tourniquet, and alcohol swabs for medical play. This play involves examination of equipment, performing procedures on dolls or puppets, and games or stories. Teaching sessions should take place before the procedure so that children will have time to assimilate the information and feel adequately in control and again after insertion of the IV line, to allow them to talk about the procedure and ventilate their feelings about the experience. It is best to prepare preschoolers shortly before the planned procedure because they become overly anxious if they are told too far in advance. Evaluation of the intervention usually is based on how the child behaved and felt during the procedure.[39]

In 1980 only 16% of pediatric hospitals taught coping techniques for procedures; now nearly half do.[33] Dolls the size of a 3- to 4-year-old child, in both sexes and with different skin tones and facial features, are available for preprocedure teaching of cutdown and shunt procedures, urethral catheter insertion, intramuscular injection, IV line insertion, and drain and traction sites. The doll can break bones; the chest can be opened to visualize the contents, and there is a hernia in the groin of the male doll. Because fantasies and misconceptions are quite possible, the dolls should be used with supervision and with the explanation that this is a doll.[32]

Consider children with myelomeningoceles, who must learn self-catheterization because of a neurogenic bladder. The goal is to promote continence and prevent renal deterioration and to significantly decrease the incidence of bacteriuria. Girls have to be able to perform the

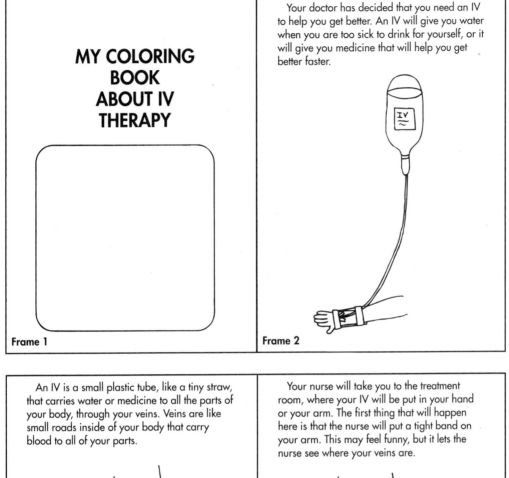

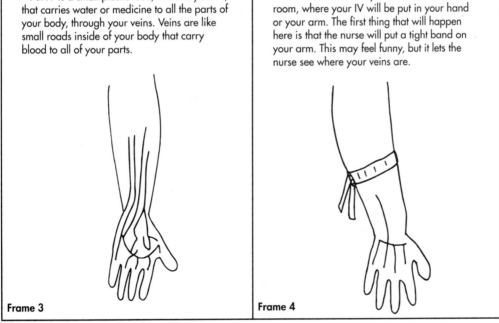

Figure 8-1   Sample educational tool designed for use with children scheduled to undergo intravenous therapy. (Thompson V: An IV therapy teaching tool for children, *Pediatr Nurs* 20:351-355, 1994.)

Continued

After we have decided where your IV will go, the nurse will clean off that spot with some alcohol. Alcohol kills germs. The alcohol may feel cold and smell funny, but it will not hurt.

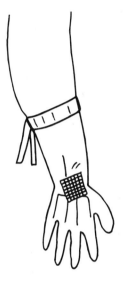

Frame 5

After the vein is picked, and the spot cleaned off, the hard part comes. A needle will be put under your skin and into your vein. This part hurts, but it is a short hurt. Some boys and girls have said that it feels like a hard pinch, or like a bee sting. The nurse will tell you before putting the needle in. It is OK to cry, or squeeze the nurse's hand when it hurts, but it is very important that you hold very still during this part.

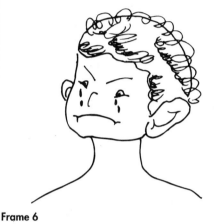

Frame 6

After the IV is in place in your vein, the needle is taken out, and the small plastic tube will stay in your vein. The hurting part is over now. The IV will be taped in place, and you will have a small, soft board taped to your hand or arm. This will help the IV to stay in place while it is needed.

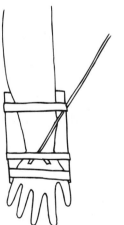

Frame 7

Some patients need to get water or medicine all of the time. The bottle of medicine will hang on a pole that looks like this. You can roll this pole with you wherever you go. You can go to the bathroom, or to the playroom, when you are feeling better. The machine on the pole may beep sometimes. Ask your nurse what it sounds like. Some children think that it sounds like a Nintendo game. When it beeps it means that the nurse needs to look at your IV or that you need a new bottle of medicine.

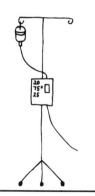

Frame 8

Figure 8-1, cont'd   For legend see p. 183

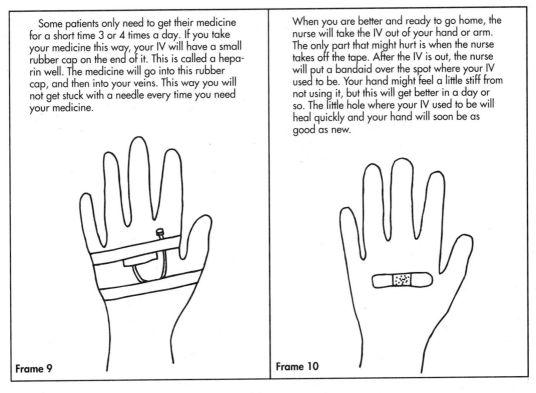

Some patients only need to get their medicine for a short time 3 or 4 times a day. If you take your medicine this way, your IV will have a small rubber cap on the end of it. This is called a heparin well. The medicine will go into this rubber cap, and then into your veins. This way you will not get stuck with a needle every time you need your medicine.

When you are better and ready to go home, the nurse will take the IV out of your hand or arm. The only part that might hurt is when the nurse takes off the tape. After the IV is out, the nurse will put a bandaid over the spot where your IV used to be. Your hand might feel a little stiff from not using it, but this will get better in a day or so. The little hole where your IV used to be will heal quickly and your hand will soon be as good as new.

Frame 9

Frame 10

Figure 8-1, cont'd   For legend see p. 183

psychomotor skills of washing hands, gathering equipment, removing garments, washing the perineum, lubricating the catheter, spreading the labia and inserting the catheter, draining the bladder, removing the catheter, and washing the catheter and hands. Teaching involves an anatomically correct doll placed in the child's lap face forward, guiding the child to become proficient in use of the catheter with the doll and then with herself. Appropriate reinforcement is important.[36]

Or consider preparing 4- to 8-year-old children for a magnetic resonance imaging (MRI) procedure with its narrow bore tube and noise for a period of time. Because sedation and anesthesia can be as frightening as the procedure, an alternate play therapy preparation was developed. Teaching involved explaining the procedure in age-appropriate terms. Photos of children or a teddy bear undergoing MRI emphasize what the examination entails and what the child is required to do. A small model of a magnetic resonance imaging unit including sliding table top and light and a tape recording of the noise allows children to act out the examination and play with plastic figures representing themselves, the radiographers, and nurses. A color-in storybook of a visit to the MRI unit through the eyes of a child is used. Although apparently no control group was studied, the authors believe there has been a dramatic decrease in the number of failed MRI examinations.[34]

Some children with chronic illnesses may have no adult supervision on return home from school, and community-based programs on self-care for these children are fairly numerous. Parents report that many after-school day-care programs will not take a child with a chronic illness.

Box 8-7   *Assessment of the Child's Readiness for Self-Care*

1. What is the child's cognitive developmental level? Is the child capable of solving problems in a rational manner? Can this child read well enough to follow written instructions and write well enough to take messages?
2. Is the child able to follow instructions related to aspects of self-care and to record behavior and signs?
3. Is the child socially mature? Can the child demonstrate the ability to judge right from wrong? Can he or she resist peer pressure? Does the child show respect for the rights of others?
4. Is the child overly shy or fearful? Can the child tolerate separations without excessive fear or upset?
5. Does the child have self-discipline?
6. Can the child entertain himself or herself?
7. Does the child take responsibility for home chores?
8. Does the child know basic first aid?
9. Does the child know what to do in case of an emergency (e.g., fire, police)?
10. How well does the child understand his or her illness?
11. Does the child have the knowledge and manual dexterity to safely carry out treatments?
12. Can the child manage during a medical emergency?
13. Can the child distinguish between a real medical emergency and a more trivial problem?
14. Can the child handle unusual and unexpected situations without excessive fear and upset?

From Holaday B and others: Chronically ill children in self-care: issues for pediatric nurses, *Pediatr Health Care* 7:256-263, 1993.

Self-care education programs are important and, if the children are ready for them, have potentially positive effects, such as developing maturity, self-reliance, decision-making ability, and responsibility.[18] Negative consequences of children's self-care are obvious, and parents worry about emergencies and security. Because cognitive, social, and emotional development rates differ with each child, it is best not to identify an exact age at which children with a chronic illness can begin self-care. Instead the provider and parents need to jointly assess the child's maturity levels, knowledge of the illness, and ability to perform medical treatments. Boxes 8-7 and 8-8 provide assessment tools for this purpose and guidelines for a self-care training program.

The child's motivation is perhaps the most important predictor of success in self-care programs. Children need not only to be comfortable with their ability to perform treatments and to manage their illness but also to know how to follow important rules without testing the limits and how to get help.[18] Physically, children should be able to safely manipulate medical equipment, avoid injury, manage locks, and operate relevant appliances and equipment. They

also need the ability to tolerate separation from adults without loneliness, fear, or self-destructive behavior.

The training program described in Box 8-9 should run over a 4- to 5-week period to give children the time to develop required skills. Children learn best from active participation, including skill rehearsal and role-playing, rather than from passive observation of adults modeling behaviors. Booster (review) sessions are needed periodically. Providers can also explore other training opportunities in their communities, including whether health information is available over latchkey telephone hotlines.[18]

National Standards and Tested Programs

Certification of child life specialists is available through the Child Life Certifying Commission.

SUMMARY

Pregnancy, parenting, and child development offer many opportunities for teaching that will make a real difference in people's lives, yet little evidence is found to indicate whether these op-

Box 8-8 — Self-Assessment for Parents of Children in Self-Care

1. How many days per week and hours per day will the child be in self-care?
2. Will the child be able to maintain friendships with other children?
3. Are your health care providers (e.g., physician, nurse) aware of the fact that your child is in self-care?
4. Have you developed clear in-home rules that the child is to follow?
5. Is an older sibling going to care for the ill child? How does the sibling feel about this? Is the sibling prepared to care for the ill child?
6. How do you plan to monitor the child's safety, activities, and status when the child is home alone?
7. Do you have a neighbor who is willing to periodically check on things?
8. Do you have a designated neighbor to help in case of an emergency?
9. Have you purchased any types of special entertainment devices (e.g., VCR, computer, radio) to keep the child entertained while at home alone?
10. Will the child have to prepare a snack or meal? Can the child do this safely?
11. What types of safety devices (e.g., first aid kit, smoke and burglar alarms) have been purchased to protect the child?
12. Have you specified what activities the child is allowed to take part in while home alone?
13. Is the child motivated for self-care?
14. Have you taught your child the self-care skills needed to manage the illness when at home alone? Do you believe your child can correctly and safely perform these activities?
15. Does the child have the necessary support from parents, siblings, or neighbors to carry out a self-care regimen?
16. Have you taught your child what to do in case of an emergency? A medical emergency? Does the child know the role of police, fire fighters, paramedics, and 911?
17. Can the child safely operate household appliances (e.g., stove, microwave, fans, heater)?
18. Does you child know basic first aid?

From Holaday B and others: Chronically ill children in self-care: issues for pediatric nurses, *Pediatr Health Care* 7:256-263, 1993.

Box 8-9 — Guidelines for a Self-Care Training Program

I. Management of chronic illness
  1. Knowledge of disease and its management
    a. Symptom discrimination
    b. Effects and side effects of medications
    c. Treatments
  2. Self-care skills related to disease
    a. Self-monitoring and self-recording of data by child about condition
    b. Processing and evaluating of information the child gathers about himself
    c. Decision making with respect to child's selecting the most appropriate action from among potential solutions
    d. Self-instruction on the use of self-statements by child to prompt, direct, or maintain performance
    e. Panic control

II. Safety
  1. Safety rules and prevention of injury
  2. How to safely use household appliances
  3. Handling household emergencies ranging from power failure to personal injury
  4. First aid for home accidents
  5. Discriminating between safe and unsafe play activities
  6. How to use 911
  7. Traveling safely to and from school
  8. Taking care of the key
  9. Protection from abduction and molestation

III. Self-care/child care
  1. Safe and nutritious snack preparation
  2. Telephone skills
  3. Child care techniques
  4. Family rules
  5. Activities for after school
  6. Time management
  7. Ways to cope with fear

From Holaday B and others: Chronically ill children in self-care: issues for pediatric nurses, *Pediatr Health Care* 7:256-263, 1993.

portunities are exploited. Much work remains to be accomplished in the development of standards of practice and tested programs.

 Study Questions

1. Because children who have been critically ill may be at increased risk for a respiratory or cardiac event at home, it is important that the parents learn basic life-support skills. What learning conditions are essential so that the parents are competent and feel confident in providing this care for their child?

2. Federal law now requires that health care providers give to parents of children receiving immunizations standardized written information about many aspects of the vaccines and the diseases they may prevent. Thus parents are given vaccine information pamphlets (VIPs) that must contain the information necessary to meet statutory requirements, and frequently they are long. Concerns that these VIPs might frighten parents and deter them from having their children immunized have proved to be unfounded; however, some parents feel overwhelmed with information.[6] Are you surprised by the concerns of providers? What could be done to make the mandated information more accessible to parents with little formal education?

3. A summary of an article by Brent and others[3] on breastfeeding in a low-income population shows that it is the consensus of the international pediatric community that breastfeeding is the optimal form of infant nutrition. Because women from low-income groups have a much lower incidence of breastfeeding and the rates of infant mortality and morbidity among inner-city poor children are high, the authors believe it is extremely important to reverse this trend. Women who planned to breastfeed were counseled about management; women who planned to bottle-feed were counseled on the benefits of breastfeeding to mother and infant. The program, which used a lactation consultant, was successful in increasing the incidence and duration of breastfeeding in an inner-city, low-income population. Are you surprised by the methods or the findings in this study?

4. A nurse describes her work with a premature baby and his mother. Identify the learning principles involved.

"One of our mothers was frightened and unsure about holding her baby. Stating that she didn't know how and was afraid that he would choke, the mother would try to feed her son, but then quickly hand him over to the nurse. As the developmental specialist, I sat down with the mother and refused to let her hand her son over. Instead, I encouraged her to watch his mouth, counting his breaths and watching his sucking and swallowing. I suddenly noticed that her baby had stopped sucking and was staring at her face, scanning the outer edges of her head in an arch. I whispered to her to look at her baby's face. When she saw the intense focus and clear interest in his face, she melted and was enthralled. As she smiled, her baby continued to look at her. I suggested that she remain still so that he could scan her face. From that moment on, her behavior changed. She began to watch him closely and then asked him if he was ready to eat. When she saw the clear, alert look, she knew he was ready. She even learned that if she shifted her face away, he could suck more easily and that if she brought it back during his breaks, he rested and relaxed while gazing at her. No longer was she afraid."

Learning Principles

From VandenBerg KA: What to tell parents about the developmental needs of their baby at discharge, *Neonatal Network* 18:57-59, 1999.

5. The Back to Sleep campaign has disseminated the message that infants should sleep in a supine position. Studies found decreases in the prone sleep positioning from 70% in 1992 to 24% in 1996 and in rates of sudden infant death syndrome (SIDS) from 1.2 to 0.74/1000 live births. A more recent telephone survey of African-American, Hispanic, Asian, and American Indian parents from inner cities in the northcentral United States found that although 80% of these parents had heard of sleep position recommendations, 40% still preferred prone positioning. Parents feared that choking would occur in the supine position and felt their infants slept better on their stomachs. The authors indicated that more efforts are needed to convince parents who disagree with and resist recommendations.[20] How would you do this?

References

1. American Academy of Pediatrics: Child life programs, *Pediatrics* 91:671-673, 1993.
2. American Academy of Pediatrics: The role of home-visitation programs in improving health outcomes in children and families, *Pediatrics* 101:486-489, 1998.
3. Brent NB and others: Breast-feeding in a low-income population, *Arch Pediatr Adolesc Med* 149:798-803, 1995.
4. Broome ME, Lillis PP, Smith MC: Pain interventions with children: a meta-analysis of research, *Nurs Res* 38:154-158, 1989.
5. Brooten D and others: Functions of the CNS in early discharge and home follow-up of very low birthweight infants, *Clin Nurse Spec* 5:196-201, 1991.
6. Clayton EW, Hickson GB, Miller CS: Parents' responses to vaccine information pamphlets, *Pediatrics* 93:369-372, 1994.
7. Cohen MH: The triggers of heightened parental uncertainty in chronic, life-threatening childhood illness, *Qual Health Res* 5:63-77, 1995.
8. Corrarino JE, Walsh PJ, Anselmo D: A program to educate women who test positive for the hepatitis B virus during the perinatal period, *Am J Matern Child Nurs* 24:151-155, 1999.
9. DasEilen R, Reifman A: Effects of Brazelton demonstrations on later parenting: a meta-analysis, *J Pediatr Psychol* 21:857-868, 1996.
10. DeWalle HEK and others: Effect of mass media campaign to reduce socioeconomic differences in women's awareness and behavior concerning use of folic acid: cross sectional study, *Br Med J* 319:291-292, 1999.
11. Dracup K, Doering LV, Moser DK, Evangelista L: Retention and use of cardiopulmonary resuscitation skills in parents of infants at risk for cardiopulmonary arrest, *Pediatr Nurs* 24:219-225, 1998.
12. Eidelman AI, Hoffmann NW, Kaitz M: Cognitive deficits in women after childbirth, *Obstet Gynecol* 81:764-767, 1993.
13. Enkin M, Keirse MJNC, Renfrew M, Neilson J: *A guide to effective care in pregnancy and childbirth*, New York, 1995, Oxford University Press.
14. Fennell DC, Fishel AH: Parent education: an evaluation of STEP on abusive parents' perceptions and abuse potential, *J Child Adolesc Psychiatr Nurs* 11:107-120, 1998.
15. Goldenberg RL, Rouse DJ: Prevention of premature birth, *N Engl J Med* 339:313-320, 1998.
16. Gottesman MM: Enabling parents to "read" their baby, *J Pediatr HealthCare* 13:148-151, 1999.
17. Hart S, Field T, Nearing G: Depressed mothers' neonates improve following the MABI and a Brazelton demonstration, *J Pediatr Psychol* 23:351-356, 1998.
18. Holaday B and others: Chronically ill children in self-care: issues for pediatric nurses, *J Pediatr Health Care* 7:256-263, 1993.
19. Jellinek M and others: Facing tragic decisions with parents in the neonatal intensive care unit: clinical perspectives, *Pediatrics* 89:119-122, 1992.
20. Johnson CM and others: Infant sleep position: a telephone survey of inner-city parents of color, *Pediatrics* 104:1208-1211, 1999.
21. Jones EG, Badger TA, Moore I: Children's knowledge of internal anatomy: conceptual orientation and review of research, *J Pediatr Nurs* 7:262-268, 1992.
22. Jones LC: A meta-analysis study of the effects of childbirth education on the parent-infant relationship, *Health Care Women Int* 7:357-370, 1986.
23. Krebs TL: Clinical pathway for enhanced parent and preterm infant interaction through parent education, *J Perinat Neonat Nurs* 12(2):38-49, 1998.
24. Leitch DB: Mother-infant interaction: achieving synchrony, *Nurs Res* 48:55-58, 1999.
25. Levy SR, Iverson BK, Walberg HJ: Adolescent pregnancy programs and educational interventions: a research synthesis and review, *J Soc Health* 3:99-103, 1983.
26. Lowe NK: Maternal confidence in coping with labor; a self-efficacy concept, *J Obstet Gynecol Neonatal Nurs* 20:457-463, 1991.

27. McCrindle BW and others: An evaluation of parental concerns and misperceptions about heart murmurs, *Clin Pediatr* 34:25-31, 1995.

28. Moore ML, Freda MC: Reducing preterm and low birth-weight births: Still a nursing challenge, *Matern-Child Nurs* 23:200-208, 1998.

29. Moser DK, Dracup K, Doering LV: Effect of cardiopulmonary resuscitation training for parents of high-risk neonates on perceived anxiety, control and burden, *Heart Lung* 28:326-333, 1999.

30. Moynihan P, Naclerio L, Kiley K: Parent participation, *Nurs Clin North Am* 30:231-241, 1995.

31. Mullen P, Ramirez G, Groff JY: A meta-analysis of randomized trials of prenatal smoking cessation interventions, *Am J Obstet Gynecol* 171:1328-1334, 1994.

32. O'Brien E: Use of the Zaadi Doll to provide health education to children and families, *J Pediatr Nurs* 10(4):266-267, 1995.

33. O'Bryne K, Peterson L, Saldana L: Survey of pediatric hospitals' preparation programs: evidence of the impact of health psychology research, *Health Psychol* 16:147-154, 1997.

34. Pressdee D, May L, Eastman E, Grier D: The use of play therapy in the preparation of children undergoing MR imaging, *Clin Radiology* 52:945-947, 1997.

35. St. James PS, Shapiro E, Waisbren SE: The resource mothers program for maternal phenylketonuria, *Am J Public Health* 89:762-764, 1999.

36. Segal ES, Deatrich JA, Hagelgans NA: The determinants of self-catheterization programs in children with myelomeningoceles, *J Pediatr Nurs* 10:82-88, 1995.

37. Sheikh L, O'Brien M, McCluskey-Fawcett K: Parent preparation for the NICU-to-home transition: staff and parent perceptions, *Children's Health Care* 22:227-239, 1993.

38. Sherwen LN, Scoloveno MA, Weingarten CT: *Nursing care of the childbearing family*, ed 2, Norwalk, CT, 1995, Appleton & Lange.

39. Thompson V: An IV therapy teaching tool for children, *Pediatr Nurs* 20:351-355, 1994.

Chapter 9

Patient Self-Management for the Rheumatic Diseases

GENERAL APPROACH

A firm theoretical base for patient education in rheumatic disease care has been developed during the past 15 years. Education in self-management has enabled patients to control their symptoms and to become partners in care with their health care providers.[1,2] A large variety of organized programs, planned according to educationally and psychologically valid principles and implemented consistently by trained personnel, have produced desirable changes in knowledge, behavior, and health outcome in patients with arthritis—over and above the medical treatment and incidental education to which they have been exposed. As a result, national and international dissemination of programs and standards for patient education in arthritis management is in progress.[3] Programs for other rheumatic diseases are following a similar model.

The model for arthritis education and the research base to support it were developed largely in the 1980s. Early advances in chronic disease education occurred in diseases with significant mortality and strong links between behaviors and disease outcomes. The preceding chapters on heart disease, asthma, and diabetes describe these developments. The toll of arthritis is found more in disability and discomfort than in death, and most forms of the rheumatic diseases are not preventable and are only partially responsive to treatment. There are 105 recognized rheumatic conditions, many of them rare. Osteoarthritis of the hands, weight-bearing joints, and the back affects 12% of the U.S. population between the ages of 25 and 74 years. The most common symptoms are musculoskeletal pain, loss of function, and consequent decreased ability to perform daily activities and work. The systemic inflammatory diseases affect about 3 million persons; examples include rheumatoid arthritis, systemic lupus erythematosus, and ankylosing spondylitis.[3]

Elements of care include medication for pain and inflammation; prescribed exercise for strength, endurance, and range of motion; rest; joint protection; modalities such as ice, heat, and splints; and joint surgery in selected patients. Outcome goals commonly considered important include improvement or maintenance of function, employability, and psychosocial status and control of pain, symptoms, and disease activity.[3] Patients must learn to constantly readjust their regimen according to changing disease activity. The education programs that most affect health status and behavior emphasize the development of a daily routine of self-management activity and give attention to coping with physical exercise, developing self-efficacy, and achieving success in problem solving.[11] The unpredictable course and varying disease activity may cause patients to view their disease as uncontrollable, which in turn may cause them to experience anxiety and depression, leading to increased perception of pain and decreased efforts to cope. The need to avoid this spiral makes it particularly important that these patients develop self-efficacy.[18]

EDUCATIONAL APPROACHES AND RESEARCH BASE

Behaviors thought to affect the health and psychological status of persons with arthritis include exercise, relaxation, joint protection, and adherence to medication regimens. Educational techniques already tested, with generally positive results, include interactive computer, telephone, and mail versus in-person classes. Almost no study has been undertaken on patient education by direct caregivers within the context of clinical care.

The Arthritis Self-Management Program (ASMP) is perhaps the best-known model program and one whose effectiveness has been well studied. It is taught 2 hours a week for 6 weeks and includes content on pathophysiology, medications, personal exercise and pain-management programs, nutrition, appropriate use of joints, and communication with physicians. Its iterative development since 1978 has been constantly improved through research and its strong theoretical base. Early studies found that individuals who felt they had control improved.[10] The medical interventions for arthritis have, for the most part, limited benefits. Because of the chronic nature of arthritis, persons with this disease must learn to manage and cope with it on a day-to-day basis. Their ability to succeed in this task commonly differentiates those who are incapacitated from those who continue to lead full and active lives in the face of equal disease severity.[11] Randomized trials have shown that ASMP increases self-efficacy, self-management behaviors, exercise, and use of cognitive pain management techniques to decrease pain, and decreases ambulatory visits to physicians. Longitudinal cohort studies have demonstrated that these effects con-

tinue without formal reinforcement for as long as 4 years. Recent study of a 3-week version of the ASMP has found that it is not as effective as the 6-week version.[13]

Behavioral learning theory, with its emphasis on self-efficacy, has served as a prime theoretical base for the ASMP. The leaders teaching the course are individuals with arthritis, and thus they serve as models for solving problems. The program also strongly emphasizes successful adoption of new behaviors and provides regular feedback. Skills mastery is aided by contracting for some self-management behavior the patient wants to develop for the following week, with a minimal confidence level of 70%. The contract script is shown in Box 9-1. Course materials contained in *The Arthritis Helpbook* were written with an emphasis on modeling, showing real persons with whom participants could identify. Participants are taught to use positive self-talk, to identify the negative ways they think about the disease and their self-help behaviors, and then to consciously change these to more positive behaviors.[10] Measurement of progress is accomplished in part by the Arthritis Self-Efficacy Scale, which appears in Box 4-13.

Most research on patient education to date has been undertaken on relatively few of the rheumatic diseases and for populations that are predominantly white and relatively well educated.[3] Several reviews of this literature may be found in Appendix C. The most recent review concludes that medical care, including the use of medications, can offer a 20% to 50% improvement in reported symptoms of arthritis. Data from patient education studies suggest that a further improvement of 15% to 30% is attainable through patient education interventions.[7] The one review that provides a meta-analysis summarizes 15 studies and shows moderate effect sizes of psychoeducational interventions on pain, depression, and disability.[15]

Research on the ASMP shows the following results.

1. In randomized trials the ASMP improves behaviors, self-efficacy, and aspects of health status.

Box 9-1   *Contract Script*

I. Deciding What One Wants to Accomplish

Ask the person, "What will you do this week?" It is important that the activity come from the participant and not you. This activity does not have to be something covered in class—just something that the participant wants to do to change behavior. Do not let anyone say. "I will try . . . " Each person should say, "I will . . . "

II. Making a Plan

This is the difficult and most important part of contracting. Part I is worthless without part II.

The plan should contain all of the following elements:

1. Exactly what is the participant going to do (i.e., how far will you walk, how will you eat less, what relaxation techniques will you practice)?
2. How much (i.e., walk around the block, 15 minutes, etc.)?
3. When will the participant do this? Again, this must be specific (i.e., before lunch, in the shower, when I come home from work).
4. How often will the activity be done? This is a bit tricky. Most participants tend to say every day. In contracting, the most important thing is to succeed. Therefore, it is better to contract to do something four times a week and exceed the contract by actually doing it five times than to contract to do something every day and fail by only doing it 6 days. To insure success, we usually encourage people to contract to do something 3 to 5 days a week. Remember that success and self-efficacy are

as important, or maybe even more important, than actually doing the behavior.

III. Checking the Contract

Once the contract is complete, ask the participant "Given a scale of 0 to 100, with 0 being totally unsure and 100 being totally certain, how certain are you that you will (repeat the participant's contract verbatim)?"

If the answer is 70 or above, this is probably a realistic contract and the participant should write it on his or her contract sheet.

If the answer is below 70, then the contract should be reassessed. Ask the participant: "What makes you uncertain? What problems do you foresee?" Then discuss the problems. Ask other participants to offer solutions. YOU should offer solutions LAST. Once the problem solving is completed, have the participant restate the contract and return to repeat part III, checking the contract.

• • •

NOTE: This contracting process may seem cumbersome and time-consuming. However, it does work and is well worth the effort. The first time you contract with a group, plan 2 to 3 minutes per person. Contracting is a learned skill. Your participant will soon be saying "I will _____ four times this week before lunch and am 80% certain I can do this." Thus, after two or three contracting sessions, contracting should take less than a minute per participant.

From Lorig K, Gonzalez V: The integration of theory with practice: a 12-year case study, *Health Educ Q* 19:355-368, 1992; reprinted from Lorig K: *Arthritis self-management leader's manual*, rev ed, Atlanta, 1984, Arthritis Foundation.

---

2. Formal reinforcement appears to improve the long-term outcomes of the ASMP.
3. The effects of the ASMP last for as long as 4 years without formal reinforcement.
4. The mechanism by which the ASMP affects health status appears to be more closely linked to changes in self-efficacy than to changes in behaviors.
5. The ASMP is an intervention that can

be and has been disseminated widely. In 1984 the Arthritis Foundation began to distribute it throughout the United States, and in more recent years its use has been encouraged internationally.[11]

Evidence indicates that 4 years after participation in the ASMP, patients' pain declined a mean of 20% and their visits to physicians by 40%, while physical disability increased 9%. Estimated 4-year savings were $648 per person for patients with rheumatoid arthritis and $189 per osteoarthritis patient.[12]

Relapse prevention in patients who are attempting to cope with persistent pain from rheumatoid arthritis should be part of a self-management program. Figure 9-1 provides a model of this process. Early warning signs include an increase in pain, disruption in sleep patterns, and lack of response to a usual medication regimen. Interpersonal situations, such as a visit from out-of-town relatives, and intrapersonal events, such as increased depression or

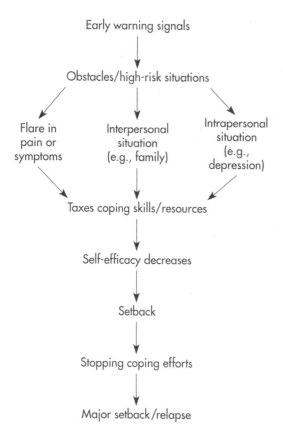

Figure 9-1 Model of relapse process in coping with pain. (From Keefe FJ, Van Horn Y: Cognitive-behavioral treatment of rheumatoid arthritis pain; maintaining treatment gains, *Arthritis Care Res* 6:213-222, 1993.)

anxiety, may overwhelm the patient's perceived ability to control pain or other symptoms with previously successful coping strategies. To help identify high-risk situations that are likely to lead to relapse, patients can be asked to describe past setbacks. Through self-monitoring and cognitive rehearsal of previous relapse episodes, patients can pinpoint specific early warning signs of relapse and can rehearse how to cope with different relapse situations.[8]

Spousal training appears to be useful. A study of spouse-assisted pain-coping skill intervention found patients to have significantly lower levels of pain, psychological disability and pain behavior, better marital adjustment, and self-efficacy than did patients in conventional pain coping skills training without spouses or an arthritis education spousal support control condition. This intervention is based on the notion that spouses can learn how to prompt and positively reinforce a patient's efforts to cope with arthritis pain. Spouses are trained in three sets of coping skills: (1) attention diversion—relaxation, imagery, and distraction (how to focus on sights and sounds in one's physical environment and how to use backward counting to distract oneself from pain); (2) activity—rest cycling and pleasant activity scheduling; and (3) cognitive restructuring—identifying and changing self defeating pain-related cognitions. The couple learns through behavioral rehearsal, mutual goal setting, and practicing these skills in settings in which pain has been a problem such as an extended shopping trip at a large mall.[9]

Arthritis self-management education has been used as a model to develop programs for other rheumatic diseases such as fibromyalgia. This syndrome is characterized by widespread musculoskeletal pain and multiple tender points, severe fatigue, sleep disturbance, and stiffness. Because the etiology of fibromyalgia is unknown, treatment is largely symptomatic and unstandardized. Self-management education programs include information on the fibromyalgia syndrome; physical training; cognitive-behavioral therapy, including self-efficacy training, relaxation, and coping techniques; and communication with providers and family.[2] A recent study of a 6-week exercise and education program for these patients showed improvement in their physical function, sense of well being, and fatigue level that was partially sustained at 3 months.[6]

For all education in the rheumatic diseases, it is important to note that unless educational treatments attend to creating an appropriate level of self-efficacy, they may increase awareness of the disease process without developing a corresponding confidence to cope with it.[8]

COMMUNITY-BASED EDUCATION AND EDUCATION OF SPECIAL POPULATIONS

The ASMP, originally developed at Stanford University, was designed to be community-based—to be held in settings such as libraries, senior centers, churches, and shopping malls.[10] The ASMP is endorsed by the Arthritis Foundation and sponsored by local chapters throughout the United States and other countries. Some persons either may choose not to participate in the ASMP or may not have access to it; however, several home-study programs have been developed and tested.

One home-study program, "Bone up on Arthritis" (BUOA), contains six lessons presented on audiocassette tapes and in booklets, which can be used when and where clients choose. BUOA is intended to be easily implemented within a community, with a community-based intervener acting as facilitator and coordinator. Each BUOA participant is matched with a resource person who teaches classes to small groups or distributes the lessons through the mail and who serves as a local information and referral source. The program has been tested on a rural population, which showed improved scores on all outcome measures (self-care behavior, helplessness, pain, dysfunction, and depression).[5] Programs using phone contact have been found to be successful as have totally mail-delivered self-management programs.[4,14]

Learning About Rheumatoid Arthritis (LARA) is a written individualized instruction program tested on an urban population and shown to be effective.[16] It uses performance measures of outcome, for example, asking participants to drink from a coffee mug, carry a handbag or flight bag (handle over the shoulder or elbow), move a pot with a handle from one flat surface to another 2 feet away, get up from a chair (use of two hands), and slide objects across the floor instead of carrying them. It will be important to investigate the cost-effectiveness of these various educational programs, as well as to understand their instructional effectiveness and access for persons in various living situations.[16]

Much work is required to understand how best to help persons from a variety of special groups attain the benefits of the self-management programs described here. For example, generalizability of self-efficacy theory across cultures still needs further study.[10]

Folk models—the tacit beliefs that are commonly held and communicated among lay members of a group and that are frequently at odds with the expert's set of beliefs—need to be understood for a variety of groups. A study of a folk model of arthritis among middle-class older adults found that commonly mentioned causes of arthritis were damp and cold weather, which was said by some to cause "frozen joints"; a diet of too much calcium, which leads to deposits in joints; and injury, overuse, or misuse of joints.[17] It is important for those who wish to communicate with persons about arthritis to have an understanding of the kinds of knowledge and beliefs individuals have about it.[16] No description of a folk model of arthritis for minorities or low-income groups could be located.

NATIONAL STANDARDS AND TESTED PROGRAMS

The Arthritis Foundation, which has played a major role in this field, has adopted four of the more successful programs and has used trained leaders to disseminate them nationwide.

Patient education standards for the rheumatic disease field are shown in Appendix D. As with the diabetes field, these are essentially process standards—that is, they do not set targeted levels of outcome standards.

SUMMARY

Inasmuch as the ASMP has been the most widely available program, it serves as an excellent model of patient education. Well grounded in both theory and research and currently widely disseminated, it is community based, uses trained lay leaders, and is sufficiently standardized to be replicable. It appears that the success of the ASMP depends more on strengthening or changing psychological attributes such as self-efficacy than on the performance of a particular behavior or techniques.[12] Health care providers have also defined patient education standards.

 Study Question

1. Wynne[19] found that only one third of patients receiving nonsteroidal anti-inflammatory drugs (NSAIDs) remembered receiving information about potential side effects. This lack of knowledge was associated with hospital admission for acute gastrointestinal bleeding. More than one third of those patients had suffered epigastric pain and most had continued to comply fully with NSAID therapy, apparently unaware of a possible link. How should such a problem be handled by a managed care organization?

References

1. Burckhardt CS: Arthritis and musculoskeletal patient education standards, *Arthritis Care Res* 7:1-4, 1994.
2. Burckhardt CS, Bjelle A: Education programmes for fibromyalgia patients: description and evaluation, *Ballieres Clin Rheumatol* 8:935-955, 1994.
3. Daltroy LH, Liang MH: Arthritis education: opportunities and state of the art, *Health Educ Q* 20:3-16, 1993.
4. Fries JF, Carey C, McShane DJ: Patient education in arthritis: randomized controlled trial of a mail-delivered program, *J Rheum* 24:1378-1383, 1997.
5. Goeppinger J and others: From research to practice: the effects of the jointly sponsored dissemination of an arthritis self-care nursing intervention, *Appl Nurs Res* 8:106-113, 1995.
6. Gowans SE, deHueck A, Voss S, Richardson M: A randomized controlled trial of exercise and education for individuals with fibromyalgia, *Arthritis Care Res* 12:120-128, 1999.
7. Hirano PC, Laurent DD, Lorig K: Arthritis patient education studies, 1987-1991: a review of the literature, *Patient Educ Couns* 24:9-54, 1994.
8. Keefe FJ, Van Horn Y: Cognitive-behavioral treatment of rheumatoid arthritis pain; maintaining treatment gains, *Arthritis Care Res* 6:213-222, 1993.
9. Keefe FJ and others: Spouse-assisted coping skills training in the management of osteoarthritic knee pain, *Arthritis Care Res* 9:279-291, 1996.
10. Lorig K, Gonzalez V: The integration of theory with practice: a 12-year case study, *Health Educ Q* 19:355-368, 1992.
11. Lorig K, Homan H: Arthritis self-management studies: a twelve-year review, *Health Educ Q* 20:17-28, 1993.
12. Lorig KR, Mazonson PD, Homan HR: Evidence suggesting that health education for self-management in patients with chronic arthritis has sustained health benefits while reducing health care costs, *Arthritis Rheum* 36:439-446, 1993.
13. Lorig K and others: Arthritis self-management program variations: three studies, *Arthritis Care Res* 11:448-454, 1998.
14. Maisiak R, Austin J, Heck L: Health outcomes of two telephone interventions for patients with rheumatoid arthritis or osteoarthritis, *Arthritis Rheum* 39:1391-1399, 1996.
15. Mullen PD and others: Efficacy of psychoeducational interventions on pain, depression, and disability in people with arthritis: a meta-analysis, *J Rheumatol* 14(suppl 15):33-39, 1987.
16. Neuberger GB and others: Promoting self-care in clients with arthritis, *Arthritis Care Res* 6:141-148, 1993.
17. Rice GE, Young LH: A folk model of arthritis, *Health Values* 18(2):15-27, 1994.
18. Taal E and others: Group education for patients with rheumatoid arthritis, *Patient Educ Couns* 20:1677-1687, 1993.
19. Wynne HA, Long A: Patient awareness of the adverse effects of non-steroidal anti-inflammatory drugs (NSAIDS), *Br J Clin Pharmacol* 42:253-256, 1996.

Chapter 10

Other Areas of Patient Education Practice

A number of areas of patient education practice are developing slowly (mental health), are in decline because of philosophical changes (adherence), were developed years ago and are now stable (preprocedure and postprocedure preparation), or are predominantly dealt with in public health education interventions (acquired immunodeficiency syndrome [AIDS] education). Others such as genetics education and education for patients with neurological problems are newly developing. There are many other areas in which patient education practice could be helpful to patients but that have not been developed with a research base and a body of literature that describes assessment, intervention strategies, and programs of education in the field. For example, there is very little focus on men's health outside of major disease categories, and the same is true for older adults, especially those with chronic illness.

Homeless populations could benefit tremendously from community-based education focused on staying well and dealing with health problems associated with their lifestyle. May and Evans[47] describe education provided by volunteers, including nurses, in 13 urban shelters. Health problems for which education was provided included mental health, alcohol and drug concerns, injuries, skin disorders, high blood pressure, infection, and dental health. Education about human immunodeficiency virus (HIV) risk reduction, prevention of pregnancy, parenting skills, and instruction in first aid would also be helpful in these areas.

This chapter describes several fields of patient education practice that are in various stages of development.

MENTAL HEALTH

General Approach

The mental health field has developed what it calls "psychoeducation," which refers to training individuals in psychological knowledge or skills. A component of the learning process in therapy,[39] it is also used to refer to programs that in other fields are called patient education. Originally used with persons with schizophrenia, this model is now applied to individuals with depression, to those with serious mental illness, to those with obsessive-compulsive disorder, and to persons with addiction disorders.

Educational Approaches and Research Base

Psychoeducation provides knowledge and skill development and support for individuals with psychiatric illness, as well as for their families.

The family is especially important because the environment it creates can influence the course of illness and recovery for the patient and because family members themselves need help in coping with the negative effects of the illness. The purposes of patient and family psychoeducation include ameliorating symptoms of the illness; reducing family burden and stress; helping participants acquire new coping, social, and communication skills that will improve their quality of life; enhancing treatment compliance; and relapse prevention and warning.[15]

Typical program topics include specific mental illness diagnosis and causes, symptoms, medications, stress management, goal setting and self-esteem, and highly structured problem solving. A topical outline of one program is shown in Box 10-1.[34]

It is important not only to provide information but also to teach and model specific management skills for dealing with an illness. The group leader for a psychoeducational group needs to be able to tolerate the slow pace and frequent repetitions of content as well as patients' internal states of depression.

Psychoeducation can help families move beyond shame and stigma and develop the skills and knowledge to meet professionals on an equal footing.[31] Psychoeducation often focuses heavily on teaching basic life skills that patients need to negotiate day-to-day living. Many patients have problem-solving as well as self-care deficits, skills not addressed in traditional treatment programs. A sufficiently large, accumulated research base for psychoeducation could not be located. Clusters of current studies for disorders show what can be accomplished.

For the population with severe dementia, such as those with Alzheimer's disease (AD), educational support groups have long been available for caregivers. During the early stages of dementia caregivers are more likely to benefit from a structured, time-limited educational group to gain the information necessary to provide care. They need to understand the functional impact of dementia; the need to accommodate care to the

---

Box 10-1 *Topical Outline for Patient and Family Psychoeducation*

BOTH PATIENTS AND FAMILY	PATIENTS	FAMILY
Nature of illness, etiology, treatment	Monitoring stress; balancing stimulation with caution about adding stressors	Maintaining simple, structured, consistent environment
Relationship of illness and stress		Management of specific behavioral problems
Identification of early symptoms of acute episodes of illness	Self-regulation of specific symptoms of illness	Importance of low-key, noncritical attitude and communication
Medications—their purpose, importance	Learning to understand others; empathy development	Including the patient in activities
Aftercare visits—using staff for consultation on problems	Developing social and leisure skills; balancing with constructive activity	Importance of developing own life
Communication and problem-solving skills	Learning to live with stigma	Support groups for families; advocacy for mentally ill
	Self-help groups for the mentally ill	

From Holmes H and others: Nursing model of psychoeducation for the seriously mentally ill patient, *Issues Ment Health Nurs* 15:85-104, 1994.
NOTE: Education is tailored to the needs of the individual patient and family but includes information in these topical areas when they are assessed as appropriate.

receiver's cognitive, emotional, and behavioral dysfunction; the need for caregiver self-care; legal and financial planning; and the role of community support groups. In later stages of the illness caregivers may prefer to participate in an ongoing support group.[20]

Recent research findings seem to indicate that the causes of death for persons with AD vary with the level of cognitive impairment close to the time of death. Illnesses potentially amenable to treatment caused death at all levels of AD but more so early in the course of the disease. Cognitive impairment may make patients less able to recognize and report symptoms of medical problems, which means that caregivers must be well educated to note these problems early.[39]

Depression affects 5% of the population each year. Older women with depression are a special population for whom education is useful in conjunction with other therapies. Not only can knowledge and skills be taught that can prevent depressive symptoms from becoming severe enough to require hospitalization but education can also function as a tool for perspective transformation. Participants learn that they are not the problem but that they suffer from a role-determined social-identity deficit, which can be altered. Education has been incorporated into traditional therapeutic interventions to overcome self-destructive thinking habits and to develop communication skills, particularly assertiveness. Education is also a primary intervention tool, including the use of stimulation to avoid boredom, learning why and how social deficits can cause depressive symptoms, and learning how to construct a satisfactory social self.[7]

Maynard[48] describes content and sequence for psychoeducational group meetings for women with depression (Table 10-1). The program is based on the belief that attaining skills to better manage life events can help prevent depressive symptoms from becoming severe enough to require hospitalization. Note that, as with other examples common in the literature, the content and sequence should be preceded by a clear set of behavioral outcome goals.

Family members who live with a member with depression have varying educational needs as they work through the adjustment. At stage 1 family members often lack information about symptoms and treatment alternatives. At stage 2 they need to learn techniques to facilitate communication, including talking about symptoms of worsening depression with the depressed member and avoiding making the depression worse. They also need to learn how to monitor medication adherence without causing conflict. Stage 3 involves developing new ways of relating to the ill member such as setting limits and how and when to shift the sense of responsibility to the ill member.[1]

Prevention of relapse is a prime educational goal for persons with bipolar disorder or with schizophrenia. Perry and others[57] taught patients with bipolar disorder (manic-depressive disorder) to identify early symptoms of relapse, which are frequently idiosyncratic to the patient and usually occur 2 to 4 weeks before full relapse. This approach did not work with depressive cycles but did significantly extend time between manic relapses, in comparison to a control group. Persons with schizophrenia learn the relationship between illness and stress, including its link to relapse; medication taking; legal issues including patient rights; identification of early symptoms of acute episodes; and communication, problem-solving and negotiation skills.[40] Macpherson, Jerrom, and Hughes[44] found a subgroup of about one third of patients who were unable to learn adequately to give informed consent. Patients hospitalized with acute psychotic conditions have successfully been educated about their medications with computer-based instruction.[45] Persons with chronic mental illness have a higher prevalence of medical illnesses and higher mortality rates than the general population. They are expected to manage their own medical care even though the symptoms of their disorders—hallucinations, delusions, paranoia, and withdrawal from depression—may interfere with their ability to seek health care and to follow through with recommendations. Fre-

| TABLE 10-1 | Content and Sequence for Psychoeducational Group Meetings |

Meeting No.	Topic	Content
1	Depression	Do get-acquainted exercises; provide overview of the sessions; state group objectives and ground rules; discuss the holistic approach to depression; give information about depression (i.e., nature of depression, symptoms of depression, causes of depression, differences in depression between women and men, and social factors related to depression in women); and give information about medication for depression (i.e., benefits and side effects, limitations of medications, and how to talk with the physician about medications).
2	Relationship of thoughts to depression	Discuss the role of thoughts in feelings, particularly depression; discuss irrational beliefs and steps in changing cognitive patterns; identify personal negative self-statements and irrational beliefs; and discuss the theory of learned helplessness.
3	Role of social factors in depression	Discuss how current social expectations of women influence feelings; discuss realistic and unrealistic expectations women have of themselves; discuss the concept of multiple roles and identify number of roles each woman has; discuss expectations others have for women; identify factors in society that are oppressive for women and discuss how they affect their lives; identify which factors can be changed; and discuss marital and parenting relationships.
4	Goal setting	Share importance of goal-setting and steps in goal-setting; share steps to take in setting goals; and discuss types of goals.
5	Self-esteem	Share goals set over previous week; teach information related to self-esteem, including the nature of self-esteem, factors in development of self-esteem, and self-ideal; and share techniques for improving self-esteem based on awareness of self and self-messages, affirmations to substitute positive messages, and action to change behavior.
6	Understanding family of origin	Discuss family structure, messages received during childhood, and kinds of relationships between family members; discuss how childhood messages continue to influence adult life; discuss how to give up old messages and old hurts; discuss verbal, physical, and sexual abuse in the family; and discuss consequences and methods of handling abuse.
7	Assertiveness	Give information about characteristics of assertive, passive, and aggressive behaviors; identify and discuss basic rights; and discuss and practice skills for accepting and giving criticism, communicating needs, and saying no.
8	Stress management	Provide information about stress and its role in depression; discuss physiologic and psychologic responses to stress; and teach stress management strategies.
9	Caring for the body	Teach the importance of diet, exercise, rest, and other preventive health practices; give information about such practices as breast self-examination; and discuss relationship of health practices to depression.
10	Review and terminate	Teach role of social support and methods to increase social networks; discuss what each woman has gained from the meetings; discuss long-term goals; and share positive feelings and experiences.

From Maynard C: Psychoeducational approach to depression in women, *J Psychosoc Nurs* 31(12):9-14, 1993.

quently, lack of knowledge, home, family, or network of friends are barriers to self-care for general health problems.[24]

ADHERENCE TO PRESCRIBED REGIMENS

General Approach

Adherence to a regimen prescribed by a provider has been a prevailing goal of patient education for some time. Previously referred to as "compliance," the concept itself came under attack as moralistic and inappropriate in some patient care situations, particularly when the regimen had to be adjusted to fit the patient's changing condition. Errors in taking or not taking prescribed medications have been documented on a widespread basis. In most studies at least one third of patients failed to comply with instructions, and in some the rate is 50% or higher. Both clinical judgment on the part of the provider and self-report on the part of the patient are known to be inaccurate. Clear instructions, including the use of icons (pictures depicting instructions) (see example in Figure 10-1), simplified regimens, reminder pill containers and calendars, telephone follow-up, tailoring the regimen to the patient's lifestyle, and involving a significant other are all known to be helpful in attaining adherence.[6]

Although the goal of adherence to a prescribed regimen is still legitimate, there are several caveats. First, it is not always clear that the regimen will accomplish the benefits expected, even if the patient reliably follows it. Second, judging patients by whether they adhere to medical authority is now widely understood to be paternalistic and assumes an authority providers do not have. Most medication recommendations require some degree of independent patient judgment and accommodation. At the least, regimens should be jointly developed around treatment goals shared by the patient and the provider and constructed so that they are convenient and reflect the patient's assessment of benefit from and burden of the regimen. Perhaps self-management to a jointly specified set of behaviors and outcomes is a more satisfactory alternate goal.

Educational Approaches and Research Base

Box 10-2 summarizes adherence-enhancing educational and behavioral interventions.

More than a decade ago Posavac and others[59] reviewed 58 studies evaluating the effectiveness of programs to increase compliance with medical treatment regimens. The mean effect size was 0.47, with lesser impact as the amount of lifestyle changes required by the treatment regimen increased. The most successful interventions involved improving the facility providing care and

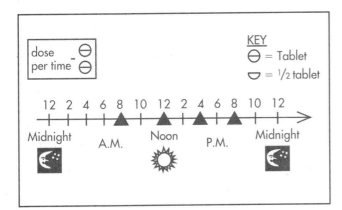

Figure 10-1 Example of nonintegrated icon. (From Morrow DG and others: Icons improve older and younger adults' comprehension of medication information, *J Gerontol* 53(4):240-254, 1998.)

Box 10-2 *Adherence-Enhancing Interventions*

Educational Strategies to Enable Patients to Implement and Maintain Regimen

- Provide verbal instruction in small amounts, specific to activity; deliver over time
- Dispense limited amounts of printed instructions to reinforce verbal information
- Use material at patient's reading/comprehension level
- Dispense materials over time
- Assess level of patient's understanding; encourage questions
- Focus on activities of the regimen, not on the disease
- Augment verbal instructions with demonstrations
- Utilize other instructional media (e.g., videotapes, interactive computer programs)
- Provide opportunities for practice and return demonstration (e.g., counting pulse, taking nitroglycerin, selecting foods from a menu)
- Refer to community resources for additional skill development (e.g., YMCA for exercise class, American Heart Association for food shopping tours, hospital for cooking classes)

Behavioral Strategies to Enhance Adherence

- Modeling of behavior via word, action, video; reference model must be similar in ability (e.g., demonstrate exercise in cardiac rehabilitation session; select food from a restaurant menu)
- Tailor regimen to fit patient's lifestyle (e.g., develop medication schedule to accommodate work schedule; recommend diet changes with sensitivity to cultural food preferences and available resources)
- Goal setting: Make goals proximal, attainable, very specific (e.g., walk eight blocks three times/week for the next month; reduce milk fat to 1%; reduce meat portion to 4 oz)
- Self-monitoring: Record activities related to goal and review with provider at next visit; use for self-review to identify patterns threatening adherence; use for problem solving

- Reinforcement (administered by provider or patient [self-reinforcement]): Review self-monitor records, provide praise for attempts and progress in meeting goals; patient can use to reinforce self for progress made
- Problem-solving: Review threats to adherence; identify problems; anticipate potential problems; identify solutions; select a solution and test it; rehearse how potential problems might be managed
- Cuing: Set up system of reminders to take medicine, exercise (e.g., set out walking shoes; place a reminder sticker in obvious place about a bedtime medicine)
- Habit building: Pair an activity with an established habit (e.g., place pill bottle next to morning juice glass or toothpaste; bedtime medication by clock radio)
- Contracting: Make a written agreement between patient and provider concerning how/when patient will reach set goal; usually involves a reward when goal is achieved; uses incremental steps in reaching goal; specifics included in contract
- Social support: Enlist assistance of significant support systems at home, work, and social environment; invite attendance at exercise, cooking classes, and follow-up appointment; involve others in behavior change plan
- Self-efficacy enhancing: Provide opportunities for successful performance (performance mastery is most influential); give feedback and praise; use verbal persuasion; instill self-confidence; set short, specific goals; practice self-regulation through continuous or episodic self-monitoring, followed by self-evaluation and self-reinforcement; develop skills and enhance knowledge

From Burke LE, Dunbar-Jacob J: Adherence to medication, diet, and activity recommendations: from assessment to maintenance, *J Cardiovasc Nurs* 9:62-79, 1995.

helping patients to incorporate the treatment regimen into their daily routine. More recently Morris and Schulz[54] completed a nonquantitative review of the patient-compliance literature and concluded that after decades of research very little consistent information is available. One major reason for this lack of understanding is that compliance research has been dominated by the perspective of the health care professional. Future research needs to investigate the patient's decision-making process and the reasons for those decisions. Although the conclusions of the authors of these two reviews differ somewhat, each provides a valid perspective.

Obtaining a more useful body of research for understanding adherence issues is important. In addition to increased costs of treatment and the deaths that might have been delayed, in older adults alone nonadherence has been linked to 23% of nursing home admissions and 10% of all hospital admissions.[55] Outcome-oriented definitions of adherence differ from process-oriented ones. Although it is important to take medication safely (process), it is possible to obtain a satisfactory therapeutic outcome without taking the medication exactly as prescribed. Morris, Tabak, and Gondek[53] found that in the past 12 years the percentage of patients receiving written information about their medications has moved from 5% to 15% in the physician's office and from 16% to 59% at the pharmacy. Boards of pharmacy in 40 states now require that pharmacists offer to counsel patients about their medications.

Community-Based Education and Education of Special Populations

Adherence education takes place wherever care is given, including in ambulatory and community settings.

Cultural issues clearly play a role in adherence. An interesting study of Cambodian adults with minimal formal education, who were receiving public assistance and utilizing an ambulatory clinic in Seattle, found two thirds of the group to be noncompliant with instructions to take their medications.[63] Some of this resistance can be attributed to concern about the effects of Western medication on "internal strength" and Cambodian ideas about pharmacokinetics—in other words, culturally conceived compliance. These individuals made considerable effort to comply with therapy but did so in a manner consistent with their underlying understanding of how medicines and the body work. They believed that Western drugs were "strong medicine" (in comparison with herbal medicine) that might interfere with the body's "internal strength," and so they stopped taking them when they felt weak. For the same reason they feared taking two different medications at the same time. They believed that in some cases higher doses yielded faster results and that in the absence of symptoms medication should be discontinued. Once these cultural ideas are understood, cultural noncompliance is predictable and can be addressed systematically.

There is also some evidence that certain populations, such as those with diabetes, have a considerably increased rate of depression, which is associated with less adequate adherence to self-care and poorer glycemia control.[22] Because somatic illnesses may be associated with an increased prevalence of depression, treatment of the depression may be an important way to increase adherence.

PREPROCEDURE AND POSTPROCEDURE EDUCATION

General Approach

Preprocedure and postprocedure education encompass a wide variety of medical treatments, including surgery. A relatively strong research base has developed around the use of sensory information (what the patient will see, hear, feel, smell, and taste) during the procedure and procedural information (description of what will be done during the procedure) to help patients minimize their emotional reactions, increase their coping strategies, and have a better outcome from the procedure. The optimal amount of each kind of information has not been established.

Self-regulation theory, a cognitive theory that explains human behavior as an outcome of information processing, is the basis for research on preparatory teaching. A schema (mental image based on prior experience) serves as a framework for organizing input as an experience progresses, and teaching sensory and procedural information helps to develop the schema about the event.

Educational Approaches and Research Base

An example of a preoperative program is the Preoperative Total Joint Assessment and Education Program at the University of Pittsburgh.[60] Because nearly all patients undergoing joint procedures are admitted on the day of surgery, the program is offered in conjunction with pretesting for the procedure on an outpatient basis 2 to 4 weeks before surgery. Content focuses on postoperative care, including exercises, wound care, and pain management. Included also is information about the following possible complications and their prevention:

- Respiratory problems (coughing, deep breathing, use of spirometer)
- Deep vein thrombosis (elastic stockings and a sequential compression device)
- Wound care (dressings, signs and symptoms of infection)
- Pain management (patient-controlled analgesia, epidural analgesia, and medications as needed)
- Comfort measures (relaxation techniques, breathing exercises)
- Antibiotic therapy (including coverage for future invasive procedures)

Patients are provided with the total joint orthopedic clinical pathway, which highlights critical events and corresponding time.[60] Special care related to total knee and total hip arthroplasty procedures includes hip reflexion precautions, use of adaptive equipment such as an elevated toilet seat, and guidelines for exercise and sexual activity after surgery. Patients see the physical therapist to learn about assistive devices, gait training, and transfer techniques, in-cluding appropriate weight bearing, and consult the occupational therapist to help gain independence in activities of daily living. The addition of specific learning objectives would be helpful.

Many other examples of preoperative teaching programs are available. A randomized controlled trial found that patients who received a preoperative video were 2 to 16 times more likely to be able to recall appropriate knowledge than were those receiving usual care. The video relieves caregivers of step-by-step explanations of the procedure and allows them to focus on individual concerns and needs of a patient.[19] In another randomized controlled trial Bondy and others[4] found that mailing a video and pamphlets to the patient's home to provide anesthetic-focused patient education for total hip and total knee replacement surgery diminished the preoperative anxiety in comparison with the normal procedure of using a clinical pathway and a visit with an anesthetist. The video showed the sequence of events before, during, and after anesthesia and explained benefits and possible side effects. Such an outcome is important because it can decrease the need for sedation to relieve anxiety and pain.[4]

Information about patient-controlled analgesia (PCA) is a portion of the operative teaching plan. PCA allows patients to receive a continuous or bolus administration of an analgesic and to administer it when they believe it is necessary. This method is also used for obstetric patients and for those with cancer pain. Studies find that structured instruction provided a more efficient way to learn about pain management with the use of PCA than did incidental teaching[65] (Table 10-2). Patients need to know about the preventive approach to pain management and about the lockout interval between doses; a pattern of an excessive number of unmet demands for medication may indicate incorrect use of the pump or inadequate understanding.

PCA is most frequently initiated in the recovery room when patients are emerging from general anesthesia and may not have been planned preoperatively. Inclusion of PCA education in all preoperative education would solve this problem.[69] Those who have been formally educated

TABLE 10-2   Questionnaire to Evaluate PCA Instruction

Directions: Please read the following statements and circle the number that best represents your experience after surgery when using the PCA pump. If you agree with the statement, circle (1); if you disagree with the statement, circle (2).

	Agree	Disagree
Part I: Use of the PCA Pump		
1. I was receiving pain medicine because the PCA pump provides continuous administration of pain medicine.	1	2
2. The only time I received pain medicine was when I gave it to myself.	1	2
3. I knew I could never overdose myself because the PCA pump controls the amount of medicine I receive.	1	2
4. If I didn't get pain relief after I pressed the control button of the PCA pump, I waited 10 minutes before I pressed the button again.	1	2
5. I only received pain medicine when I pressed the button on the PCA pump.	1	2
6. If I didn't get pain relief after many tries at pressing the control button on the PCA pump I waited until my doctor visited to tell him (her).	1	2
7. If I had pain I pressed the control button of the PCA pump to receive additional pain medicine.	1	2
8. If I didn't get pain relief after I pressed the control button of the PCA pump, I called the nurse for a "pain shot."	1	2
9. I know I had to keep the number of times I self-administered pain medicine to a minimum so I wouldn't become sleepy or drowsy.	1	2
10. I didn't press the control button of the PCA pump when I had pain because I was afraid I would overdose myself.	1	2
11. I knew if I used the PCA pump to self-administer pain medicine I would not become drowsy and sleepy.	1	2
12. I knew I had to call a nurse if I didn't get pain relief after many tries of pressing the control button of the PCA pump.	1	2
Part II: Management of Pain		
1. I never worried about giving myself an overdose when I administered pain medicine using the PCA pump.	1	2
2. One of the reasons I hated to cough or deep breathe is because I couldn't get optimal pain relief using the PCA pump.	1	2
3. The reason I would use the PCA pump again is because I liked the feeling of control I had over my pain.	1	2
4. I had difficulty keeping free of pain when I used the PCA pump to administer the pain medicine.	1	2
5. One of the reasons I hated to move in bed is because I couldn't relieve my pain using the PCA pump.	1	2
6. I felt drowsy and sleepy when I used the PCA pump to relieve the pain.	1	2
7. I was able to get optimal pain relief using the PCA pump before I coughed and did deep breathing.	1	2
8. If I didn't get pain relief after my first try with the PCA pump, I didn't try again because I was afraid I would overdose myself.	1	2
9. I was able to keep relatively free of pain when I administered the pain medicine using the PCA pump.	1	2
10. One of the reasons I was able to move freely while in bed is because I was able to reduce my pain using the PCA pump.	1	2
11. I was alert and awake while I used the PCA pump to control my pain.	1	2
12. I would never use a PCA pump again to control my pain.	1	2

From Timmons ME, Bower FL: The effect of structured preoperative teaching on patients' use of patient-controlled analgesia (PCA) and their management of pain, *Orthop Nurs* 12:23-31, 1993.

had lower pain intensity scores.[38] This is problematic because there is a temporary decrease in cognitive ability in the immediate postoperative period, which is to be expected because some of the drugs used were developed especially to produce amnesia of the intraoperative episode. Studies have shown that PCA can yield higher levels of patient satisfaction with less sedation, shorter lengths of stay, and fewer complications.[68] A patient handout about PCA is shown in Figure 10-2.

Because ambulatory surgery patients go home 1 to 2 hours postoperatively, it is important to assess their learning ability; patients may believe they are back to normal when they are not.[27] Hotlines for discharged surgical patients are operated by protocol to give sound and consistent advice. Postoperative concerns about which patients call include activity, bowel movements and voiding, cough, pain, fever/chills, medications, nausea and vomiting, wounds, tight dressings and casts, and feeling faint and dizzy.[11]

Investigators have examined preparation for a variety of stressful events such as gastroendoscopy, orthopedic cast removal, pelvic examination, surgery, radiation therapy, and colposcopy. Conclusions are that (1) the sensory information alone is superior to procedural information alone, (2) either is superior to a control condition, but (3) a combination of sensory and procedural information is the most effective preparatory strategy.

Table 10-3 describes sensations associated with cardiac catheterization as they were experienced by at least 40% of the patients in two different settings.[9] Box 10-3 shows a script developed for preparatory sensory information for cardiac catheterization, which is based on the sensations described in the study.

Some investigators have identified the need to tailor the type and amount of information according to the coping style of the patient: "Blunters" avoid information that will intensify the psychological impact of the procedure and "monitors" seek information.[21] A study of individuals undergoing cardiac catheterization found that a videotape containing procedural and sensory information in a modeling format was better for monitors, whereas a procedural modeling video was the optimal preparatory treatment for blunters (Table 10-4).[17] The effectiveness of preparatory information interventions in reducing anxiety in patients undergoing cardiac catheterization is supported by a number of studies. This intervention enables patients to form accurate expectations about the impending procedure rather than anticipating it in threatening or unrealistic terms.[31]

Summaries of research on procedure/operative teaching were among the first to be completed; six are shown in Appendix C. One reviewer found that offering both procedural information and emotional support was more effective than offering either alone.[55] From nearly 200 studies, Devine[18] found statistically reliable and positive effects of this kind of teaching on recovery, pain, psychological well-being, and satisfaction with care. Positive cost-relevant effects have been obtained across a wide range of patients, treatment providers, settings, and historical periods.

HIV-AIDS AND SEXUALLY TRANSMITTED DISEASE (STD) PATIENT EDUCATION

General Approach

Controlling the AIDS epidemic continues to depend heavily on educating people in ways to avoid becoming infected. Of necessity, this information must be widely available in communities, particularly in those with high risk factors. Issues of education and informed consent are extremely important in testing. Much less has been written about educating persons with AIDS (PWAs) in how to take care of themselves when their test results are positive for HIV or after they are sick. The mass media have been very influential in shaping attitudes about AIDS.

Educational Approaches and Research Base

As with nearly all other diseases, knowledge alone is insufficient to bring about necessary behavior changes. Most interventions to date have used social learning theory. Individuals

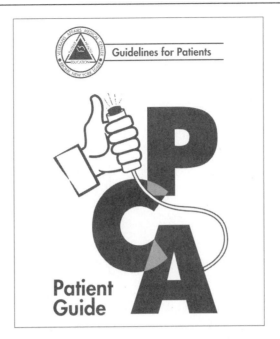

What Is PCA?

"PCA" is patient-controlled analgesia. This means **you** have control of your pain medicine.

When you need pain medicine, instead of calling the nurse, you can push your PCA button. A pump will give you pain medicine through your IV when you think you need it.

We care about your comfort! If you have any questions, please ask your doctor or nurse.

How Much Medicine Will I Receive?

The doctor will program your PCA pump to deliver an amount of pain medicine that is safe for someone of your size, age, and illness.

The pump is programmed with a safe amount of medicine. A safe time limit between doses is also set, so you cannot get too much.

When you press and release the PCA button, the pump will beep and give you some medicine. If you don't hear that beep, the "lock-out time" has not yet passed. Wait a few minutes and try again.

Watching Over Your Pain Treatment

The nurses and doctors need your help to know how the medicine is working. Use this scale to rate your pain.

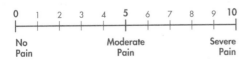

When you improve and have less pain, you will be switched to pain pills. You will no longer need the PCA pump.

What About Side Effects?

Sometimes, side effects may occur to PCA patients:

- Nausea
- Feeling sleepy
- Itchy feeling
- Hard to pass urine

If you are bothered by any of these side effects, or if your IV hurts, tell your nurse and doctor. The staff will be checking your pump. They will also check to see if you are sleepy or breathing slowly.

Also, pain medicine can make you sedated (sleepy). Remember that **you** are in control. It's up to you to balance your pain control and sleepiness. Try to keep awake enough to move, breath deeply, and care for yourself as much as you can. This will help you heal faster.

Safety Rules

1. You are the **only** person who should press the PCA button. Your family, friends, or hospital staff are not to press the button.

2. Always get help walking if you feel dizzy or very sleepy.

3. Do **not** eat if you feel very sleepy. Wait until you are more awake so you won't choke.

Figure 10-2 Sample patient handout about PCA. (Courtesy Bronx Veterans Affairs Medical Center, Bronx, NY.)

| TABLE 10-3 | Procedure for Cardiac Catheterization with Associated Sensations |

| | Sensations | |
Phase of Procedure	Medical Center	Rural Hospital
Phase 1—Patient is placed on table, undressed, and partially covered with a cloth. Right and left groin are washed with soap and water. Groin area is shaved and swabbed with Betadine.	Coldness in groin area; buzzing and humming (machine noise); seeing tubing, lights, monitors, and clocks; seeing doctors and nurses	Coldness in groin area; wet feeling in groin
Phase 2—Cardiac monitor is attached. Sterile drapes are put down. Physician locates pulse in right groin. Needle is inserted to numb area with Xylocaine.	Burning in groin; needlestick in groin	Stinging in groin; needlestick in groin
Phase 3—Small incision is made in the groin and enlarged with hemostats. Physician palpates artery and inserts needle into artery.	Pressure in groin; pain in groin	Pressure in groin
Phase 4—Guidewire is inserted over needle. Dilator is inserted and removed.	Pressure; pushing; pain in groin	Pressure
Phase 5—Sheath is inserted. Physician moves table to see, on fluoroscopy, the location of the tip of the wire. Guidewire is removed and needle flushed with heparin. Catheter is inserted and visualized on fluoroscopy.	Popping, buzzing, clicking (machine noises); seeing knobs, screens (equipment); pressure; pushing	Pressure
Phase 6—Monitor is observed for heart pressures; pressures recorded. Dye is injected using injector machine. Dye transit is observed on fluoroscopy.	Hot, burning feeling (mostly traveling from upper body downward); background talking; seeing camera, lights, monitor	Hot, burning feeling (mostly upper body downward); moist, wet
Phase 7—Guidewire is reinserted, catheter is removed, second catheter is inserted. Catheter insertion visualized on fluoroscopy. Dye is injected by hand. Dye transit is observed on fluoroscopy.	Pain, pressure (chest and back); equipment noise; seeing equipment	Pain, pressure in chest
Phase 8—Guidewire is reinserted, catheter is removed, third catheter is inserted. Catheter insertion visualized on fluoroscopy. Dye is injected by hand. Dye transit is observed on fluoroscopy. Catheter is removed. Guidewire is removed. Occlusive pressure is applied to groin.	Pain, pressure (chest and back); equipment noise; seeing equipment	Pain, pressure (chest and back)
Phase 9—Sheet is removed, patient is moved to stretcher, and stretcher is moved to hallway. Occlusive pressure is applied for 20 minutes.	Pressure; back pain	

From Cason CL, Russell DG, Fincher SB: Preparatory sensory information for cardiac catheterization, *Cardiovasc Nurs* 28:41-45, 1992.

Box 10-3	*Preparatory Sensory Information for Cardiac Catheterization*

Just before you are taken to the catheterization lab you may be given a sedative. This will relax you, but you will be awake during the procedure. You may also be given an antihistamine to decrease the chance of a reaction to the dye. When you get to the lab, you will see x-ray equipment, monitors, and hospital staff dressed in surgical clothing. The room will be cold and you will hear fans and motors running. You will lie on your back on the examining table during the entire procedure. Because the table is hard, you may feel some discomfort. If you do, tell the doctor. Your clothes will be removed and you will be partially covered with a cloth. The lab technicians will clean the groin with soap and water, shave it, and swab it with Betadine. The Betadine will feel cold and will leave a yellowish color that will wash off your skin. The lab technicians will put patches on your chest and attach wires so they can watch your heart rhythm during the procedure. You will be covered with a special sheet from neck to foot. The doctor will check for a pulse in your groin area and numb the area with Xylocaine. When he or she gives you the Xylocaine, you will feel a needlestick, followed by a burning or stinging sensation. Once the area is numb, you mainly will feel pressure in the groin as the doctor makes a small incision and inserts the catheter. While the doctor guides the catheter up to the heart, the lights in the room periodically will be turned on and off, and you will hear a popping or clicking noise. The doctor will move the table to see where the catheter is by looking at the monitor. When the catheter reaches the heart, a machine will inject dye through the catheter. You will feel a burning or hot sensation, which you may feel anywhere in your body. Most people feel the burning in their faces, shoulders, chests, and down to their bottoms. Some describe the feeling as a hot flash or as if they had urinated or are sitting in warm water. It lasts only a few seconds. The doctor will then change catheters and inject more dye by hand. You may then feel pressure in your groin and tightness or heaviness in your chest. Some people have chest discomfort. If you do, be sure to tell the doctor. At the end of the procedure, the doctor will remove the catheter and place a bandage on your groin. You will be moved from the examining table to a stretcher and taken to a waiting area for about 20 minutes. The doctor or nurse will hold the bandage to your groin to keep it from bleeding. You will feel pressure in the groin and may feel some discomfort from lying on the table for such a long time. When the doctor is sure that you will not have any problems, you will be taken back to your room.

From Cason CL, Russell DG, Fincher SB: Preparatory sensory information for cardiac catheterization, *Cardiovasc Nurs* 28:41-45, 1992.

must become skilled in preventive behaviors, and those behaviors must be reinforced by their peers. They must also have the materials they need, such as condoms. In addition to education, people must have strong negotiating skills to maintain preventive behavior in pressured social relationships. They must be rigorously tested to learn if they can maintain these behaviors, and they must be confident in their ability to avoid risky behaviors.[3]

Since the AIDS epidemic began, educators have produced thousands of brochures and pamphlets to educate the public. Such material is useful because it is portable and inexpensive, and it can be shared and be referred to repeatedly. However, as with other areas of education, much of this literature is written at a higher reading level than the target population has mastered. For example, distributing brochures in family planning clinics is one viable option for teaching women about preventing HIV infection. Yet one study showed that the mean reading level of brochures was equivalent to grade 9.9, and the formal education of 18% of the women seen in Virginia family planning clinics fell below this level.[67] Recall that most individuals read several grade levels below the last grade they completed. The mean reading level of brochures targeted to adolescents and to minority women was lower than the average. Yet only 16% of adolescents, 6% of minority women, and 12% of women who spoke English as a second language had educa-

TABLE 10-4	Videotapes on Procedural Modeling and Procedural-Sensory Modeling	
Preparatory Information Treatment	**Visual Information**	**Auditory or Printed Information**
Procedural modeling videotape	Patient is on a stretcher just outside the cath lab. Staff members wheel the patient into the cath lab and (1) cover patient with a drape sheet, (2) remove patient's gown, (3) help patient transfer from a stretcher to x-ray table, and (4) place a pillow under patient's head.	Accompanying "voice-over" by patient: "The staff members assisting with my cath wheeled me into the cath lab next to a narrow bed—called an x-ray table. They covered me with a light sheet to protect my privacy and slipped off my hospital gown. I was helped off the stretcher and onto the cath table and I was asked to lie as still as possible throughout the procedure."
Procedural-sensory modeling videotape	As above.	As above, but with this addition: "When I was on the table I had a chance to look around the room. Next to the table were the x-ray cameras which would photograph the inside of my heart and chest. Overhead were TV screens which would be used to monitor my progress. I also noticed beeping signals, which the doctor said were sounds from the heart monitor. Another thing I noticed was that the staff members were dressed in masks and gowns to prevent the spread of germs. I mentioned to them that I was a bit cool, but the doctor said I'd be warmer in a couple of minutes when they covered me with sterile sheets."

From Davis TMA and others: Preparing adult patients for cardiac catheterization: informational treatment and coping style interactions, *Heart Lung* 23:130-139, 1994.

tional attainment equal to or exceeding the reading level of the brochures targeted for their group. Expert assistance with adult literacy problems can usually be obtained from the local school district office.

When individuals are notified of HIV positivity, counseling and education are crucial. These persons must be helped to cope emotionally and should not be allowed to leave the notification session until they can repeat the information they have been given. They must know how to recognize important symptoms and how to avoid infecting others.

Because 80% of women with HIV infection are of reproductive age, testing frequently occurs in obstetrical and neonatal settings. The benefits of HIV antibody screening include the possibility of treatment for both mother and infant. If there is a loss of confidentiality, serious discrimination in housing, employment, insurance, child care, and family support is quite possible in a group already at risk of discrimination because of race or poverty. In a study in San Francisco, most women understood that they had given permission for the test but did not understand its clinical implications and recalled few risks; 78% of those tested did not return to learn their test results. These findings clearly raise questions about the adequacy of the informed consent obtained.

Community-Based Education and Education of Special Populations

Systems of technology for delivering education about AIDS in the community can be very helpful. A number of AIDS hotlines offer confidential telephone call-in services. One specialized computer network provides nurse-supervised information, decision support, and communication services to home-dwelling PWAs.[5] An electronic encyclopedia, which includes more than 200 pages of information relevant to living at home with AIDS, was designed to help PWAs enhance their self-care, understand illness-specific issues, and promote home-based management of their illness. The decision-support module guided users in an analysis of a self-defined decision problem, helping the user focus on the values and trade-offs that occur when making difficult choices. The public communication area functions as a support group. Instructions about self-care or messages encouraging hope can be retained and reviewed for as long as an individual desires. Such a network is an example of how innovative technologies can be used to deliver scarce nursing resources to persons in the community.

Other vulnerable populations may be seen in community-based organizations, such as day hospitals or partial hospitalization programs for individuals with prolonged mental illness.[64] These persons may have cognitive deficits that interfere with acquiring knowledge about HIV and AIDS, as well as impairments in impulse control and judgment that increase their risk of exposure to the disease through intravenous drug use or sexual activity. They are frequently at high risk for the disease and need to be taught preventive behaviors.

Finally, a study of poor African-American women seeking care in an inner-city prenatal clinic found that use of condoms in the previous year was significantly related to perceptions of susceptibility.[25] Items measuring elements of the health belief model are shown in Table 10-5. The findings suggest that messages emphasizing the ubiquity of risk, especially in demographically high-risk populations, may be particularly appropriate and effective.

A second study of the same population found significant deficits in understanding of treatment, whereas transmission was much better understood.[35] Such a finding should not be surprising because most educational messages from public health sources have emphasized transmission. The knowledge test used in this study can be found in Table 10-6. Although knowledge is only a portion of what is necessary to adopt protective behavior against the AIDS virus, it is important to learn whether basic knowledge is being disseminated to vulnerable populations. Haitian women in Miami were confused about the meaning of positive versus negative, the concept of antibody, and the concept of window period between exposure and presentation of antibodies.[69]

African-American and Hispanic women are disproportionately affected by AIDS and STDs. An intervention with objectives to recognize risk, to commit to changing behavior, and to acquire skills may be found in Box 10-4. Notice that it is behavioral in orientation. This intervention is specific to women since they face barriers to change related to power imbalances in their relationships with men. This intervention showed significantly decreased rates of chlamydial infection and gonorrhea in comparison with a control group that received standard counseling about STDs.[62]

Self-care education programs for patients with AIDS and their families are increasingly using designs similar to those for programs found to be successful for persons with arthritis, asthma, and diabetes. Development of self-care skills and confidence to manage this chronic illness are the target outcomes. Knowledge is useful as it relates to these goals. One trial of self-management education with men with late-stage HIV disease

TABLE 10-5	Distribution of Responses to the Health Belief Model Items

Scale	% Strongly Agree/Agree
Susceptibility Scale	
You can't get AIDS because your sexual partner(s) is (are) very clean.	25.0
You are not the kind of person who is likely to get AIDS.	25.0
You are less likely than most people to get AIDS.	43.6
Given your lifestyle, there is a chance you could get AIDS.	44.3
You're afraid you could get AIDS from your sexual partner(s).	41.3
Mean = 3.19, *SD* = 0.74, Range = 1 to 5	
Severity Scale	
AIDS is a life-threatening disease.	98.6
You are not worried about getting AIDS.	28.2
AIDS is not as bad as venereal disease (VD).	5.5
AIDS can be cured if treated early.	8.3
You are afraid of getting AIDS.	83.6
Your body could fight off AIDS because you are very healthy.	8.3
Mean = 4.08, *SD* = 0.50, Range = 1 to 5	
Barriers Scale	
The quality of your sex life would suffer if you did all the things that are important to protect yourself from getting AIDS.	33.2
Protecting yourself against AIDS would be hard to do, given your lifestyle.	10.4
If you tried hard to protect yourself against AIDS, it would be a hassle.	10.6
It would be embarrassing for you if you were to do all the things you have to do to protect yourself from getting AIDS.	11.6
Mean = 2.18, *SD* = 0.69, Range = 1 to 5	
Benefits Scale	**% Rated Very Effective**
Refuse to have sex with casual sexual partners if they don't agree to use a condom (rubber).	81.5
Avoid sex with men who have many sexual partners.	84.8
Refuse to have sex with anyone who is infected with the AIDS virus.	89.2
Refuse to have sex with a man who shoots drugs, because he could have the AIDS virus.	88.0
Mean = 3.75, *SD* = 0.37, Range = 1 to 4	

From Gielen AC and others: Women's protective sexual behaviors: a test of the health belief model, *AIDS Educ Prev* 6:1-11, 1994.

TABLE 10-6   Knowledge of Routes of Transmission

Women who have had certain experiences are more likely to be infected with the AIDS virus than other women. But not everybody agrees on what experiences put women at increased risk of AIDS. For each of the following, please tell me whether you think a woman having had this experience would make her a lot more likely, a little more likely, or no more likely to get AIDS.

	A Lot More Likely (%)	A Little More Likely (%)	No More Likely (%)	Don't Know (%)
Getting a blood transfusion?	49	40	10	1
Being around someone with AIDS?	6	15	79	<1
Having sex with a lot of different partners without using a condom?	96	4	<1	0
Deep kissing or French kissing a person who has AIDS?	23	31	42	4
Sharing needles when shooting drugs?	99	1	1	0
Having a sexual partner who had frequent blood transfusions?	55	36	6	2
Having anal intercourse?	58	24	8	11
Touching someone with AIDS?	1	8	89	1
Having a sex partner who had AIDS or had a positive test for the AIDS virus?	92	7	1	<1
Having a sexual partner who shoots up drugs?	90	9	<1	<1
Having a sexual partner who was bisexual (he had sex with a man)?	86	11	2	1
Having ever had a disease or an infection spread by sex?	33	41	22	6

	True (%)	False (%)	Don't Know (%)
Knowledge of HIV Antibody Test			
The AIDS virus test is done by taking a sample of blood.	92	3	6
The AIDS virus test can tell you if you have the disease AIDS.	76	20	4
If an AIDS virus test comes back positive, it means that the person can give AIDS to someone else.	86	11	3
If a person's AIDS virus test comes back positive, it means that the person has been infected with the AIDS virus.	91	6	3
If an AIDS virus test comes back negative, it means the person can never get AIDS.	1	98	1
If an AIDS virus test comes back negative, it means that no sign of the virus has shown up yet.	85	13	3

From Kass NE and others: Pregnant women's knowledge of the human immunodeficiency virus: implications for education and counseling, *Women Health Issues* 2:17-25, 1992.

Continued

TABLE 10-6 Knowledge of Routes of Transmission—cont'd	True (%)	False (%)	Don't Know (%)
Knowledge of Treatments			
Doctors can help people with the AIDS virus feel better and live longer.	40	51	9
There is a drug that a pregnant woman who has the AIDS virus can take to keep her baby from getting the AIDS virus.	4	67	30
There is a drug that can cure babies who get AIDS from their mothers.	5	73	22
Doctors can help babies who have AIDS feel better and live longer.	33	53	14
Knowledge of Vertical Transmission			
A pregnant woman who has the AIDS virus can give AIDS to her baby.	98	1	1
If a pregnant woman's AIDS virus test comes back positive, it means that her baby will definitely have AIDS.	61	28	11
If a newborn's AIDS virus test is positive it means that the mother must be infected with the AIDS virus.	83	12	5
If a newborn's AIDS virus test is positive it means that the baby's father must be infected with the AIDS virus.	58	31	11
All newborns with a positive AIDS virus test are infected with the AIDS virus.	79	15	6

From Kass NE and others: Pregnant women's knowledge of the human immunodeficiency virus: implications for education and counseling, *Women Health Issues* 2:17-25, 1992.

showed a decrease in symptom severity and an increase in self-efficacy with opposite findings in the control group. The intervention included sessions of small group education (10 to 15 members) led by a PWA and a health professional. The self-care skills developed were interpreting and acting on symptoms; using and adhering to medication regimens, which are now very complex for these patients; dealing with fatigue, depression, and helplessness; communicating with providers; accessing services; and learning how to exercise, eat well, and prepare food. Role-playing and other forms of highly interactive teaching and modeling of those who have excellent self-management skills were used.[26] Besides education in caregiving skills, families need help in dealing with feelings of stigma and isolation, anger, the patient's dementia, and financial and legal concerns. They learn by rehearsing skills such as talking with their loved one about a living will.[58]

THE ELDERLY

Special teaching/learning demands of elderly persons have been incorporated into earlier chapters but are highlighted here. Staff must be alert to be sure that the training needs of these patients and their caregivers are adequately addressed. For example, unplanned hospital readmission within 30 days of discharge is considered a sentinel event for poor quality of teaching. Factors associated with this premature readmission include an age of 80 years or older, five or more comorbidities, lack of documented patient or family education, and a history of depression.[46] Patients who participate in programs that address these factors through validation of patient and care-

Box 10-4	*Content and Objectives of the Intervention**

Session 1. Recognition of Risk

1. Increase awareness that minorities are disproportionately affected by AIDS and other sexually transmitted diseases (diagrams). Discuss risk as a community problem related to poverty, not skin color.
2. Address myths. For African-American participants, address the belief that the human immunodeficiency virus was purposely planted in the African-American community.
3. Address the belief that disease is "dirty" and encourage acceptance of responsibility for infection. Begin building feelings of self-efficacy and power to control one's life.
4. Discuss the selection of sex partners, and show that there is no way to judge who is safe.
5. Provide information about sexually transmitted diseases: their transmission, behavior that increases the risk of acquisition, symptoms (color illustrations of signs and lesions), and consequences for women and fetuses.
6. Increase awareness of personal risk by associating the current sexually transmitted disease with future infection (including HIV). Emphasize the effect on families (videotapes of actual persons with AIDS).

Session 2. Commitment to Change

1. Provide information about the prevention of sexually transmitted diseases and the importance of early treatment, full compliance with treatment protocols, and observation of symptoms in partners. Discuss the avoidance of douching.
2. Particularly for African-American participants, extend the proscription against sharing eating utensils (to prevent disease) to a proscription against having unprotected sex.
3. Teach what to ask partners about current behavior and history.
4. Teach the use and erotic application of condoms (practice on plastic models of the penis).

5. Discuss barriers to condom use and how to overcome them.
6. Discuss what women want from a relationship, what they derive, and why they may tolerate poor behavior from partners. Discuss unprotected sex that results from misplaced trust and low self-esteem or from the desire to avoid conflict, violence, or loss of a partner. For African-American participants, discuss the dearth of available men.
7. Teach decision-making skills and emphasize that everyone has the power to make decisions (videotapes).

Session 3. Acquisition of Skills

1. Increase skills for communicating and negotiating about sex, particularly condom use, stressing ways to minimize threats to male self-esteem (videotapes, handouts, and discussion).
2. For Mexican-American participants, facilitate recognition that sexual enjoyment is appropriate for women. Discuss how to use the concept of "machismo" to convince men to be responsible lovers.
3. Teach basic skills to deal with sexual dysfunction resulting from condom use.
4. Raise feelings of self-efficacy in communication about condom use (videotapes and role play with a male facilitator).
5. Increase skills in erotic application of condoms through additional practice.
6. Identify and discuss triggers to unsafe sex.
7. Set goals.
8. Facilitate bonding and mutual support within the group.
9. Acknowledge problems of economic and physical survival (information on local resources).
10. Encourage the sharing of information with others to build a support network for risk reduction.

From Shain RN and others: A randomized controlled trial of a behavioral intervention to prevent sexually transmitted disease among minority women, *N Engl J Med* 340:93-100, 1999.
*Items shown in parentheses are examples of teaching materials or techniques.
AIDS, acquired immunodeficiency syndrome; *HIV,* human immunodeficiency virus.

giver learning, phone follow-up and coordination, and home services show significantly fewer readmissions and shorter length of stay than do control groups whose care, including subsequent hospitalizations, costs twice as much.[56]

Some education focuses on sustaining functioning. A significant body of research shows that memory training improves memory functioning (meta-analysis effect sizes of 0.66 and 0.73). This training uses follow-up (booster sessions).[49] Fall prevention education for community-dwelling elderly patients teaches exercise and home safety and develops fall prevention self-efficacy.[61]

Patient education for older adults offers several obvious challenges, but as yet has not developed into a full-fledged field of practice in terms of a research base and standards of practice. Much of the existing literature has focused on issues regarding learning, especially deficits in memory, increased cognitive response time, and sensory function declines with age. Perhaps an equally relevant focus should be on empowerment and self-management of disability. Researchers have reported significant correlations between autonomy, active involvement, achievement motivation, and health.[50]

Yet there is an inclination on the part of some professionals to use a paternalistic approach to care, thereby undermining older adults' autonomy. Older adults with a positive mindset (characterized by optimism, positive attitudes about self and self-care, and determination to remain independent) have been noted to remain independent despite the severity of their medical problems. The more paternalistic and biomedically oriented the professional, the greater the patient's perception of being misunderstood, which in turn undermines his or her self-confidence. On the other hand, one study shows that the health care professionals involved believed they had fulfilled their goals for care despite the patient's experience of threatened autonomy and undermined care goals.[51]

Clark and others[13] presented another perspective on the educational tasks for older adult patients. Many older adults face the need to successfully self-manage chronic illness, to make decisions about their care, to perform activities aimed at management of their condition, and to apply skills to maintain adequate psychosocial functioning. All these behaviors are aimed at decreasing the impact of disease on daily life. Table 10-7 shows typical self-management tasks for five common chronic illnesses.

Very few empirical data are available that address learning needs for older adults in managing multiple comorbidities, and frequently contradictory or confusing management advice is presented. For example, recommendations for a walking program after a coronary attack may conflict with management of arthritic hips and knees. Is the patient to aggravate one condition or avoid managing it? Multiple conditions can deplete physical and mental energy for coping. Little is known about how older adults are able to access and use large, complex health care systems.

Because 80% to 90% of persons with Alzheimer's disease are cared for in their homes by family members, these caregivers' needs for support and training are evident but are frequently not met. Patients with AD have cognitive losses (memory, time sense, inability to make choices or problem solve, poor judgment, and loss of language abilities) and affective or personality losses (emotional lability, loss of tact and control of temper, decreased attention span, social withdrawal, and antisocial behavior). Caregivers must learn behavior management techniques. They can also learn to deal with a patient's lowered stress threshold by modifying environmental demands such as noise or competing stimuli, pain, or fatigue, which cause the patient to become anxious or agitated. Caregivers learn to read these cues by loss of eye contact and the patient becoming dysfunctional. Caregivers particularly need help in simplifying day-to-day tasks such as bathing and dressing.[23]

END STAGE RENAL DISEASE (ESRD)

Education of patients and caregivers to provide home dialysis was for a long time an essential part of the management of ESRD. Today dialysis is provided in centers. Some necessary education

TABLE 10-7	Common Self-Management Tasks for Five Chronic Diseases

Tasks	Heart Disease	Asthma	Arthritis	COPD	Diabetes
Recognizing and responding to symptoms, monitoring physical indicators, controlling triggers to symptoms	X	X		X	X
Using medicine	X	X	X	X	X
Managing acute episodes and emergencies	X	X	X		X
Maintaining nutrition and diet	X		X	X	X
Maintaining adequate exercise/activity	X	X	X	X	X
Giving up smoking	X	X	X	X	X
Using relaxation and stress-reducing techniques	X	X	X		
Interacting with health care providers	X	X			X
Seeking information and using community services		X	X		X
Adapting to work	X	X	X		
Managing relations with significant others	X	X	X	X	
Managing emotions and psychological responses to illness	X	X	X		X

From Clark NM and others: Self-management of chronic disease of older adults, *J Aging Health* 3:3-27, 1991.
COPD, chronic obstructive pulmonary disease; *X*, reported in a study of self-management.

remains the same—diet modification for example. Patients need basic skills to meet their protein goal, including keeping a food record, weighing and measuring protein portions, and identifying grams of protein. Lipo[43] identifies optimal teaching strategies to attain this goal: modeling of the correct behavior with demonstrations of cooking techniques; taste testing; visiting restaurants; role-playing new behaviors; and using motivational techniques such as follow-up phone calls, incentives, and feedback to patients about how they are doing. As evaluation techniques patients are asked to write down their lunch menus for the next day with the new goal for protein intake or to show the provider how much 3 ounces of a food is. The fact that sample renal educational materials available in this setting had an average reading level of eleventh grade is unfortunate but not surprising.

In the year 2000 it is expected that more than 50% of patients undergoing dialysis will be elderly. Badzek, Hines, and Moss[2] found that a majority of these patients lacked information needed for self-care and that many had diminished cognitive capacity, which can be associated both with renal failure and with advanced age. Educational programs will need to adjust to these demographic characteristics by adopting teaching methods that are repetitive and ongoing. Initiating advance care planning education as soon as dialysis begins will also be important, as many of these patients will eventually lack decision-making capacity.

Predialysis education is perhaps the newest development in this field. Although only 20% to 25% of patients are referred to a nephrologist before dialysis, predialysis programs can help with planning a timely instead of a catastrophic move to dialysis and assist with patient choice of options of no treatment or various renal replacement therapies.[42] Predialysis education programs can also focus on diet and fluid restrictions, on exercise training, and on dealing with the psychosocial impact of chronic renal failure.

A trial found that patients receiving one such intervention had a better mood and experienced less anxiety and functional disability than did patients in the control group. An important goal of such programs is for the patient to attain as high a quality of life as possible, and predialysis programs should be followed by other educational programs as the patient starts dialysis.[37] Apparently, patient education for the early to middle stages of renal disease and for patients in transition to renal replacement therapy are still unusual. Several studies have shown that patients who receive this education have the potential to delay the initiation of ESRD treatment and a better potential for rehabilitation, in addition to decreased cost of treatment and decreased hospital time at initiation of treatment. Early education is believed to be appropriate for patients with a creatinine clearance of 50 to 80 ml/min. After the cause of renal disease is established and treated, the educational approach should focus on methods to delay progressive deterioration of renal function.[32]

GENETIC TESTING

The mapping of the human genome has resulted in expansion of genetic screening for conditions such as breast cancer, colon cancer, cardiovascular diseases, and Alzheimer's disease in addition to the increased use of screening in prenatal care as described in Chapter 8. These tests are now heavily marketed to primary care providers, but it is clear that the expansion of this field has hardly begun and will dramatically increase the need for competent patient education. This is perhaps especially true because it is not uncommon for providers to misinterpret test results, and it is difficult for patients to understand the concepts of probability, false-positives or false-negatives, and incomplete penetrance.[12]

As a field, genetic counseling has developed a tradition of nondirective counseling drawn from the fields of psychoanalysis and psychodynamic therapy. Directive counseling is believed to be a form of persuasive coercion as is spending more time on one option or on its negative or positive aspects. Against a historical backdrop of the eugenics movement, it is especially important in this field to promote client autonomy and self-directedness. Genetic counseling is very labor intensive and expensive. Genetics education is necessary for the large numbers of people who may be considering being screened or who need to manage risks identified by screening. It is also combined with genetic counseling in clinical situations. Both genetic counseling and education should serve to provide a framework by which clients might think through the problem facing them and arrive at their own decisions.[36]

Some beginning work in testing the comparative effectiveness of educational and counseling interventions has been done. Cystic fibrosis (CF) provides a good example. Because almost 500 different mutations that can cause CF have been described to date, general population carrier screening cannot detect all carriers. The usual screening practice focuses on the six most common mutations, which detects fewer than 85% of carriers who have a Northern European background, and a lower percentage of individuals from other backgrounds. The limitations of screening require strong education.[14] Both video and written approaches can work.

Chevront and others[10] tested the comparative efficacy for relatives of persons with CF of pretest education and genetic testing in a clinical setting from a certified genetic counselor versus pretest education delivered in patients' homes which required them to send in a buccal sample for testing. These two interventions were equally effective on measures of knowledge, anxiety, and affect. This kind of research helps to provide answers about effective ways to reach large numbers of individuals who will need genetic education.

NEUROLOGICAL ILLNESSES

For some neurological illnesses there is a long history of patient education; for others there is a new focus on it. For example, educational materials about low back pain are commonly available, usually following the traditional biomedical model of knowledge of spinal anatomy, biomechanics, and pathological changes; avoidance of activities that aggravate pain; good posture; and back-specific exercises including bending and lifting.[8] These materials and skills may also be taught through back schools or as programs in primary care settings, focused on prevention of back injury or relieving pain once injury is present. Ongoing concern about the efficacy of this treatment is supported by a recent study. In a randomized controlled trial of education to prevent low back injury among 4000 postal workers, Daltroy and others[16] found no reduction in the rate of low back injury or time off from work for this problem.

Literature on the learning needs of individuals with spinal cord injury is limited and focuses primarily on inpatient rehabilitation. Ongoing educational programs to address the issues faced by these patients should include how to prevent or manage bladder and kidney problems, pain and spasticity, bowel problems, pressure ulcers, contractures, and autonomic dysreflexia; fertility and family planning issues; exercise and nutrition; weight control; and stress reduction.[29]

A million people in the United States have Parkinson's disease, which slowly progresses over 5 to 20 years or more. Patients must learn compensation techniques such as new methods for getting in and out of bed and chairs, using the bathroom, and navigating stairs and uneven floor surfaces.[66] Other examples of areas of patient education practice that require developing are readily available. An initial study of education for patients with Parkinson's disease focused on improving functional outcomes by using an educational strategy that sought to improve self-efficacy and optimism.[52] Results showed decreases in visits to physicians, hospital days, and sick days, as well as stabilization of symptoms in the intervention group.

The literature documents that in many chronic diseases long-term patient outcomes are affected by factors such as exercise, lifestyle, risk factors, side effects of medications and their management, interaction with comorbid disease conditions, social and spousal support, depression,[22] and self-efficacy. Many of these are potentially amenable to patient education interventions and have been successfully altered both in patients with other disease states and in normal subjects.

Among persons with epilepsy, 60% to 75% will become free of seizures with appropriate treatment. The patient must learn how to: maintain antiepileptic drug therapy; avoid factors that precipitate seizure activity; and keep a complete seizure calendar (description of seizure activity, missed medicine doses and adverse effect, potential precipitating factors, and concomitant medications or illnesses). Safety and first aid, driving, pregnancy and parenting issues also must be addressed.[30]

Finally, each year hundreds of thousands of Americans sustain mild traumatic brain injuries (TBIs). It is not uncommon for these patients to have attention/concentration problems for several weeks, months, or longer after the injury. Many patients who seem "normal" at discharge later experience headaches, dizziness, blurred vision, slow or foggy thinking, memory problems, depression, anxiety, and decreased tolerance for frustration. Many patients and families do not receive education about the meaning of these symptoms or how to manage them.[41] Those with more severe TBIs who require intensive care and eventually rehabilitation, also require family education at each stage, including management of patient behavioral and emotional changes. Such education should contribute to prevention of decompensation in the vulnerable family.[33]

SUMMARY

This chapter describes areas of patient education practice that range from those that are just developing to those with a stable research base, the findings of which should be widely applied in practice. Yet there are many other patient problems for which education could be very useful. The postscript that follows Chapter 11 and summarizes Part II of this book further details some of these opportunities.

Box 10-5 | *Goals for Teaching Home Mechanical Ventilation Care*

1. Maintain Clear Airway

Education related to:
Tracheostomy care, suctioning, tube change
Signs of infection
Proper hydration for thin, clear secretions
Chest physiotherapy and augmented cough
Medication administration bronchodilators
  and antibiotics
Mobility

**2. Maintain Adequate Oxygenation
and Ventilation**

Education related to:
Proper use and maintenance of mechanical
  ventilator
Use of manual resuscitation bag
In-line nebulized medications

**3. Perform Skills to Maintain Cleanliness
and Maximum Strength and Flexibility**

Education related to:
Bathing, shampooing, shaving
Mouth care
Management of bowel and bladder
  elimination
Range of motion, strength and flexibility
  exercises

**4. Prevent Irritation, Infection, and Skin
Breakdown**

Education related to:
Turning, positioning
Transfer, ambulation
Tracheostomy stoma care, PEG site care

5. Maintain Adequate Nutrition and Hydration

Education related to:
Feeding
Flushing, declogging tube
Assessing hydration/dehydration
Recognizing and dealing with diarrhea and
  constipation

**6. Maintain Effective Coping with Home Care
for Both Patient and Caregivers**

Education related to:
Recognition of coping skills found to be useful
  in past experiences
Communication
Resources for counseling, networking with
  others
Other care options available

From Glass C, Grap MJ, Battle G: Preparing the patient and family for home mechanical ventilation, *MedSurg Nurs* 8: 99-107, 1999.
PEG, percutaneous endoscopic gastrostomy.

 Study Questions

1. A survey of 25 leaflets and fact sheets on prostatectomy found that while only 6 discussed the possible changes in sexual sensation after transurethral resection of the prostate, 35% of patients reported a change and 12% were worried about it.[51] Why would you be concerned about this?

2. Home mechanical ventilation has emerged as a method for treating chronic stable respiratory failure, particularly from neuromuscular disease. Families spend an average of 11 hours a day providing care, which includes maintaining adequate caloric intake and a workable bowel program, responding to alarms, and developing skills for cleaning the ventilator, performing manual resuscitation in case of equipment shutdown, preventing aspiration, etc. Box 10-5 describes goals for teaching home mechanical ventilation care.[28] Critique this plan.

References

1. Badger TA: Living with depression, *J Psychosoc Nurs* 34:21-29, 1996.

2. Badzek L, Hines SC, Moss AH: Inadequate self-care knowledge among elderly hemodialysis patients: assessing its prevalence and potential causes, *ANNA J* 25:293-300, 1998.

3. Bandura A: Perceived self-efficacy in the exercise of control over AIDS infection, *Eval Program Plann* 13:9-17, 1990.

4. Bondy LR and others: The effect of patient education on preoperative patient anxiety, *Regl Anesth Pain Med* 24:158-164, 1999.

5. Brennan PF, Ripich S: Use of a home-care computer network by persons with AIDS, *Int J Technol Assess Health Care* 10:258-272, 1994.

6. Burke LE, Dunbar-Jacob J: Adherence to medication, diet, and activity recommendations: from assessment to maintenance, *J Cardiovasc Nurs* 9:62-79, 1995.

7. Burnside B, Hodgins G: The role of education in a program to treat depression in older women, *Educ Gerontol* 18:483-496, 1992.

8. Burton AK and others: Patient educational material in the management of low back pain in primary care, *Bull Hosp Jt Dis* 55:138-141, 1996.

9. Cason CL, Russell DG, Fincher SB: Preparatory sensory information for cardiac catheterization, *Cardiovasc Nurs* 28:41-45, 1992.

10. Chevront B and others: Psychosocial and educational outcomes associated with home- and clinic-based pretest education and cystic fibrosis carrier testing among a population of at-risk relatives, *Am J Med Genet* 75:461-468, 1998.

11. Chewitt MA, Fallis WM, Suski MC: The surgical hotline, *J Nurs Adm* 27(12):42-49, 1997.

12. Cho MK, Arruda M, Holtzman NA: Educational material about genetic tests, *Am J Med Genet* 73:314-320, 1997.

13. Clark NM and others: Self-management of chronic disease of older adults, *J Aging Health* 3:3-27, 1991.

14. Clayton EW and others: Teaching about cystic fibrosis carrier screening by using written and video information, *Am J Hum Genet* 57:171-181, 1995.

15. Daley DC, Bowler K, Cahalane H: Approaches to patient and family education with affective disorders, *Patient Educ Counsel* 19:163-174, 1992.

16. Daltroy LH and others: A controlled trial of an educational program to prevent low back injuries, *N Engl J Med* 337:322-328, 1997.

17. Davis TMA and others: Preparing adult patients for cardiac catheterization: informational treatment and coping style interactions, *Heart Lung* 23:130-139, 1994.

18. Devine EC: Effects of psychoeducational care for adult surgical patients: a meta-analysis of 191 studies, *Patient Educ Counsel* 19:129-142, 1992.

19. Done ML, Lee A: The use of a video to convey preanesthetic information to patients undergoing ambulatory surgery, *Anesth Analg* 87:531-536, 1998.

20. Farran CJ, Keane-Hagerty E: Interventions for caregivers of persons with dementia: educational support groups and Alzheimer's Association support groups, *Appl Nurs Res* 7:112-117, 1994.

21. Garvin BJ, Huston GP, Baker CF: Information used by nurses to prepare patients for a stressful event, *Appl Nurs Res* 5:158-163, 1992.

22. Gavard JA, Lustman PJ, Clouse RE: Prevalence of depression in adults with diabetes, *Diabetes Care* 16:1167-1178, 1993.

23. Gerdner LA, Hall GR, Buckwalter KC: Caregiving training for people with Alzheimer's based on a stress threshold model, *Image* 28:241-246, 1996.

24. Getty C, Perese E, Knaub S: Capacity for self-care of persons with mental illnesses living in community residences and the ability of their surrogate families to perform health care functions. *Issues Ment Health Nurs* 19:53-70, 1998.

25. Gielen AC and others: Women's protective sexual behaviors: a test of the health belief model, *AIDS Educ Prev* 6:1-11, 1994.

26. Gifford AL and others: Pilot randomized trial of education to improve self-management skills of men with symptomatic HIV/AIDs, *J Acquir Immune Defic Syndr Hum Retrovirol* 18:136-144, 1998.

27. Girard N: Anesthesia and learning: the mind-body connection, *Semin Perioper Nurs* 3:121-133, 1994.

28. Glass C, Grap MJ, Battle G: Preparing the patient and family for home mechanical ventilation, *Med-Surg Nurs* 8:99-107, 1999.

29. Hart KA, Rintala DH, Fuhrer JM: Educational interests of individuals with spinal cord injury living in the community: medical, sexuality and wellness topics, *Rehabil Nurs* 21(2):82-90, 1996.

30. Hausman SV and others: Epilepsy education: a nursing perspective, *Mayo Clin Proc* 71:1114-1117, 1996.

31. Hayes R, Gantt A: Patient psychoeducation: the therapeutic use of knowledge for the mentally ill, *Soc Work Health Care* 17:53-67, 1992.

32. Hayslip DM, Suttle CD: Pre-ESRD patient education: a review of the literature, *Adv Ren Replace Ther* 2:217-226, 1995.

33. Holland D, Shigaki CL: Educating families and caretakers of traumatically brain injured patients in the new health care environment: a three phase model and bibliography, *Brain Inj* 12:993-1009, 1998.

34. Holmes H and others: Nursing model of psychoeducation for the seriously mentally ill patient, *Issues Ment Health Nurs* 15:85-104, 1994.

35. Kass NE and others: Pregnant women's knowledge of the human immunodeficiency virus: implications for education and counseling, *Women Health Issues* 2:17-25, 1992.

36. Kessler S: Psychological aspects of genetic counseling. IX. Nondirectiveness revisited, *Am J Med Genet* 72:164-171, 1997.

37. Klang B and others: Predialysis patient education: effects on functioning and well-being in uraemic patients, *J Adv Nurs* 28:36-44, 1998.

38. Knoerl D and others: Preoperative PCA teaching program to manage postoperative pain, *MedSurg Nurs* 8:25-33, 36, 1999.

39. Kukill WA and others: Causes of death associated with Alzheimer disease: variation by level of cognitive impairment before death, *J Am Geriatr Soc* 42:723-726, 1994.

40. Landsvert SS, Kane CR: Antonovsky's sense of coherence: theoretical basis of psychoeducation in schizophrenia, *Issues Ment Health Nurs* 19:419-431, 1998.

41. Lawler KA, Terregino CA: Guidelines for evaluation and education of adult patients with mild traumatic brain injuries in acute care hospital setting, *J Head Trauma Rehabil* 11(6):18-28, 1996.

42. Levin A and others: Multidisciplinary predialysis programs: quantification and limitations of their impact on patient outcomes in two Canadian settings, *Am J Kidney Dis* 29:533-540, 1997.

43. Lipo J: Teaching pre-end stage renal disease patients, *Top Clin Nutr* 12(1):51-56, 1996.

44. Macpherson R, Jerrom B, Hughes A: A controlled study of education about drug treatment in schizophrenia, *Br J Psychiatry* 168:709-717, 1996.

45. Madoff SA and others: Computerized medication instruction for psychiatric inpatients admitted for acute care, *MD Comput* 13:427-441, 1996.

46. Marcantonio ER and others: Factors associated with unplanned hospital readmission among patients 65 years of age and older in a Medicare managed care plan, *Am J Med* 107:13-17, 1999.

47. May KM, Evans GG: Health education for homeless populations, *J Community Health Nurs* 11:229-237, 1994.

48. Maynard C: Psychoeducational approach to depression in women, *J Psychosoc Nurs* 31(12):9-14, 1993.

49. McDougall GJ Jr: Cognitive interventions among older adults. *Annu Rev Nurs Res* 17:219-240, 1999.

50. McWilliam CL and others: A new perspective on threatened autonomy in elderly persons: the disempowering process, *Soc Sci Med* 38:327-338, 1994.

51. Meredith P and others: Comparison of patients' needs for information on prostate surgery with printed materials provided by surgeons, *Qual Health Care* 4:18-23, 1994.

52. Montgomery EB and others: Patient education and health promotion can be effective in Parkinson's disease: a randomized controlled trial, *Am J Med* 97:429-435, 1994.

53. Morris LA, Tabak ER, Gondek K: Counseling patients about prescribed medication: 12 year trends, *Med Care* 35:996-1007, 1997.

54. Morris LS, Schulz RM: Patient compliance—an overview, *J Clin Pharmacol Ther* 17:283-295, 1992.

55. Mumford E, Schlesinger HJ, Glass GV: The effects of psychological intervention on recovery from surgery and heart attacks: an analysis of the literature, *Am J Public Health* 72:141-151, 1982.

56. Naylor MD and others: Comprehensive discharge planning and home follow-up of hospitalized elders, *JAMA* 281:613-620, 1999.

57. Perry A and others: Randomised controlled trial of efficacy of teaching patients with bipolar disorder to identify early symptoms of relapse and obtain treatment, *Br Med J* 318:149-153, 1999.

58. Pomeroy EC, Rubin A, Alker RJ: A psychoeducational group intervention for family members of persons with HIV/AIDs, *Fam Process* 35:299-312, 1996.

59. Posavac EJ and others: Increasing compliance to medical treatment regimens: a meta-analysis of program evaluation, *Eval Health Prof* 8:7-22, 1985.

60. Roach JA, Tremblay LM, Bowers DL: A preoperative assessment and education program: implementation and outcomes, *Patient Educ Counsel* 25:83-88, 1995.

61. Schoenfelder DP, Van Why K: A fall prevention program for community dwelling elders, *Public Health Nurs* 14:383-390, 1997.

62. Shain RN and others: A randomized controlled trial of a behavioral intervention to prevent sexually transmitted disease among minority women, *N Engl J Med* 340:93-100, 1999.

63. Shimada J and others: "Strong medicine": Cambodian views of medicine and medical compliance, *J Gen Intern Med* 10:369-374, 1995.

64. Steiner J, Lussier R, Rosenblatt W: Knowledge about risk factors for AIDS in a day hospital population, *Hosp Community Psychiatry* 43:734-735, 1992.

65. Timmons ME, Bower FL: The effect of structured preoperative teaching on patients' use of patient-controlled analgesia (PCA) and their management of pain, *Orthop Nurs* 12:23-31, 1993.

66. Vickers LF: An interdisciplinary home healthcare program for patients with Parkinson's disease, *Rehabil Nurs* 23:286-299, 1998.

67. Wells JA and others: Literacy of women attending family planning clinics in Virginia and reading levels of brochures on HIV prevention, *Fam Plann Perspect* 26:113-115, 131, 1994.

68. Wholihan D: A patient education tool for patient-controlled analgesia, *Oncol Nurs Forum* 24:1801-1804, 1997.

69. Wingerd JL, Page JB: HIV testing among Haitian women: lessons in the recognition of risk, *Health Educ Behav* 24:736-745, 1997.

Patient Education and Health Policy

Over the years patient education has been commonly regarded as a private matter between provider and patient, usually physician and patient, because for many years this was the only relationship acknowledged to have the authority to provide information to patients. This chapter addresses the development of public policy that is increasing pressures on providers to be responsible for delivering information to patients. The policy mechanisms used are varied—incentives, threat of direct regulation if providers do not voluntarily fulfill their role in informing patients, and potential sanctions attached to institutions in which providers practice.

The ultimate question is whether these mechanisms of public policy work to ensure that patients obtain the information and skills they need. These efforts are part of a slow trend toward support of patient autonomy—enabling patients to make their own decisions—and away from the paternalistic culture of the medical profession in which all information flow to patients is controlled according to medical values. Because patient education falls outside the biomedical model, it has been viewed as discretionary and marginal. Increasingly, those who make public policy see it otherwise. Indeed, a growing body of research focused on investigating the

relationship between education and health suggests lack of education as a significant risk factor for poor health.

REGULATION OF HEALTH INFORMATION

The following examples illustrate policy mechanisms being used in the attempt to ensure that patients receive appropriate education.

National Introduction of Diabetes Teaching Programs in Germany

Although patient education has been widely accepted as an integral part of diabetes therapy for years, in many countries only a very limited number of persons with non–insulin-dependent diabetes mellitus (NIDDM) receive adequate structured education. In the United States a long struggle has taken place to arrange reimbursement for provision of diabetes education as a professional service.

Since 1991 nearly all German insurance funds cover physician fees for structured diabetes education programs and provide reimbursement for the costs of teaching materials provided to patients. A prerequisite for this remuneration is completion of a specific postgraduate training course by both the physician and the office staff. Figure 11-1 shows the organization of the program's implementation. The training course for office-based physicians and their staffs follows the guidelines developed by the German Diabetes Association. It includes microteaching of techniques and preparation in basic methods of adult education. Although each team pays a significant fee for the seminar, by April 1995 more than 13,000 physicians and their staffs had participated in the training courses. Most teaching of patients is delivered by nonphysician providers, and programs for patients are similar to those described in Chapter 7.[3]

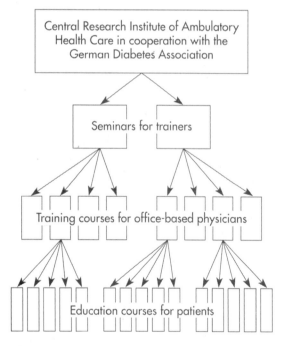

Figure 11-1 Organization of nationwide implementation of structured treatment and education program for NIDDM patients in Germany. Central Institute is responsible for quality control and organization for trainer seminars for trainers (diabetologists and their diabetes educators) (1.5 days). (From Joergens V, Gruesser M: Three years' experience after national introduction of teaching programs for type II diabetic patients in Germany: how to train general practitioners, *Patient Educ Counsel* 26:195-202, 1995.)

Initial evaluation of this program showed that, after provider participation, the quality of diabetes care improved substantially: significant weight reduction occurred in patients, a relevant decrease of the prescription of oral antidiabetic agents was achieved, and metabolic control improved significantly. Cost savings in the care of persons with diabetes are expected as a result of decreases in rates of amputation, diabetic coma, and hospitalization. The number of patients participating in the program is to be monitored throughout Germany.[3]

Information About Advanced Directives

The Patient Self-Determination Act (PSDA), passed by the U.S. Congress in 1991, requires health care institutions that receive Medicare funds to inform patients at the time of admission about their rights and privileges in connection with life-support measures. Advance directives (ADs), such as living wills and durable powers of attorney for health care, are seen as ways for patients to provide direction to caregivers if patients should not be able to speak for themselves. Under the PSDA, provider organizations also are required to document whether patients have ADs, to implement policies to recognize ADs, and to educate their staff and communities about them.

The assumption underlying the PSDA is that persons will execute ADs if they are given sufficient information and encouragement. A growing body of research indicates that this assumption is simplistic. For example, persons older than 60 years are not executing ADs in significant numbers despite high levels of familiarity and understanding. Intervention studies have been shown to produce modest increases in use of ADs.[2] Yet the desired outcome from the AD movement is to help patients to knowledgeably make their own decisions about whether to have an AD and, if so, what to put in it.

Patients and families frequently need time to deal with losses and with conflicts among family members. There is a belief that providers will abandon patients with ADs at some level. At the time of admission patients are often anxious, in pain, and depressed and cannot attend to information about ADs. In reality, many people need a teaching/counseling process to assist them with the decision about whether to develop an AD and what it will say. They need repeated explanations and discussions of options with a health care provider, as opposed to being informed by an admitting clerk that they can have an AD. It should be acknowledged that some patients defer action because their present perceived state of affairs does not urgently call for an AD or they are confident that they can rely on others and prefer the informality of decision making by family members. Indeed, intensive interventions, including repeated efforts to persuade patients to complete an AD, could be seen as coercive.

Box 11-1 provides an example of a comprehension test for ADs, cardiopulmonary resuscitation, and artificial nutrition and hydration. An understanding of these issues is important to support end-of-life decision making. Responses to open-ended questions were recorded verbatim.[5] What are the implicit learning objectives represented by this test? Is the questionnaire complete in testing the skills represented in the implicit objectives? What is the usefulness of such an instrument? Would you use it clinically?

Information About Prescription Drugs

Although information about prescription drugs has been regulated for a long time, recent trends reflect stronger efforts to ensure that patients receive relevant information. Two recent lines of regulation reflect this goal. The first is directed toward pharmacists, and the second is directed at the manufacturers of prescription drugs.

The Omnibus Reconciliation Act of 1990 (OBRA '90) contains several regulations regarding prescription drugs, including requiring pharmacists to offer counseling about these medications to patients whose care is funded by Medicaid. In fact, most states have adopted requirements for pharmacists to counsel all patients. In some instances written counseling is sufficient. The following information is to be included: route; dosage; duration; special direc-

tions and precautions; common severe side effects, adverse effects, or interactions (including their avoidance and action required if they occur); techniques for self-monitoring drug therapy; storage; and action to be taken in the event of a missed dose.[4]

For many years the Food and Drug Administration (FDA) has regulated written information that comes with prescription drugs, known as patient package inserts (PPIs). As recently as the 1960s, physicians were viewed as the sole dispensers of such information. In 1980 the FDA proposed, on a pilot basis, a regulation that required mandatory patient information for 10 drugs or classes of drugs. Many physicians, pharmacists, and drug manufacturers opposed this program, contending that it would encourage self-diagnosis, produce adverse reactions in patients through suggestion, adversely affect liability of health care providers and manufacturers, interfere with the physician-patient relationship, impose unnecessary burdens on manufacturers and pharmacists, and increase the costs of prescription drug products.[6]

The FDA suggested that PPIs could reduce inappropriate drug use and promote their optimal use. The proposed regulations requiring PPIs for most prescription drug products were revoked in 1982, with the expectation that the private sector would voluntarily distribute patient information. Such programs for distribution of drug information currently exist through physician organizations, the American Association of Retired Persons, and the United States Pharmacopeia.[6] In August of 1995 the FDA again proposed regulations for prescription drug labeling and medication guide requirements. The thrust of these regulations was to require standards for drug distribution and quality, to enhance patients' ability to understand the benefits and risks of treatment, and to use the drugs effectively. The voluntary program endorsed in the 1980s is judged to have made minimal progress in improving the distribution of drug information to patients. The information that actually reaches most patients is found to focus primarily on how to use the medication, with little precautionary

Box 11-1   *Patient Comprehension Questionnaire*

(a) Open-ended and
(b) Yes-or-No Questions

1. (a) What is an advance medical directive (often called a living will)?
   (b) Does an advance medical directive:
      Indicate a person's wishes about medical treatments?*
      Indicate the physician's opinions about medical treatments?

2. (a) When is the information a patient provides in the advance medical directive used?
   (b) Is the information a patient provides in the advance medical directive used when the patient:
      Enters the hospital for routine surgery?
      Comes for a routine check-up?
      Is unable to communicate?*
      Is unable to make decisions?*

3. (a) Why is the advance medical directive important?
   (b) Is the advance medical directive important because:
      It serves as a guide for family, friends, and physicians?*
      It helps with planning preventive health care measures?

4. (a) When is cardiopulmonary resuscitation (CPR) used?
   (b) Do physicians use CPR when:
      A patient has a stroke?
      A patient stops breathing?*
      A patient's heart stops beating?*
      A patient has dizziness?

5. (a) When physicians give CPR, what exactly do they do?
   (b) Does CPR involve:
      Giving the patient medications through an IV?
      Pressing on the patient's chest?*
      Bandaging the patient's chest?

Giving the patient artificial breathing?*
Taking x-rays of the patient's chest?
Giving the patient an electric shock?*
Measuring brain waves?
Inserting a heart catheter?

6. (a) What is artificial breathing?
   (b) Does artificial breathing involve:
      Providing oxygen through a face mask?
      Insertion of a tube into a windpipe?*
      Connecting the patient to a breathing machine?*
      Asking the patient to breathe rapidly?

7. (a) What is artificial feeding and fluids?
   (b) Is artificial feeding and fluids:
      A kind of antibiotic?
      A form of nourishment?*

8. (a) When do patients need to receive artificial feeding and fluids?
   (b) Do patients need to receive artificial feeding and fluids when:
      They are unable to eat or swallow enough food to stay alive?*
      They have a pain in their stomach?

9. (a) How are artificial feeding and fluids given to a patient?
   (b) Are artificial feeding and fluids given to patients:
      As a pill?
      Through a tube?*
   (c) Can artificial feeding and fluids be given to a patient through a tube that goes:
      Into a vein?*
      Into the liver?
      Into the lung?
      Through the skin to the stomach?*
      Through a catheter to the bladder?
      From the nose to the stomach?

From Moore KA and others: Elderly outpatients' understanding of a physician-initiated advance directive discussion, *Arch Fam Med* 3:1057-1063, 1994.
*Indicates the correct response is yes.

Box 11-2	*Socioeconomic Status and Health—Possible Mediational Variables Based on Personal Health Behaviors and Psychological and Cognitive Constructs*

PERSONAL HEALTH BEHAVIORS	PSYCHOLOGICAL AND COGNITIVE CONSTRUCTS
Diet and nutrition	Social support
Exercise	Anxiety
Smoking	Depression
Seat belt use	Health locus of control
Life stresses	Learned helplessness
Efficiency in use of medical services	Sense of coherence
Health insurance status	Self-efficacy
Use of preventive medical services	Optimism
Coping skills	Time preference
Problem-solving skills	Health knowledge

From Pincus T, Callahan LF: Associations of low formal education level and poor health status: behavioral, in addition to demographic and medical explanations? *J Clin Epidemiol* 47:355-361, 1994.

or adverse drug information, and it varies highly in quality.[1]

Time will tell whether the same objections raised two decades ago will be overcome in a political climate that favors giving patients wider access to drug information.

RELATIONSHIP BETWEEN EDUCATION AND HEALTH

Associations between higher socioeconomic status (SES) and better health have been reported for more than 150 years. Formal education is one component of SES, correlated with income and occupation, as well as with working and living conditions. Box 11-2 lists possible mediational variables in this relationship. Low educational attainment is associated with high levels of infectious disease, many chronic noninfectious diseases, self-reported poor health, shorter survival when sick, and shorter life expectancy.[7] Those who have analyzed these relationships conclude that high educational attainment improves health directly through development of skills and information to help people deal with the stresses of life and indirectly through engendering a sense of personal control.[8]

Perhaps because the standard medical model does not incorporate these elements, they have been neglected. Related to the psychological and cognitive constructs listed in Box 11-2 is the serious impact of lack of functional literacy on the receipt of proper health care. The entire health care system assumes adequate literacy skills, for example, to read and understand labels on medication containers, appointment slips, informed consent documents, health education materials, health insurance forms, and instructions pertaining to diagnostic tests. More specifically, those skills might include knowing how to take a medication four times a day, how to take a drug on an empty stomach, how many pills of a prescription should be taken, how many times a prescription can be refilled, or when the next appointment is scheduled. If patients cannot understand the forms, low literacy may also be an access barrier to receiving Medicaid assistance.[9]

This constellation of skills might be called functional health literacy—the ability to use reading, writing, and computational skills at a level adequate to meet the needs of everyday situations. Functional literacy varies by context and setting; the literacy skills of a patient might be adequate at home or at work but marginal or inadequate in a health care setting. A study of two urban public hospitals found that many patients (20% to 60%) lack some of these skills.[9] In a Los Angeles public hospital, 11% of English-speaking and 33% of Spanish-speaking patients could not read well enough to understand preparation instructions—written at a fourth-grade level—for an upper gastrointestinal tract radiographic procedure. In an Atlanta public hospital, 43% of patients could not fully comprehend the "Rights and Responsibilities" section of the Medicaid application.

Patients are frequently discharged from a clinic and given only brief oral instructions, with health care providers assuming that they can read and understand important materials such as prescription bottles and appointment slips. This incorrect assumption certainly results in poorer health outcomes or adverse reactions among patients with low literacy skills. The problem is particularly acute among older adult patients. In the two public hospitals cited in the preceding paragraph, 48% to 81% of patients aged 60 years or older had inadequate functional health literacy.[9]

Thus adults with limited literacy face formidable problems in using the health care system. Even though appropriate availability of information and the opportunity to use it have increasingly been regulated, the needs of this group have not been seriously incorporated into mainstream health practice or the regulations governing it; nor have any measures been enforced. For example, the FDA's proposed rules for medication guide requirements do not address the extent of low literacy or illiteracy among the population.[1]

In our literacy-dependent society, lack of adequate patient education available to all the people we serve should be seen as a serious remediable deficit—a lack that stands in the way of achieving the health care outcomes and contributes to what many see as unjust differences among social classes.

SUMMARY

Slowly, but not very surely, patient education is moving from being perceived as a private matter managed by a patient's provider to being regulated by public policy. This chapter has provided several examples of the growing governmental regulation of this field, as well as highlighting an area in which well-designed and enforced regulation might serve to improve health care outcomes and ensure their more just distribution.

References

1. Department of Health and Human Services, Food and Drug Administration: Prescription drug product labeling; medication guide requirements; proposed rule, 21 Code of Federal Regulations Part 201, *Fed Regis* 60:44182-44252, 1995.
2. High DM: Advance directives and the elderly: a study of intervention strategies to increase use, *Gerontologist* 33:342-349, 1993.
3. Joergens V, Gruesser M: Three years' experience after national introduction of teaching programs for type II diabetic patients in Germany: how to train general practitioners, *Patient Educ Counsel* 26:195-202, 1995.
4. Molzon JA: What kinds of patient counseling are required? *Am Pharm* NS32(3):50-57, 1992.
5. Moore KA and others: Elderly outpatients' understanding of a physician-initiated advance directive discussion, *Arch Fam Med* 3:1057-1063, 1994.
6. Nightingale SL: Written patient information on prescription drugs, *Int J Technol Assess Health Care* 11:399-409, 1995.
7. Pincus T, Callahan LF: Associations of low formal education level and poor health status: behavioral, in addition to demographic and medical explanations? *J Clin Epidemiol* 47:355-361, 1994.
8. Ross CE, Wu C: The links between education and health, *Am Soc Rev* 60:719-745, 1995.
9. Williams MV and others: Inadequate functional health literacy among patients at two public hospitals, *JAMA* 274:1677-1682, 1995.

Postscript to Part II and New Directions

Chapters 5 through 10 describe the best-developed areas of patient education practice, and Chapter 11 addresses the pressures in public policy to ensure that essential information reaches patients. The obvious question—How well are we doing in patient education?—is never asked. A review of these chapters elicits several observations and new directions for the field.

1. In most instances, minority populations are heavily burdened by the diseases around which these educational programs have been organized. Yet we know very little about cultural models and educational approaches that are most effective with these populations.
2. Nearly all the indirect evidence available indicates that patient education is not accessible to significant portions of the population. Although the problem has been documented for a long time, persons with low or no literacy must be presumed to have very little access to the large number of printed materials used.
3. Each field of practice in patient education has developed with different strengths rather than according to some grand model. All deal with self-

management. For example, cancer education focuses on self-assessment, especially breast self-examination, monitoring of symptoms, and pain management. Cardiac education focuses heavily on alteration of risk factors. Structures for quality management also differ. Diabetes education has opportunities both for accreditation of programs and certification of practitioners. In asthma and arthritis education, standardized tested programs have been developed.
4. What patients need to learn has little to do with what is instructionally possible, but rather with how the medical system is organized to deliver care. Almost no focus on longitudinal learning over a lifetime or over the course of self-management of a health care problem yet exists. Education still is not viewed as a long-term investment.
5. A wide variety of behavioral change models is available to guide interventions. Clear guidelines for use of these models may be found in Box 1.[8] (Most have been reviewed in previous chapters.) Most patient education must incorporate methods that are known to change behavior.

Box 1	*Guidelines for Provider Counseling Actions as Suggested by Health Behavior Change Theories*

1. Cognition and Information-Processing Models

Assess the extent to which the patient has thought about the issues and how much information he/she has previously received on the topic.

Present information based on patient's previous experience with the behavior change.

Stress important information first.

Provide both sensory and procedural information.

Provide written information based on the patient's educational level.

Check for comprehension of material and fit with previous schema.

2. Health Belief Model

Assess the patient's perceived susceptibility and severity of the outcome and frame the health message according to these perceptions.

Elicit perceived barriers to the health-behavior change in question and discuss how to overcome these barriers.

Assess the perceived benefits for engaging in the behavior and incorporate these benefits as reinforcers for behavior.

3. Theory of Reasoned Action

Determine whether the patient thinks family members and friends endorse the behavior.

Highlight the social pressure to engage in the behavior if it exists.

Provide examples of similar others who are currently engaging in the behavior.

Use specific examples of behaviors when assessing behavioral intentions.

4. Social Cognitive Theory

Increase self-efficacy for the behavior.

Provide opportunities for the patient to master the necessary skills.

Model or provide models of the targeted behavior.

Ask the patient to rehearse the behavior and provide feedback on his/her performance.

Address previously failed attempts and explore individual and environmental factors that may have contributed to these unsuccessful attempts.

Explore successes with other health behavior changes and techniques employed that may generalize to the targeted behavior change.

Increase outcome expectancies for the behavior.

Provide information to the patient on the efficacy of the behavior.

Arrange for the patient to meet a similar other who has experience with the behavior and endorses its effectiveness.

5. Behavior Modification

Determine whether a skill or performance deficit exists.

Teach the patient the necessary skills to engage in the behavior.

From Elder JP, Ayala GX, Harris S: Theories and intervention approaches to health-behavior change in primary care, *Am J Prev Med* 17:275-284, 1999.

6. Virtually all chronic disease management programs now include education focused on developing mastery and confidence and continued contact over time. These programs provide practice and feedback in new skills, including decision making and problem solving in real-life situations and attention to emotional and role management in addition to medical management since fear, anger, frustration, and depression are not uncommon.[13]

7. One widespread but untested assumption is that patient education does not have negative side effects. Conversely, there is almost no focus on the ethics of patient education, including when it is morally required and what conditions constitute manipulation as well as other important questions.

| Box 1 | *Guidelines for Provider Counseling Actions as Suggested by Health Behavior Change Theories—cont'd* |

5. Behavior Modification—cont'd

Reduce punishment for pro-health behavior. Reduce reinforcement for health-damaging behavior.

Agree on positive reinforcers to be used as behavior change occurs.

Agree on negative reinforcers to be used when behavior change does not occur.

Reinforce the behavior by inquiring about its performance.

6. Self-Management

Teach the patient how to monitor his/her own behavior.

Help the patient to become aware of internal cues for the behavior he/she is attempting to extinguish.

Decide on alternative, competing behaviors in which the patient can engage.

Identify, with the patient, external cues for the behavior.

Teach the patient how to use external cues to reinforce appropriate behavior or strategies to reduce the likelihood of engaging in inappropriate behavior.

7. Interpersonal and Social-Support Theories

Convey empathy and understanding for the difficulties of behavior change.

Provide a private setting in which to repeat and clarify instructions and assess resistance to change.

Schedule follow-up visits to evaluate the patient's progress and demonstrate commitment to provide support during the change process.

Engage the family in the targeted behavior. Address the entire family to gain commitment from all members for support of the behavior change.

8. Transtheoretical Model

Assess the patient's stage of change by minimally assessing whether he/she is currently engaging in the behavior or whether he/she has thought about possible changes to improve his/her health.

Use motivational interviewing techniques such as expressing empathy, providing a menu of options and avoiding argumentation.

Persons in the precontemplation stage should be made aware of the consequences for not engaging in health-behavior change, be provided the opportunity to share their feelings about their condition and discuss how their behavior affects the rest of the family.

People who are contemplators should be taught to closely monitor their motivations for engaging in the health-behavior change and explore their ambivalence and reasons they think change might be beneficial.

Individuals in the preparation stage should be asked to verbalize a commitment to change both to themselves and to their family members.

Action-stage individuals and those in the maintenance stage should work with the provider to set up rewards for appropriate behavior and stress-management techniques and establish supportive relationships.

8. Almost all policy documents focus on the right to information, completely ignoring the fact that education is necessary to use the information.

9. Most standards for patient education are process oriented, rather than outcome directed, and do not judge patient learning against a standard of achievement that is known to optimally affect quality of life and health status. Although the accumulated meta-analyses of research show great promise for beneficial outcomes from patient education, only meager evidence exists for how it is carried out. A badly needed next step in the development of patient education as a field of study and as a service is regular use of well-validated outcome measurement tools.

10. Changes in information technology make information easily available on the Internet. In addition, computer-based support systems have been designed to provide multiple learning opportunities. The Comprehensive Health Enhancement Support System (CHESS) provides information services (database of common questions and answers, instant library and personal stories of those who have struggled with a particular health crisis, consumer guide to services, and links to other World Wide Web sites), support services (discussion groups, ask an expert service), problem-solving services, and self-monitoring and guid-ance services. CHESS is now available on the Internet with modules developed for breast cancer, HIV/AIDS, heart disease, Alzheimer's disease, sexual assault, and substance abuse. Each module is built on extensive studies of patients' needs and has been shown to be effective with impoverished minority women as well as with other groups.[10]

11. The number of self-tests continues to increase. Figure 1 provides brief information about a self-test for chlamydia. Vaginal introital specimens are self-collected using only an instructional booklet.[16]

12. Quality improvement methods frequently require patient education. For

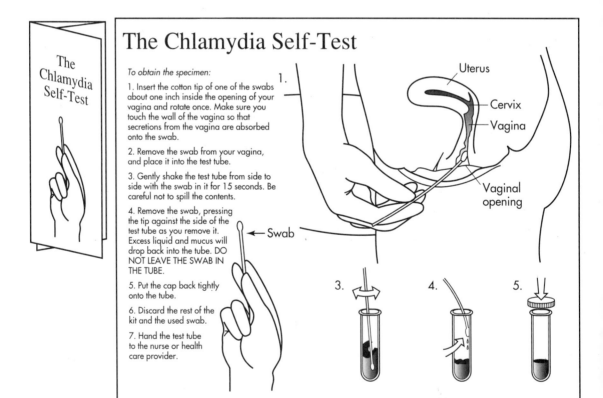

Figure 1 Polymerase chain reaction self-test instruction booklet used in this study. (From Polaneczky M and others: Use of self-collected vaginal specimens for detection of *Chlamydia trachomatis* infection, *Obstet Gynecol* 91:375-378, 1998.)

example, Wiley and others[19] found that many nurseries lack neonatal jaundice protocols, tracking systems, and parent education. Hyperbilirubinemia requiring phototherapy is the most common reason for hospital readmission of neonates.

EMERGING AREAS OF PATIENT EDUCATION

End of Life and Informed Consent

Patient education programs are newly developing in end-of-life care, and informed consent is increasingly seen as an educational issue, not just an issue of disclosure of information.

The quality of end-of-life care is now a central issue in health care. Patient education emphasizing patients' rights to accept or refuse medical treatments and to complete advance directives is central to this effort. Table 1 describes common treatments for sustaining life[2]; yet, as many as 75% of patients lack decision-making capacity when choices about life-sustaining interventions need to be made. Educational interventions can increase the rate of advance directive completion particularly when individuals have repeated opportunities to discuss their personal goals and beliefs with health care providers and to receive help in completing the document.[11,14]

Informed consent is both a legal and an ethical concept requiring disclosure of the nature of the proposed treatment, its benefits and risks and those of the alternatives including the option of no treatment, and patient decision about what course to take. Informed consent to participate in research is more stringent than that for treatment, must be voluntary, and must include explanation of a subject's freedom to withdraw from the study at any time without detrimental effect on continued access to treatment.

Despite these requirements, there are no widely accepted criteria for determining the quality of the patient's understanding or decision making, and there is a lack of standardized tools by which to evaluate comprehension of informed consent information. The focus is frequently on the legal requirements for disclosure of information as opposed to assuring that patients understand well enough to make an informed choice. There is, however, a growing body of literature that describes how patient education can contribute to reaching the patient autonomy goals of informed consent. Examples from a number of situations follow.

- For persons with schizophrenia, neuroleptic medication may be the most effective for preventing relapse. However, because there is a serious risk of tardive dyskinesia that may be irreversible with this treatment, patient understanding for informed consent is essential. Other studies with these patients suggest that psychiatric symptoms such as hallucinations and delusions do not necessarily interfere with competency. More than half of these patients required repeat instructions and more than a third required three or more educational sessions until they gave correct responses.[20]

- Achieving informed consent for genetic testing requires facing several difficulties. Genetic issues affect the entire family rather than a single individual. The probabilistic nature of genetic predictions is hard to understand, and the relevance of population statistics for an individual remains largely unknown. Understanding seems to be directly correlated with the amount of time spent with a patient.[15]

- For high-risk procedures and those of uncertain benefit the focus must be on patients achieving understanding to allow them to make voluntary choices. For example, because infertility treatment requires healthy patients to take significant risks such as multiple pregnancy, ovarian hyperstimulation, and emotional and financial costs, the process of obtaining informed consent for such a high-risk procedure must be rigorous. Men considering prostate specific antigen (PSA) testing

TABLE 1	Describing Common Treatments for Sustaining Life		
Treatment	**Benefits**	**Drawbacks**	**End of Life Decisions**
Cardiopulmonary resuscitation (CPR)	• Involves several treatments used to restart a heart and to provide artificial respiration when breathing has stopped. • Most useful in the event of a potentially reversible heart or lung problem.	• CPR can include electric shock to the chest and connecting the person to a machine called a ventilator by putting a tube down the windpipe. • CPR can be quite traumatic. If you do not respond to it quickly you could suffer irreversible brain damage or eventually die.	• CPR was not designed to revive you if you have advanced cancer or are in shock due to a severe infection. • CPR should not be used to keep you alive for a few hours or days if you are hopelessly ill. It will only prolong your suffering.
Artificial ventilation	• A ventilator can take over your breathing and support your lungs until they recover enough to breathe again on their own. • A "trial period" on the respirator may be beneficial if you have disease such as emphysema. Some people choose to live on a respirator for long periods of time.	• The tube that is placed down your throat can cause some discomfort. If you are "intubated," you cannot talk or eat orally. • You might become machine dependent if your lungs are unable to function again.	• If you decide not to accept a respirator or do not wish to live out your life on a machine, you can be kept comfortable on medication and oxygen. • You may indicate to your physicians that if a "trial period" does not help, you do not want to continue on a respirator. Of course, you DO want to be kept very comfortable until you die.

From Brandenburg M, Gifford J: Developing a multidisciplinary brochure to teach patients and families about life-sustaining treatments, *Dimens Crit Care Nurs* 16:328-332, 1997.

TABLE 1	Describing Common Treatments for Sustaining Life—cont'd		
Treatment	**Benefits**	**Drawbacks**	**End of Life Decisions**
Feeding tubes	• If you are unable to eat, a feeding tube can be put into your stomach or small bowel to provide nutrition. • If you are ill but expected to recover, feeding tubes can be very helpful in providing nutrition needed for healing.	• It is a common belief that hopelessly ill patients will "starve to death" unless placed on a feeding tube. In reality, you will not feel hungry or thirsty if you suffer from an advanced disease such as cancer, Parkinson's or Alzheimer's. • By providing your body with foods and liquids, feeding tubes may actually extend a painful life beyond what you would wish. Without liquids you will usually die in a few days.	• Most people choose not to be kept alive by a feeding tube if their quality of life would be very poor, with no chance of improvement or recovery. • If you choose not to have a feeding tube or to use a feeding tube on a trial basis and your illness is hopeless, you can be kept very comfortable with medication.
Dialysis	• When your kidneys no longer work, you can be attached to a machine to clean your blood of toxic substances that normally accumulate. • Some people choose to live for years with artificial dialysis treatments.	• Dialysis can be physically draining. • Hemodialysis usually has to be done three times a week and takes three to four hours each time.	• Dialysis for the hopelessly ill may only prolong the dying process. • Without dialysis, if you have kidney failure, you usually slip into a coma and die peacefully.

also must give informed consent. Reasons for this recommendation and proposed content to be included in the education for informed consent may be seen in Box 2.[3]

- Because there is a shortage of donor organs for transplantation, DeJong and others[7] have suggested that the request for donation must be done sensitively and in a way that assures family understanding on which to base a decision. Research has shown that a family is more likely to consent when members are given time to understand and accept their relative's death before the organ donation request is made. The concept of brain death is con-

fusing to many. A family communication protocol may be found in Figure 2.

- The informed consent process for the Diabetes Control and Complications Trial (DCCT) was very carefully planned to assure an informed decision to participate. The trial was randomized, long term (8 to 10 years), complex, and demanding, and adherence to the protocols was essential to the trial's outcome of understanding how the treatment regimen related to development and progression of vascular complications in persons with insulin-dependent diabetes mellitus. Box 3 describes the multiple modes of presentation

---

| Box 2 | *Proposed Content for Informed Consent for PSA Screening* |

Basic Minimum

1. False positive prostate-specific antigen (PSA) test results can occur.
2. False negative PSA test results and false negative biopsies of the prostate can occur.
3. Nobody knows whether regular PSA screening will reduce the number of deaths from prostate cancer.

Conversation

1. The PSA test is a blood test for prostate cancer.
2. Done together, the digital rectal examination and the PSA test can screen for prostate cancer.
3. The PSA screening test can detect prostate cancer sooner than the digital rectal examination alone.
4. An elevated PSA test result may lead to other tests to see whether prostate cancer is present.
5. The risk of getting prostate cancer is higher in a man who is older, has a family history of prostate cancer, or is African American.
6. Prostate cancer may grow slowly and not cause any symptoms. That is why prostate cancer may not kill older men. They may outlive this cancer and die from something else.
7. A man over age 70 is less likely to die from prostate cancer even though he is at higher risk to have it.

Brochure

1. The PSA screening test is controversial.
2. There are advantages and disadvantages to taking the PSA test. One disadvantage is that a man could end up worrying about what an elevated PSA test result means.
3. Done together, the PSA and digital rectal examination, are most appropriate for men who have more than 10 years left to live.
4. A man with early prostate cancer can choose watchful waiting, radical prostatectomy, or radiation therapy.
5. There are side effects from prostate cancer treatment such as impotence, incontinence, narrowing of the urethra (strictures), trouble urinating, and rectal scarring.
6. Nobody knows whether treating prostate cancer early is helpful or whether one treatment is better than another.
7. Although a man thinking about taking the PSA test can consult a doctor, he should make the final decision himself.

From Chan EYC, Sulmasy DP: What should men know about prostate-specific antigen screening before giving informed consent? *Am J Med* 105:266-271, 1998.

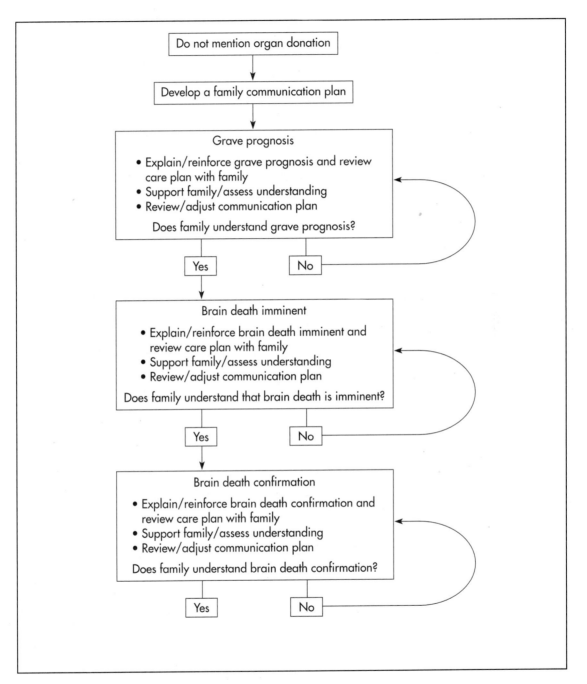

Figure 2   Family communication protocol for explaining brain death. (From DeJong W and others: Requesting organ donation: an interview study of donors and nondonor families, *Am J Crit Care* 7:13-23, 1998.)

Box 3	*Components of Informed Consent Education Program*

Information Materials

A 25-minute audiovisual presentation describing the study purpose, design, treatment group procedures, risks, benefits, and screening procedures.

A dictionary of tests and terms used in the DCCT.

A handbook covering the study in more depth than the audiovisual presentation.

Interview

An interview that assessed the volunteer's past adherence to diabetes care, including the ability to keep appointments and follow prescribed diet, glucose monitoring, and insulin regimen.

Behavioral Tasks

A set of study-related behavioral tasks to be performed at home over 2 weeks, which was then evaluated for adherence.

Self-Predictors of Adherence

An assessment of the degree of confidence the volunteer had regarding carrying out study required behaviors.

An assessment of the volunteer's expectations regarding personal adherence to study required behaviors.

Knowledge Tests

A knowledge test to determine the volunteer's understanding of the study questions, design (including randomization), risks and benefits, and requirements.

Informed Consent

A consent form for randomization and participation in the trial.

Family Questionnaire

A 20-item questionnaire administered to determine level of understanding of family members who had participated in screening process.

From DCCT Research Group: Implementation of a multicomponent process to obtain informed consent in the Diabetes Control and Complications Trial, *Control Clin Trials* 10:83-96, 1989.

---

and repetition during the informed consent process, which were expected to enhance retention of information. The behavioral tasks simulated features of the study protocol. This allowed potential participants to experience what it would be like to be in the study and the staff to assess whether they could be skilled in these tasks.[6]

- Others have described education and documentation of patient understanding managed by computer. At various points the program asks questions of patients, records their answers, and provides additional instruction if an answer is incorrect.[17]

Although informed consent is a longstanding legal and ethical requirement, there appears to be renewed interest in the contribution patient education can make in assuring patients' ability to truly understand their options.

Symptom Interpretation

Although much of patient education deals with symptom recognition and management, usual approaches seem not to have been very helpful. Improving this practice is important, and several approaches may be useful. The typical adult experiences at least one somatic symptom every 4 to 6 days and obviously interprets and deals with it, frequently without the help of a health professional. One approach to help patients distinguish serious symptoms is to teach them about the range of bodily symptoms occurring in healthy people.[1]

A second approach is physiological. A clear example occurs with asthma. Some studies have found that 15% of subjects are unable to perceive severe airway obstruction. These patients can be taught to use an objective index of pulmonary obstruction such as peak flow rate, especially if it has been previously determined that their scores are highly related to standard pulmonary measures. By providing patients with the experience of breathing through a range of air flow resistance levels, sensitivity to air flow variation can be taught. Such education can be personalized according to baseline sensitivity.[5,12]

As indicated in Chapter 7, a similar approach for blood glucose awareness training (BGAT) has been used with patients with insulin-dependent diabetes to more accurately detect their blood glucose (BG) fluctuations through symptom perception. BGAT education involves rating BG on the basis of symptoms, self-monitoring BG values, and plotting on an error grid to provide immediate feedback concerning estimation accuracy. Such training has led to consistent improvement in BG estimation accuracy with fewer auto crashes and better metabolic control in comparison with a control group. Periodic booster training is necessary to sustain these improvements.[4] Because the results of the DCCT recommended keeping the BG value very close to the normal limit, patients with a history of hypoglycemia need to take part in a structured teaching and treatment program for BGAT.[9]

Yet a third approach broadens understanding of relevant emerging symptoms beyond "common" symptoms and has been best studied with myocardial infarction. Ruston and others[18] found that patients who did not delay getting treatment ("nondelayers") knew about a wide range of symptoms including sweating, nausea, pains in the arms and neck, and breathing problems. Patients who delayed getting treatment ("delayers") generally knew only about chest and arm pain, while most extended delayers were unsure about symptoms. This is congruent with assessing an individual's concept of what having a heart attack would be like. Many thought it would be a dramatic and sudden event with collapse and death, whereas they were still able to function and relieve their symptoms to some extent.

SUMMARY

This postscript has summarized trends in patient education including significant new developments.

References

1. Barsky AJ, Borus JF: Somatization and medicalization in the era of managed care, *JAMA* 274:1931-1934, 1995.
2. Brandenburg M, Gifford J: Developing a multidisciplinary brochure to teach patients and families about life-sustaining treatments, *Dimens Crit Care Nurs* 16:328-332, 1997.
3. Chan EYC, Sulmasy DP: What should men know about prostate-specific antigen screening before giving informed consent? *Am J Med* 105:266-274, 1998.
4. Cox D and others: A multicenter evaluation of blood glucose awareness training-II, *Diabetes Care* 18:523-528, 1995.
5. Creer TL, Levstek DA, Winder JA: Home monitoring of lung function measures. In Kotses H, Harver A, editors, *Self-management of asthma*, New York, 1998, Marcel Dekker.
6. DCCT Research Group: Implementation of a multicomponent process to obtain informed consent in the Diabetes Control and Complications Trial, *Control Clin Trials* 10:83-96, 1989.
7. DeJong W and others: Requesting organ donation: an interview study of donors and nondonor families, *Am J Crit Care* 7:13-23, 1998.
8. Elder JP, Ayala GX, Harris S: Theories and intervention approaches to health-behavior change in primary care, *Am J Prev Med* 17:275-284, 1999.
9. Fritsche A, Stumvoll M, Renn W, Schmulling R-M: Diabetes teaching program improves glycemic control and preserves perception of hypoglycemia, *Diabetes Res Clin Pract* 40:129-135, 1998.
10. Gustafson DH and others: Empowering patients using computer based health support systems, *Qua Health Care* 8:49-56, 1999.
11. Hanson LC, Tulsky JA, Danis M: Can clinical interventions change care at the end of life? *Ann Intern Med* 126:381-388, 1997.

12. Kotses H: Individualized asthma self-management. In Kotses H, Harver A, editors, *Self-management of asthma*, New York, 1998, Marcel Dekker.

13. Lorig K, Chronic disease self-management, *Am Behav Scientist* 39:676-783, 1996.

14. Luptak MK, Boult C: A method for increasing elders' use of advance directives, *Gerontologist* 34:409-412, 1994.

15. Miller CK and others: The Deaconess Informed Consent Comprehension Test: an assessment tool for clinical research subjects, *Pharmacotherapy* 16:872-878, 1996.

16. Polaneczky M and others: Use of self-collected vaginal specimens for detection of *Chlamydia trachomatis* infection, *Obstet Gynecol* 91:375-378, 1998.

17. Rosoff AJ: Informed consent in the electronic age, *Am J Law Med* 25:367-386, 1999.

18. Ruston A, Clayton J, Calnan M: Patients' action during their cardiac event: qualitative study exploring differences and modifiable factors, *Br Med J* 316:1060-1065, 1998.

19. Wiley CC, Lai N, Hill C, Burke G: Nursing practice and detection of jaundice after newborn discharge, *Arch Pediatr Adolesc Med* 152:972-975, 1998.

20. Wirshing DA: Informed consent: assessment of competence, *Am J Psychiatry* 155:1508-1511, 1998.

Suggested Answers to Study Questions

CHAPTER 1 THE PRACTICE OF PATIENT EDUCATION: OVERVIEW

1. Answers will vary.
2. Parts of the teaching-learning process:
   a. The assessment of readiness for learning can use the mother's comments as the baby performs, including her comment about how frantic she gets when he cries.
   b. Learning goals are developed in response to the mother's comments, such as those about crying.
   c.–d. The teaching plan (intervention) follows the outline of the demonstration of the behavior, and the materials are the live baby and the interpersonal relationship between mother and provider, which, if formed as described, can be powerfully motivating.
   e. Evaluation is not as explicitly outlined as are other elements of the teaching process; however, one can presume that it would occur during a clinical interaction while stimulating and observing the baby's behavior. The mother's learning would be evaluated by her behavior with the baby and her responses to questions asked by the practitioner.

CHAPTER 2 MOTIVATION AND LEARNING

1. The implications are that all encounters with the health care system must advance patients' understanding so that they can better manage their own health.
2. Evidence of wanting to learn is important for situations a and b.
   a. Your questions should determine the women's understanding and feelings about cancer, about preventive care in general, about manipulating their own breasts, and about the meaning of finding a lump. Some may have had instruction in the procedure and will be able to do some or all of it correctly.
   b. Some of your questions should enable you to discover the level of disability the boy is experiencing. Can he understand language and, if so, which words? How well can he grasp things and move his arms in a feeling motion? Other questions will deal with his independence and his caregiver's ability to cooperate in the training program. Does everyone in the family (including the boy) want the child to be independent? Is the caregiver patient yet precise enough to carry out a

training program? Could she interpret the boy's behavior in terms of progress toward the goal?

3. You should not be surprised by these findings; they are what you would expect given an understanding of learning theory. Among the learning principles involved are that practice improves memory, direct experience of the skill helps the parent retain more learning than does an abstract review, and successful experience with feedback increases self-efficacy for that skill.

4. a. Establishing baseline.
   b. Modeling.
   c. Setting up reinforcement; however, it would be useful to know if giving pennies for toys reinforces the child's behavior.
   d. Shaping.
   e. Contingent reinforcement.

CHAPTER 3 EDUCATIONAL OBJECTIVES AND INSTRUCTION

1. No, because the implicit (although never stated) objectives of discharge care involve observing the wound for evidence of complications, which requires being able to recognize such signs and symptoms.

2. The nurse can suggest that the mother place green peas, cereal bits, apple slices, and other similar foods on the baby's food tray to provide practice of skills he or she needs to develop. Explanation of the organizing idea should also be given to the mother to show ways in which she can aid the baby's development. The U.S. Department of Agriculture has simple large-print booklets on this subject that can be read by mothers with limited literacy. The nurse can directly facilitate learning through modeling play and vocal games with the infant during visits and through his or her own expression of pleasure. All three of these strategies can be used. If this learning goal is needed by a number of mothers, consider developing a group teaching situation.

CHAPTER 4 EVALUATION AND RESEARCH IN PATIENT EDUCATION

1. To comprehend the means of attaining asepsis in giving an injection.

2. Transfer is involved every time the evaluation task is different from the learning tasks. Such is the case with all levels of the taxonomy with the possible exception of knowledge (cognitive). It is possible to index the degree of transfer of which the learner is capable by systematic testing of a wide variety of situations that require varying degrees of transfer (on a continuum from those tasks that are very much like the original learning task to those that are very little like it).

3. Factors and action:

Possible Factors Causing Inattentiveness and Rebelliousness	Nurse Action
The complexity of the task the nurse was teaching might have been too great for the learner's ability, resulting in failure or even lack of willingness to begin learning.	Do a more careful analysis of prerequisite skills the learner possesses. If the goals are found to be too complex, break the skills into smaller units or teach the last part of the skill first (so that the learner experiences success).
The individual may be preoccupied with other life problems and therefore may not feel motivated to develop this new behavior.	Assess the accuracy of this hypothesis by talking with him and others who know him and by watching his behavior. It may be possible to create motivation by persuading him that learning the dressing skills can help him solve his other problem. Another alternative is to wait a few weeks and try again.
This may be the individual's usual response to many things.	Assess the validity of this statement. If true, it may be possible to do some teaching in spite of the inattentiveness and rebelliousness. The success of learning may alter these responses. Another alternative is teaching aimed first at altering these attitudes

4. Analyzing patient's understanding:
   a. This person may not understand how blood sugar is measured—a certain amount per standard volume of blood. Investigate this.
   b. This is likely to be indicative of affective rather than cognitive learning. Because she is in the somewhat ambiguous situation of not being insulin-dependent, she is not motivated to move beyond the lower levels of the affective domain. It is also possible that she has not progressed beyond the denial or disbelief stage of psychosocial adaptation to illness.
   c. This comment may be evaluative of either cognitive objectives or affective objectives or both. See if the rest of the conversation provides a more specific clue, and, if not, question the father yourself. The comment may mean that the man has not understood how diabetic patients accommodate activities such as hunting trips, or it may represent a seeking of verification from an experienced person that diabetic patients really can hunt and that his son can participate in such physically taxing activities.

5. The items test the objectives fairly well. It would seem unlikely that two providers would reach the same judgment inasmuch as the response, correct, is not further refined. This tool was meant to be generic for use with many different medications. Providers would find it useful to define the correct responses about the drugs they are teaching most often.

6. Perhaps *believe* is a better term than *feel* because many of these items are cognitive. This content would be better suited to multiple-choice format. As it is, after the parent completed the tool, you know very little about why he agrees or disagrees or where misconceptions may lie.

CHAPTER 5 CANCER PATIENT EDUCATION

1. The critique should include (1) whether the questions test crucial elements, especially those that are commonly misunderstood by this population, (2) whether the reading level is so high that patients cannot understand the questions, (3) whether the score would represent true knowledge, and (4) whether the objective of increasing knowledge about screening will really contribute to any important clinical objective. My judgment is that the test is flawed on each of these criteria.

2. Not likely. What you probably want to know is how women examine their breasts (have them demonstrate) and if men can draw or describe where their prostate gland is. The questions as they are currently worded will not provide this most important information.

3. From a medical perspective it seems thorough. It does not include behavioral outcomes—only topics to be taught—and there is no evidence that it represents what patients need to know.

4. It is likely too verbal—not sufficiently pictorial. At best it could be used as a reminder of the demonstration and a focus for practice to a level of confidence, using silicone models and real breasts.

CHAPTER 7 DIABETES SELF-MANAGEMENT EDUCATION

1. Learning principles include the following:
   a. The assessment pinpointed changes that needed to be made from the perspectives of all stakeholders.
   b. People who would be delivering the program became committed to it by designing it.
   c. A teaching plan made expectations for the intervention clear and helped to ensure that appropriate materials would be available to carry it out.
   d. A cadre of nurses were certified (assured to have at least minimum skills) and could be ready resources to teach others on the units.
   e. Evaluation from several perspectives (outcomes, satisfaction) provided feedback for continuous improvement.

CHAPTER 8 EDUCATION FOR PREGNANCY AND PARENTING AND EDUCATION OF CHILDREN

1. Practice to overlearning; assessment and feedback from instructor and further instruction if necessary; speaking with parents who have used these skills successfully (modeling); and at least yearly reeducation to maintain skills.

2. No, the concerns of the providers, particularly physicians, are not surprising because they frequently believe that "lay" people cannot handle technical health information. It will be necessary to develop at least one additional version of the VIP adapted to low reading level and to develop an audiotape or a videotape version for those who are illiterate.

3. Not really. One should be surprised by the ethical problem surrounding the intervention, which pays little attention to the values and informed choice of the mothers.

4. Clearly the development of self-efficacy could be one framework within which to view this interaction. Early in the vignette the mother lacked self-efficacy but gained it as she had real life experience under the coaching of the nurse. Remember how empowering self-efficacy can be; it focuses and motivates behavior. One could also use a physiological/developmental learning framework on the part of the infant, and one could use the process of parent-infant attachment as a framework.

5. It would be useful to have observational evidence that what parents report is what they actually do. It would also be useful to understand sources of disagreement further be-

fore labeling these populations as noncompliant and to check their sense of efficacy in carrying out these recommendations. Community-based interventions using parents who have had experience with this issue are likely to be persuasive. In the end, parents will make their own decisions.

CHAPTER 9 PATIENT SELF-MANAGEMENT FOR THE RHEUMATIC DISEASES

1. A prime strategy of managed care is to use education to avoid unnecessary use of expensive services and patient loss of productive time. A managed care organization will probably be monitoring such usage in its population of persons with arthritis. Become aware of the pattern reported by Wynne very early, and establish means to get this education to everyone taking NSAIDs.

CHAPTER 10 OTHER AREAS OF PATIENT EDUCATION PRACTICE

1. Not only should there be concern related to effectiveness of teaching, there should also be concern about informed consent. Unless this information was provided in another format, these pamphlets could be used as evidence that a crucial piece of information was not disclosed.

2. The plan does not consistently describe behaviors to be attained as a result of the teaching.

Additional Study Questions and Suggested Answers

ADDITIONAL STUDY QUESTIONS

1. A radiology department found a problem of excessive repeat rates on some of its x-ray series, often because of poor bowel preparation. How would you justify development of a patient education program on preparation for these tests? What level of success could you promise?

2. One always has to be aware that messages in the environment or the content and behaviors one is teaching can be biased and not supportive of the patient's well-being. For example, an analysis of menstrual-product advertisements reveals the message that menstruation is a humiliating, shameful physiological process that must be concealed and that the advertised products cleanse and deodorize.[5] Another example is the development of contraceptive technologies that make women more dependent on medical professionals for their administration and removal and frequently do not reflect women's reproductive needs or their experience in the use of various contraceptive methods.[10] In these situations, what is the patient educator's responsibility?

3. Patient package inserts (PPIs) are a prime educational tool for use of many drugs, including oral contraceptives. A study found that instructions in various brands of oral contraceptives were variable and confusing.[16] They differed in their recommendations of what to do after missing three or more pills and in what was considered the start day, including recommendations for using a backup method of contraception when first starting to use the pill. Should standards be set for these PPIs?

4. Compare the patient education standards for various disease entities contained in Appendix D. What conclusions can be drawn from the aggregate of this work?

5. Researchers in diabetes have found that self-care behaviors are often only weakly correlated with glycemic control.[9] What is the relevance of this finding for learning?

6. Studies show that feelings of control are important to psychosocial recovery from a cardiac event[14] and that disease severity is not a reliable predictor of psychosocial recovery. This is also true for other illnesses such as cancer and rheumatoid arthritis. Perceptions of control are associated with increased adherence in persons with

diabetes, patients undergoing cardiac rehabilitation, and individuals with hypertension. How can patient education be designed to develop perceived control by patients?

7. There are a number of theories of health behavior: health belief model, attribution theory, transtheoretic model of behavior change, and others. Faced with a patient education problem, how would you know which theories of behavior change to use?

8. Preparing patients to play a major role in choice of treatments is a goal of patient education. Some of the most structured work toward this goal has been done for persons choosing treatment for benign prostatic hypertrophy. Box 1 contains symptom questions and value questions that reflect the patient's perspective and thus help him make a treatment decision.[1] Construct a similar set of symptom and value questions for helping patients with another disorder make a treatment decision.

9. Patients' knowledge of epilepsy has frequently been found to be inadequate, and because medication remains the most effective means to control seizure activity, medication knowledge is important.[7] Figure 1 shows a comparison of learning needs for persons with epilepsy, as rank-ordered by patients, nurses, and physicians. Were the differences among the three groups predictable? What lessons do these differences hold for teaching persons with epilepsy?

10. Fatigue is one of the most common complaints of newly delivered mothers. Fatigue affects the postpartum woman's quality of life and can interfere with her health and well-being and with development of the mother-infant relationship. The shortening of postpartum hospital stays seems to have increased both fatigue potential and difficulty for nurses to assess and assist in managing postpartum fatigue. A self-management guide[16] for patients with post-

---

| **Box 1** | *Symptom and Value Questions* |

Symptom Questions

Over the past month or so, how often have you:
1. Had a burning feeling when you urinate?
2. Had to push or strain to begin urination?
3. Had to urinate again shortly after you were finished urinating?
4. Found you stopped and started again several times when you urinated?
5. Dribbled urine after you thought you were finished urinating?
    Ordered categorical responses: (1) not at all, (2) a few times, (3) fairly often, (4) usually, (5) always.

Value Questions

1. Suppose your urinary symptoms stayed just the same as they are now for the rest of your life. How would you feel about that?
2. Suppose a treatment cured your urinary symptoms, but after the treatment any sexual climaxes would result in retrograde ejaculation. How would you feel about your situation?
3. Suppose a treatment cured your urinary symptoms, but you were not able to have sexual erections. How would you feel about your situation?
4. Suppose a treatment cured your urinary symptoms, but you occasionally dripped urine or wet your pants slightly. How would you feel about your situation?
    Ordered categorical responses: (1) delighted, (2) pleased, (3) mostly satisfied, (4) mixed, (5) mostly dissatisfied, (6) unhappy, (7) terrible.

From Barry MJ and others: Patient reactions to a program designed to facilitate patient participation in treatment decisions for benign prostatic hyperplasia, *Med Care* 33: 771-782, 1995.

partum fatigue was developed by a process of:
a. Content development by literature review to identify sources of fatigue and suggestions for its management
b. Content validation by a panel of experts
c. Pilot testing of the guide with patients.

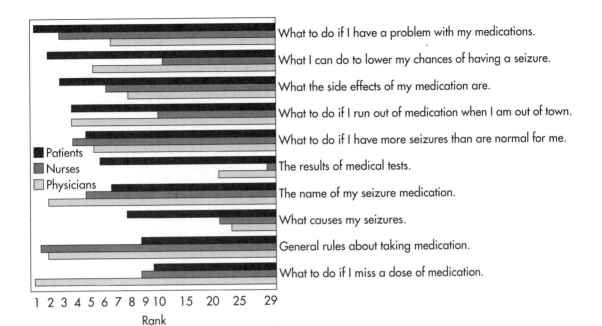

Figure 1   Comparison of the rank order of the top 10 important items for patients with the ranking of nurse and physicians. (From Dilorio C, Faherty B, Manteuffel B: Learning needs of persons with epilepsy: a comparison of perceptions of persons with epilepsy, nurses and physicians, *Neurosci Nurs* 25:22-29, 1993.)

Develop a self-management guide with a group of patients. What potential negative side effects could be associated with such a guide, and how can you guard against them?

11. Families provide 60% to 80% of the total care received by impaired older adult relatives in tasks such as helping with eating, walking, dressing, taking medications, and managing chronic health problems such as incontinence. As the number of adults older than 85 years of age increases, the need for more physical care and assistance from family members will also increase. Where do families learn how to provide aid and physical care to their members? Because caregivers of stable or chronically impaired elders typically do not qualify for any Medicare-reimbursed nursing or other support services, they strug-

gle with the responsibilities of caregiving without the benefit of any nursing assistance.

   Mahoney and Shippee-Rice[12] developed and piloted a training program for informal caregivers. The objectives are to help family caregivers achieve the following:

a. Increase their knowledge of personal care techniques and needed adaptations

b. Distinguish between normal changes associated with aging and pathological processes

c. Perform caregiving services in a more efficient manner.

d. Expand their range of caregiving skills

e. Identify the meaning of the caregiver role to themselves and their care recipients

f. Develop assertiveness techniques for use in the family system as well as in the formal caregiving system

Using this model, design and pilot a program for informal caregivers in your neighborhood.

12. Since 1981, the American Academy of Family Physicians Foundation has been developing a clearinghouse of evaluated patient education materials. The dilemma faced by busy clinicians is an overabundance of patient education materials, few of which have been appropriately evaluated. In 1989 a database describing such evaluated materials, including their cost and reading levels, became available and is now heavily used. The Materials Evaluation Questionnaire for health professionals and for patients is presented in Boxes 2 and 3.[8] What suggestions would you make for its revision?

13. For a good example of identification of a patient education need and development of a program, read the article by Yetzer and others.[18] The parts of the teaching process are clearly labeled throughout the text. Based on what you know about patient education, what additional suggestions do you have for improving this program?

14. The patient questionnaire in Box 4 was used to assess the impact of a preoperative joint replacement patient education program.[11] The authors indicate that in an effort to intervene quickly with pragmatic solutions, a dichotomous scale was chosen to focus on patients who had negative responses. Provide a critique of the tool.

15. Evaluate any teaching material for its suitability for persons with low literacy who have failing eyesight (remember that the final criterion of suitability is that persons of low literacy learn from it). Characteristics you might want to look for include the following[13]:

- Is the message behaviorally oriented and interactive?

- Is there use of stories and examples to describe difficult concepts?
- Does the material use language familiar to your patient population?
- Does it use short sentences of 12 to 15 words, alternating in length?
- Does it use techniques to draw attention to important ideas, such as arrows, underlining, bullets, boldface, and circles?
- Is there evidence that the material was pretested through focus groups, interviews, comprehension tests?
- Is the material "friendly" for aging eyes, using 14- to 18-point type on nonshiny, cream-colored paper, with black letters, written at a very low reading level?

This is an example of 9-point type.

This is an example of 12-point type.

This is an example of 14-point type.

This is an example of 18-point type.

16. Butler and Beltran[3] describe adult persons with sickle cell anemia who were dissatisfied and angry with the treatment they received and were perceived by caregivers as exaggerating their pain, seeking drugs, and being noncompliant. Would you expect that an education/support group would be helpful in resolving these issues?

17. The quiz in Box 5 is given to elders in community settings to determine the adequacy of their knowledge about urinary incontinence? Provide a critique of this tool for use in clinical practice.

18. Match the theory most identified with the following teaching approaches (theories may be used more than once).

Text continued on p. 256

Box 2	*Health Promotion Project: Materials Evaluation Questionnaire**

Directions: After reading over the material attached to this survey, please indicate your opinion by answering the questions below. If the question does not seem to apply, please circle NA. Comments are welcome. *Please* comment if you disagree or strongly disagree with any of the statements. Thank you.

Title:

Objective: In a few words, what do you think is the main purpose of this material?

	Strongly disagree	Disagree		Agree	Strongly agree	
It is designed to						
1. reinforce information.	1	2	3	4	5	NA
2. provide new information.	1	2	3	4	5	NA
3. stimulate behavior change.	1	2	3	4	5	NA

Appearance: Please rate the appearance of the material by answering each question below.

	Very low appeal	Low appeal		High appeal	Very high appeal	
4. At first glance it *attracted* my attention.	1	2	3	4	5	NA
5. It *held* my attention.	1	2	3	4	5	NA
6. Overall appearance.	1	2	3	4	5	NA
7. Quality of illustrations	1	2	3	4	5	NA
8. Use of color	1	2	3	4	5	NA
9. Typeface (large enough, attractive, etc.)	1	2	3	4	5	NA
10. Highlighting of major concepts	1	2	3	4	5	NA

Comments _____

Content: Please rate the content of the material.

	Very poor	Poor		Good	Very good	
11. Up-to-date	1	2	3	4	5	NA
12. Scientifically accurate	1	2	3	4	5	NA
13. Adequate scope for objective(s)	1	2	3	4	5	NA
14. Overall organization	1	2	3	4	5	NA
15. Logical flow of ideas	1	2	3	4	5	NA
16. Needed background given to enable understanding	1	2	3	4	5	NA
17. Summary(ies) given when needed	1	2	3	4	5	NA
18. The management of fear content	1	2	3	4	5	NA
19. Fair presentation given (e.g., avoids sexism, ethnic bias, ageism, manufacturer bias, etc.)	1	2	3	4	5	NA
20. Does the bias interfere with the intent of the item?					Yes _____ (1) No _____ (2)	

Comments _____

From Gibson PA and others: A health/patient education database for family practice, *Bull Med Libr Assoc* 79:357-369, 1991.
*For use by health professionals.

Continued

| Box 2 | *Health Promotion Project: Materials Evaluation Questionnaire—cont'd* |

Usefulness: Please respond to the statements below by circling the best response.

	Strongly disagree	Disagree		Agree	Strongly agree	
21. It is useful for its intended audience.	1	2	3	4	5	NA
22. It is believable.	1	2	3	4	5	NA
23. The material is understandable.	1	2	3	4	5	NA
24. Requires little or no explanation.	1	2	3	4	5	NA

Comments _____

Overall: Please respond to the statements below.

	Strongly disagree	Disagree		Agree	Strongly agree	
25. Overall I would recommend that physicians use this material with patients.	1	2	3	4	5	NA
26. Overall this material meets its objectives.	1	2	3	4	5	NA

Remarks: _____

Placement: Please circle all that apply.

	Strongly disagree	Disagree		Agree	Strongly agree	
27. Should be placed in the physician's waiting room.	1	2	3	4	5	NA
28. Should be placed in the exam room.	1	2	3	4	5	NA
29. Should be stored for occasional use.	1	2	3	4	5	NA
30. Other suggested settings						

Comments: _____

Please take a few seconds and complete the following:

Professional status: **Number of years**

a. Resident	❑ PGY 1	❑ PGY 2		❑ PGY 3
b. Family physician faculty	❑ under 6	❑ 6-15	❑ 16-25	❑ 26 or over
c. Practicing physician	❑ under 6	❑ 6-15	❑ 16-25	❑ 26 or over
d. R.N.	❑ under 6	❑ 6-15	❑ 16-25	❑ 26 or over
e. Other (Specify) _____	❑ under 6	❑ 6-15	❑ 16-25	❑ 26 or over

Gender:

Male _____ (1)
Female _____ (2)

Age Range:

Under 25 _____ (1)
25-35 _____ (2)
36-45 _____ (3)
46-55 _____ (4)
56-65 _____ (5)
Over 65 _____ (6)

Name _____
          (Please print)

From Gibson PA and others: A health/patient education database for family practice, *Bull Med Libr Assoc* 79:357-369, 1991.
*For use by health professionals.

Box 3	*Health Promotion Project: Materials Evaluation Questionnaire**

Directions: Please tell us what you think of the material attached to this form by answering all the questions below. For each question circle the number that best describes how you feel. If the question does not seem to apply to the material you are reviewing, please circle NA. If you wish to write comments, we would value your additional ideas.

Title: _____

Topic: _____

	Strongly disagree	Disagree		Agree	Strongly agree	
1. At first glance it *attracted* my attention.	1	2	3	4	5	NA
2. It *held* my attention.	1	2	3	4	5	NA
3. It is useful.	1	2	3	4	5	NA
4. I like the illustrations.	1	2	3	4	5	NA
5. I believe what it has to say.	1	2	3	4	5	NA
6. I would recommend it to a friend or relative to read.	1	2	3	4	5	NA
7. It is easy to understand.	1	2	3	4	5	NA
8. What it says is important.	1	2	3	4	5	NA
9. It reminds me of some things I need to think about.	1	2	3	4	5	NA
10. It gives me some new things to think about.	1	2	3	4	5	NA
11. It changes some of my thinking.	1	2	3	4	5	NA
12. It could change how I do things.	1	2	3	4	5	NA
13. Overall I recommend that doctors use this material with patients.	1	2	3	4	5	NA
14. Overall I am the right person to get this material from my doctor.	1	2	3	4	5	NA
15. Overall this material accomplishes its main purpose.	1	2	3	4	5	NA

Purpose: In just a few words, please write what you think is the main purpose of this material.

_____

_____

Comments:_____

_____

We would appreciate learning a little more about you.
( ) Male
( ) Female
Occupation _____
Years of school completed _____
Age range: ( ) Under 12
          ( ) 12-15
          ( ) 16-24
          ( ) 25-35
          ( ) 36-45
          ( ) 46-55
          ( ) 56-65
          ( ) Over 65

Thank you!

_____

From Gibson PA and others: A health/patient education database for family practice, *Bull Med Libr Assoc* 79:357-369, 1991.
*For use by patients.

| Box 4 | *Assessment of the Education Program in a Joint Replacement Center Patient Questionnaire* |

Letter

Dear

Our team is hopeful that your recent surgery is helping you to better enjoy life. To find out how you are doing since your joint replacement surgery, it is our hope that you will complete the enclosed questionnaire and return it to our office. We plan to write a research paper about the postoperative progress made by our patients. Your input would be greatly appreciated.

In gathering such information, we will be able to evaluate how our program can better serve patients before, during, and after their hospitalization. Emphasis will be on how you did once you were home. We also want to know your expectations of the surgical outcome. Did you do as well as you expected when you decided to have your operation?

We also would like to take this opportunity to say how much we enjoyed working with you and thank you in advance for helping us gather this information. We feel it will help others who are having this type of surgery know your feelings and suggestions for improvement of our program.

Sincerely,
Rhoda Lichtenstein, CRNP
Case Manager

Questionnaire

Einstein/Moss Joint Replacement Center Patient Questionnaire

1. What was the date of your surgery? _____
2. Do you feel that the preoperative teaching you received helped you fully understand:

	Yes	No
Why you needed to have this operation	___	___
How the prosthesis looked and worked	___	___
What exercises you needed to do before your admission and when you were in the hospital	___	___
What our team expected you to report, i.e., drainage, redness and heat around incision, calf pain or swelling, etc.	___	___
Any additional comments you wish to make on this question?	___	___

From Lichtenstein R, Semann S, Marmar EC: Development and impact of a hospital-based perioperative patient education program in a joint replacement center, *Orthop Nurs* 12(6):17-25, 1993.

| Box 4 | *Assessment of the Education Program in a Joint Replacement Center Patient Questionnaire—cont'd* |

3. After your admission did you:

	Yes	No
Feel the medical staff was available for the care you required	——	——
Feel the nursing staff assisted you in your care	——	——

Comments please _____
_____
_____
_____

4. Did the physical therapy department:

	Yes	No
See you on a daily basis	——	——
Help you understand the reasons behind the exercises you were doing	——	——
See that occupational therapy was part of your total program	——	——
Assign a reasonable length of time for each of your therapy sessions	——	——

	Yes	No
Too long?	——	——
Too short?	——	——
A bad time of the morning or afternoon	——	——
Too much time waiting while therapist was seeing other patients	——	——

Additional comments: Please indicate which hospital—AEMC, Willowcrest, or Moss—may have caused problems in your rehab. program.

5. Upon discharge did the physical therapy and/or social services department:

	Yes	No
Arrange outpatient therapy appointments for you	——	——
See to it that you received the necessary equipment you would need at home	——	——
Additional comments, please	——	——

6. Did you have any problems at home that were not discussed with you by the hospital staff before your discharge that our team should know about?
7. Now that the surgery and recovery periods are over, do you feel that you are able to function as much as you anticipated prior to having this operation?
8. Do you have any suggestions that would help improve our present program?

Box 5 *Incontinence Quiz*

Statements for which:

Correct Answer is "Agree"

Most people who currently have involuntary urine loss live normal lives.

Many people with involuntary urine loss can be cured and almost everyone can experience significant improvement.

There are exercises that can help control urine if one leaks when they cough, sneeze, or laugh.

Involuntary loss of urine can be caused by several easily treatable medical conditions.

Women are more likely than men to develop urinary incontinence.

Many common over-the-counter medications can cause involuntary urine loss.

Correct Answer is "Disagree"

Once people start to lose control of their urine on a regular basis they usually can never regain complete control over it again.

The best treatment for involuntary urine loss is usually surgery.

Other than pads, diapers, and catheters, little can be done to treat or cure involuntary urine loss.

Most physicians ask their older patients whether they have bladder control problems.

Most people will involuntarily or accidentally lose control of their urine on a regular basis by the time they reach age 85.

Involuntary urine loss is caused by only one or two conditions.

Involuntary loss of urine, often called a leaky bladder or urinary incontinence, is one of the results of normal aging.

Most people with involuntary urine loss talk to their doctors about it.

From Branch LG and others: Urinary incontinence knowledge among community-dwelling people 65 years of age and older, *J Am Geriatr Soc* 42:1257-1262, 1994.

Teaching Approaches	Theories
___ 1. Emphasis on seriousness of consequences of not taking a health action	a. Self-efficacy theory
___ 2. Consciousness raising	b. Transtheoretic model of change
___ 3. Reinterpretation of physiological signs and symptoms	c. Health belief model
___ 4. Relapse prevention	
___ 5. Modeling	
___ 6. Provision of cues to precipitate action	

Circle the correct answer

T F 7. A health care provider may be sued for a negative event resulting from the patient not understanding discharge instructions.

T F 8. Traditionally the goal of patient education has been compliance with the medical regimen.

19. Recent research using qualitative methods show that individuals use biomedical information selectively and incorporate it into their own experiences and sources of information, to make it "their own."

a. What philosophy of learning best describes this process?

b. What does this philosophy predict about the quality of learning that comes from such a process?

c. How should health professionals respond to such knowledge?

20. Of patients attending the minor injuries unit of a university hospital, only 18% understood that a tetanus injection would not prevent wound infection. Those who had been vaccinated in the previous year were no more knowledgeable than were others.[6] How problematic is this misconception? Should anything be done about it?

21. Piette and others[15] described a study of automated telephone assessment and self-care education with nurse follow-up to persons with diabetes. During biweekly 5- to 8-minute telephone assessments, patients interacted with the system using their

touch-tone keypad; responses were stored and determined the subsequent content of the message. During each assessment, patients reported information about self-monitored blood glucose readings, self-care, perceived glycemic control, and symptoms of poor glycemic control, foot problems, chest pain, and breathing problems. Patients also heard educational messages focusing on glucose self-monitoring, foot care, and medication adherence; reported specific barriers to self-care; and received tailored messages and advice. Each week, the automated assessment system generated reports organized according to the urgency of reported problems, and the nurse used these reports to prioritize patient contacts. On average, patients had 6 minutes of nurse telephone contact per month. In comparison with the usual care group, these patients had improved self-care and glycemic control, and decreased symptom burden.

Identify two elements of the intervention with good potential to create learning, including change in behavior.

References

1. Barry MJ and others: Patient reactions to a program designed to facilitate patient participation in treatment decisions for benign prostatic hyperplasia, *Med Care* 33:771-782, 1995.
2. Branch LG and others: Urinary incontinence knowledge among community-dwelling people 65 years of age and older, *J Am Geriatr Soc* 42:1257-1262, 1994.
3. Butler DJ, Beltran LR: Functions of an adult sickle cell group: education, task orientation, and support, *Health Soc Work* 18:49-56, 1993.
4. Clark NM, McLeroy KR: Creating capacity through health education: what we know and what we don't, *Health Educ Q* 22:273-289, 1995.
5. Coutts LB, Berg DH: The portrayal of the menstruating woman in menstrual product advertisements, *Health Care Women Int* 14:179-191, 1993.
6. Davies F, Luke LC, Burdett-Smith P: Patients' understanding of tetanus immunization, *J Accid Emerg Med* 13(4):272–273, 1996.
7. Dilorio C, Faherty B, Manteuffel B: Learning needs of persons with epilepsy: a comparison of perceptions of persons with epilepsy, nurses and physicians, *J Neurosci Nurs* 25:22-29, 1993.
8. Gibson PA and others: A health/patient education database for family practice, *Bull Med Libr Assoc* 79:357-369, 1991.
9. Glasgow RE and others: Behavioral research on diabetes at the Oregon Research Institute, *Ann Behav Med* 17:32-40, 1995.
10. Hardon AP: The needs of women versus the interests of family planning personnel, policy-makers and researchers: conflicting views on safety and acceptability of contraceptives, *Soc Sci Med* 35:753-766, 1992.
11. Lichtenstein R, Semaan S, Marmar EC: Development and impact of a hospital-based perioperative patient education program in a joint replacement center, *Orthop Nurs* 12(6):17-25, 1993.
12. Mahoney DF, Shippee-Rice R: Training family caregivers of older adults: a program model for community nurses, *J Community Health Nurs* 11:71-78, 1994.
13. Meyer J, Rainey J: Writing health education material for low-literacy populations, *J Health Educ* 25:372-374, 1994.
14. Moser DK, Dracup K: Psychosocial recovery from a cardiac event: the influence of perceived control, *Heart Lung* 24:273-280, 1995.
15. Piette JD and others: Do automated calls with nurse follow-up improve self-care and glycemic control among vulnerable patients with diabetes? *Am J Med* 108:20-27, 2000.
16. Troy NW, Daigas-Pelish P: Development of a self-care guide for postpartum fatigue, *Appl Nurs Res* 8:92-101, 1995.
17. Williams-Deane M, Potter LS: Current oral contraceptive use instructions: an analysis of patient package inserts, *Fam Plann Perspect* 24:111-115, 1992.
18. Yetzer EA and others: Development of a patient education program for new amputees, *Rehabil Nurs* 19:355-358, 1994.

SUGGESTED ANSWERS TO STUDY QUESTIONS

1. You first need to consider who loses money if the tests have to be redone because payment does constitute a reinforcer. Are patients disgusted with having to come back several times? Are other services in the hospital affected? It is likely that a good patient-education program could improve bowel preparation, probably with increasing increments of improvements as the program and its delivery are refined.

2. Constantly be aware that such messages exist and that they serve interests other than those of your patient. Teaching of such messages can be considered unethical.

3. As a step toward improving women's ability to use the pill effectively, Family Health International believes that PPIs should provide standardized, simplified instructions on using oral contraceptives.[10]

4. These standards are just a beginning because they frequently do not include evidence that following them results in improved patient outcomes at a reasonable cost. Only one (enterostomal education) includes target patient outcomes.

5. This finding may say that no matter how much patients perform self-care behaviors as taught, their diabetes is not under control, which may mean that their medical treatments do not work very well. Under these circumstances, learning and doing self-care will not be reinforced because the patient continues to get worse. This finding may also reflect faulty self-reports on the patient's part.

6. Patient education can be designed to develop feelings of control by placing the patient in a major decision-making role in choice of treatment and by concentrating on development of self-efficacy for these behaviors.

7. The research base for these models has not made clear which components or critical mass of principles are needed to achieve change and which are more or less relevant to particular problems and populations of potential learners.[4] Your best bet is to use a theory that has been shown in studies to work with the problem you are facing.

8. Answers will vary.

9. The differences reflect expected perspectives of each of the groups and show especially that patients are interested in control of their symptoms, which should not be a surprise. The lesson to be learned is that patient education should clearly address the patient's concerns, and not be constructed only from the providers' points of view. Unless this is done, patients lose interest in patient education, and satisfaction with their care frequently declines.

10.

Potential Negative Side Effects	Ways to Avoid
A serious complication that the patient does not recognize	Include those possibilities in the guide and note when to get help; have this advice validated by your panel of experts.
A feeling of lack of confidence if use of the guide does not ease the symptom	In the pilot test, verify that a wide range of users can understand and have the skills to use the guide effectively; include expected use of professional personnel if the symptoms do not abate.

11. Answers will vary.

12. Evidence about what a wide variety of patients learn from the materials.

13. It would have been helpful to obtain need-to-know behaviors from persons at various stages of recovering from amputation and to focus on development of a sense of self-efficacy in dealing with the various aspects of life with an amputation. Some of the objectives should be more focused on the actual behavior needed. For example, instead of stating that the patient should look for any red, discolored, or open areas daily, it would have been better to see if the patient could identify such areas on real amputations or at least in pictures. The use of a support group is excellent; what objectives should be accomplished through it? Would it be useful to put this process on a critical pathway to help identify benchmarks for patient progress in reaching the outcomes? It would also be helpful to have evaluation tools such as anchored scales. Although this program is a good start, persons with amputations no doubt need ongoing patient education services until they have reached optimal rehabilitation.

14. It is important that the questions are not focused on outcomes from patient education (except indirectly in Question 2); indeed, clear outcome objectives were not found in the article. Most of the questions are focused on patient satisfaction with process. This questionnaire clearly does not measure the impact of the perioperative joint replacement patient education program. "Yes-no" answers lead to socially desirable answers. Scoring on a nondichotomous scale could still have served to alert providers to patients with problems or dissatisfaction.

15. Answers will vary.

16. Perhaps. These patients were described as having disabling pain (and depended on medication to control it), depression, defenses for coping with developmental delays caused by the disease, death anxiety, and disability.[3] The education/social support group can, however, help them gain self-efficacy with a sense of control over their options, as well as the knowledge and skill base undergirding it. The support group can provide opportunities for modeling those who are coping successfully with this disease and for the emotional support of peers, which can help to ease conflicts between patients and providers.

17. Incontinence Quiz
    a. The agree/disagree response provides very limited information about what people know and is easily influenced by guessing.
    b. Develop for yourself a content grid of what people who have incontinence want to know and want to be able to do and what you think they should know

and be able to do. What is missing from this test? (In other words, compare the test against a set of learning objectives.) Questions 7 through 9 are not central to my sense of what is impotant, whereas more detail about what patients know relative to the other questions would be important.
    c. An important question should be: How much knowledge is enough? What is the outcome behavior desired? Enough to get people to treatment if they are incontinent? Without clarity about outcome and formal studies that show that particular test scores predict the outcome, it is very difficult to use the tool clinically.

18. (1) c, (2) b, (3) a, (4) b, (5) a, (6) c, (7) T, (8) T

19. a. Constructivist.
    b. That it will last, as it has been constructed to make it meaningful to that individual.
    c. Listen to it, acknowledge it, and use it unless it is dangerous.

20. Such a misconception could delay recognition of wound infection. These findings indicate failure of essential patient education. (From Davies F, Luke LC, Burdett-Smith P: Patients' understanding of tetanus immunization, *J Accid Emerg Med* 13:272-273, 1996.)

21. (1) Assessment allowing teaching targeted to each patient's needs and (2) teaching over a period of time, providing small doses of instruction over a number of months that could be incorporated into patients' daily self-care.

Appendix C

Meta-Analyses and Other Research Reviews

A number of articles summarize research on patient education. Many of these have been cited throughout this text. In the field of research summarization, a series of techniques called *meta-analysis* is now being used. These techniques select studies and extract findings by means of a rigorous procedure. The findings are then summarized across studies statistically. The goal of the procedure is to decrease the subjectivity that can be involved in traditional methods of summarization by narrative or by counting studies in which the experimental treatment does or does not show a positive effect. Increasing numbers of reviews available about patient education use meta-analysis.

Anderson KO, Masur FT III: Psychological preparation for invasive medical and dental procedures, *J Behav Med* 6:1-40, 1983.

  Psychological preparation for invasive medical and dental procedures has been based on the rationale that high levels of preprocedural fear are detrimental to patients' later adaptation. However, what constitutes an adaptive level of preprocedural concern has yet to be established. Outcome studies have used informative, psychotherapeutic, modeling, behavioral, cognitive-behavioral, and hypnotic techniques. The research, although frequently flawed, suggests that each of these approaches can be effective.

Bates TA, Broome M: Preparation of children for hospitalization and surgery: a review of the literature, *J Pediatr Nurs* 1:230-239, 1986.

  The three most commonly reported hospital and surgery preparation methods for children are hospital tours, play therapy, and filmed modeling. The research on preparation reveals that younger children tend to benefit from programs using play therapy, dolls, and puppets, whereas older children benefit from verbal explanations, diagrams, and audiovisual aids. School-aged children can be prepared several days in advance, but preschool children benefit from preparation closer to the actual event. For children with previous hospital experience, information formats with built-in coping procedures will be more beneficial in decreasing anxiety. Health care providers should allow children and parents the freedom to verbalize fears, anxieties, and questions.

Bernard-Bonnin AC and others: Self-management teaching programs and morbidity of pediatric asthma: a meta-analysis, *J Allergy Clin Immunol* 95:34-41, 1995.

  This meta-analysis, which summarizes 11 studies published between 1970 and 1991, found

261

that self-management teaching programs do not seem to reduce morbidity.

Broome ME, Lillis PP, Smith MC: Pain interventions with children: a meta-analysis of research, *Nurs Res* 38:154-158, 1989.

A combination of cognitive and affective pain management interventions was reported in more than 40% of the studies, and 70% of interventions were introduced immediately before the painful event. The pain management programs resulted in at least a 30% reduction in children's distress responses.

Brown SA: Studies of educational interventions and outcomes in diabetic adults: a meta-analysis revisited, *Patient Educ Counsel* 16:189-215, 1990.

This study expanded a 1988 summary of research on effectiveness of diabetes education. Results indicate that patients who receive diabetes patient education experience improved knowledge, self-care behaviors, metabolic outcomes, and psychological outcomes.

Brown SA: Meta-analysis of diabetes patient education research: variations in intervention effects across studies, *Res Nurs Health* 15:409-419, 1992.

Reanalysis of 73 studies from previously reported meta-analyses of diabetes patient education literature found that patient education appeared to be more effective in younger patients. For all patients, glycosylated hemoglobin levels improved between 1 and 6 months postintervention but decreased to 1-month levels after 6 months. Length of the educational intervention did not appear to influence outcomes.

Brug J, Campbell M, van Assema P: The application and impact of computer-generated personalized nutrition education: a review of the literature, *Patient Educ Counsel* 36:145-156, 1999.

This is a review of 8 studies of the impact of comprehensive computer-generated nutrition interventions based on behavior change theory. Personalized dietary and psychosocial feedback appears more likely to be read and remembered and seen as personally relevant compared with standard messages.

Burke LE, Dunbar-Jacob JM, Hill MN: Compliance with cardiovascular disease prevention strategies: a review of the research, *Ann Behav Med* 19:239-263, 1997.

This is a review (not a meta-analysis) of 46 randomized controlled studies of cognitive education and behavioral strategies to improve compliance with cardiovascular disease risk reduction. Successful strategies include signed agreements, self-efficacy enhancement, behavioral skill training, self-monitoring, and telephone-mail contact. Comparative efficacy has generally not been tested.

Devine EC: Effects of psychoeducational care for adult surgical patients: a meta-analysis of 191 studies, *Patient Educ Counsel* 19:129-142, 1992.

This is a quantitative review of 191 studies, issued between 1963 and 1989, of the effects of psychoeducational care on adult surgical patients. Statistically reliable, small-to-moderate sized beneficial effects were found on recovery, postoperative pain, and psychological distress.

Devine EC: Effects of psychoeducational care with adult surgical patients: a theory-probing meta-analysis of intervention studies. In Cook TD and others, editors, *Meta-analysis for explanation: a casebook*, New York, 1992, Russell Sage Foundation.

The large research base of controlled clinical trials of psychoeducational care administered to adult surgical patients has demonstrated that those receiving additional psychoeducational care recovered more quickly and were more satisfied with their care than were patients receiving the usual psychoeducational care provided in the setting. This finding was true in both sexes, among many different ages and types of surgery. These interventions usually took less than an hour of registered nurse time. This meta-analysis probes for support for various theories and finds some support for self regulation under stress, nonstress physiological model, and social learning theory.

Devine EC: Meta-analysis of the effects of psychoeducational care in adults with asthma. *Res Nurs Health* 19:367-376, 1996.

Thirty-one studies published between 1972 and 1993 are summarized. Psychoeducational care including education, behavioral skill development, cognitive therapy, and/or nonbehavioral support/counseling were included in this meta-analysis. Education provided demonstrable benefits in the occurrence of asthma attacks, peak expiratory flow rate, functional status, adherence to treatment regimen, utilization of health care, use of PRN medications, psychological well-being, and psychomotor knowledge of inhaler use, but not in dynamic respiratory volume. Provision of this care is well justified by the existing research.

Devine EC, Cook TD: A meta-analytic analysis of effects of psychoeducational interventions on length of post-surgical hospital stay, *Nurs Res* 32:267-274, 1983.

Forty-nine studies of the relationships between brief psychoeducational interventions and the length of postsurgical hospitalization were reviewed. The interventions were often multidimensional and included providing patients with information about procedures, pain, and sensations to expect; skills training or teaching the patient exercises to promote recovery by preventing complications or reducing anxiety; and psychosocial support by a health care provider who prepared interactions to reduce patients' anxiety or enhance their ability to cope with hospitalization. Results showed that interventions reduced hospital stay by about 11¼ days and had an effect size of 0.38 standard deviation unit (up to 0.3 standard deviation is small, 0.3 to 0.5 is moderately large, and over 0.5 is large).

Devine ED, Cook TD: Clinical and cost-saving effects of psychoeducational interventions with surgical patients: a meta-analysis, *Res Nurs Health* 9:89-105, 1986.

A meta-analysis of 102 studies was conducted to examine how psychoeducational interventions influenced recovery, pain, psychological well-being, and satisfaction with care among adult patients hospitalized for surgery. Statistically reliable and positive effects were reported on each of these four classes of outcome. The average duration of treatments included in the meta-analysis was 42 minutes. The average effect size across all measures of recovery was 0.50, which means that these interventions reliably facilitate the recovery of surgical patients.

Devine EC, Pearcy J: Meta-analysis of the effects of psychoeducational care in adults with chronic obstructive pulmonary disease, *Patient Educ Counsel* 29:167-178, 1996.

This is a meta-analysis of 65 studies of the effect of education, exercise, and/or psychosocial support (called psychoeducational care) in adults with chronic obstructive pulmonary disease, published from 1954 to 1994. Pulmonary rehabilitation (large muscle exercise and education plus a variety of psychosocial or behavioral interventions) had statistically significant beneficial effects on psychological well-being, endurance, functional status, dyspnea, and adherence. Education alone had significant beneficial effects only on accuracy of performing inhaler skills. The effects of education on health care utilization and on adherence to treatment regimen were inconclusive, suggesting the need for further research.

Devine EC, Reifschneider E: A meta-analysis of the effects of psychoeducational care in adults with hypertension, *Nurs Res* 44:237-245, 1995.

This meta-analysis of 102 studies completed between 1965 and 1993 found small to medium-sized statistically significant beneficial effects on blood pressure from patient education and psychosocial support (called psychoeducational care). Statistically significant large treatment effects were obtained on knowledge, drug compliance, and compliance with health care appointments. Twenty-five combinations of education, behavioral support, and/or psychosocial support were found with no specific combination occurring in more than five interventions. Whether these activities were actually performed by subjects, duration of treatment or direct comparison between types of psychoeducational care were rarely reported.

Devine EC, Westlake SK: The effects of psychoeducational care provided to adults with cancer: meta-analysis of 116 studies, *Oncol Nurs Forum* 22:1369-1381, 1995.

Psychoeducational care was found to have statistically significant beneficial effects in adults with cancer in relation to anxiety, depression, mood, nausea, vomiting, pain, and knowledge. Differentiating among the effectiveness of various types of psychoeducational care was problematic with the current studies.

DiFabio RP: Efficacy of comprehensive rehabilitation programs and back school for patients with low back pain: a meta-analysis, *Phys Ther* 75:865-878, 1998.

Nineteen prospective randomized controlled trials were evaluated. The average effect size for comprehensive rehabilitation programs that included back school ($d = 0.28$) was larger than the average effect size for programs that offered back school as the primary intervention ($d = -0.14$), with the former superior to back school programs in pain reduction, increased spinal mobility, and strength. Both types of programs showed reasonable success with education/compliance outcomes ($d = 0.27$ to 0.28). So existing research has found back schools to be most efficacious when combined with a comprehensive rehabilitation program. Work/vocational and disability outcomes were not improved substantially beyond control levels in comprehensive or primary back school programs. (A negative *d* index shows that the control or comparison group has superior outcomes compared with the group receiving back school.)

Dusseldorp E and others: A meta-analysis of psychoeducational programs for coronary heart disease patients, *Health Psychol* 18:506-519, 1999.

This is a meta-analysis of 37 studies of the effects of psychoeducational (health education and stress management) programs for patients with coronary heart disease. These programs yielded a 34% decrease in mortality from cardiac disease, a 29% decrease in recurrence of myocardial infarction, and significant positive effects on blood pressure, cholesterol, body weight, smoking behavior, physical exercise, and eating habits. No effects on anxiety or depression were found.

Glanz K: Compliance with dietary regimens: its magnitude, measurement and determinants, *Prev Med* 9:787-804, 1980.

Studies of patient compliance with dietary regimens for cardiovascular disease risk reduction, weight reduction, renal disease, diabetes, and other conditions were reviewed. Patient noncompliance with dietary regimens was found to be at least as frequent as noncompliance with medication regimens. Health professionals might increase their effectiveness by recognizing that nonhealth motivations may lead individuals to take appropriate actions and that social and familial influences may affect patients' willingness, desire, and ability to adhere to diets.

Glanz K: Nutrition education for risk-factor reduction and patient education: a review, *Prev Med* 14:721-725, 1985.

Studies of adult nutrition education and counseling for weight reduction, diabetes, cancer, low-fat diets, sodium-restricted diets, and renal diets were also reviewed. These studies draw on a variety of theories from communications, anthropology, education, sociology, and psychology, although before the last 15 to 20 years nutrition education was usually thought of as informational or persuasive. A wide gap exists between the development of behavioral science strategies for nutrition education and the testing of these strategies in practice. On the basis of this review, several basic educational principles for patient nutrition education should be considered in the design of all educational efforts: tailoring of both dietary regimens and educational strategies, use of social support within and outside of the health care setting, provision of skills training in addition to information, effective patient-provider communication, and attention to follow-up, monitoring, and reinforcement.

Glanz K: Patient and public education for cholesterol reduction: a review of strategies and issues, *Patient Educ Counsel* 12:235-257, 1988.

Current knowledge regarding patient and public education for cholesterol reduction lags behind the epidemiological and clinical evidence that forms the basis for controlling blood cholesterol levels.

Goeppinger J, Lorig K: Interventions to reduce the impact of chronic disease: community-based arthritis patient education, *Annu Rev Nurs Res* 15:101-122, 1997.

This is a narrative review of community-based arthritis patient education studies conducted between 1980 and 1995. It is not a meta-analysis. Twenty years of cumulative arthritis patient education research shows the effectiveness of population-focused, community-based interventions although not with low-income and minority populations.

Greenland P, Chu JS: Efficacy of cardiac rehabilitation services with emphasis on patients after myocardial infarction, *Ann Intern Med* 109:650-663, 1988.

Cardiac rehabilitation programs commonly offer education about the heart, causes of myocardial infarction, cardiac risk factors, and other general teaching designed to reassure patients with cardiac disease by making them more knowledgeable about their heart conditions. The evidence that teaching or counseling or both are helpful in cardiac programs after infarction is not conclusive.

Hansel NK: Review of oral hygiene patient education, *Patient Educ Counsel* 5:89-93, 1983.

Most attempts to improve oral hygiene practices have relied heavily on instructional approaches of the lecture-demonstration type or on such strategies combined with practice sessions in brushing and flossing. Frequently, behavior change may persist for only a short time after the preventive program ends.

Harrison JA, Mullen PD, Green LW: A meta-analysis of studies of the Health Belief Model with adults, *Health Educ Res* 7:107-116, 1992.

Meta-analysis of 16 studies of Health Belief Model (HBM) dimensions found weak effect sizes and lack of homogeneity. This indicates that it is premature to draw conclusions about the predictive validity of the HBM as operationalized in these studies.

Hathaway D: Effect of preoperative instruction on postoperative outcomes: a meta-analysis, *Nurs Res* 35:269-275, 1986.

A meta-analysis was performed on 68 studies of traditional preoperative instruction, using both physiological and psychological dependent variables. An average effect size of 0.44 was found. This result was not dissimilar to the findings of other analyses on these kinds of preoperative interventions.

Hawley DJ: Psycho-educational interventions in the treatment of arthritis, *Bailliere's Clin Rheumatol* 9:803-823, 1995.

Structured educational programs for patients with rheumatic diseases began in the late 1970s. Hawley reviews 34 clinical trials of psychoeducation for rheumatic disease performed between 1985 and 1995. While most studies of self-management education showed slight improvement, its effect on functional ability is unclear. Twenty of the 26 studies demonstrated improvement in pain. This is not a meta-analysis.

Hirano PC, Laurent DD, Lorig K: Arthritis patient education studies, 1987-1991: a review of the literature, *Patient Educ Counsel* 24:9-54, 1994.

Clinical studies have shown that medical care, including the use of medications, can offer a 20% to 50% improvement in reported arthritis symptoms. Data from patient education studies suggest that a further improvement of 15% to 30% is attainable through patient education interventions.

Hunsberger M, Love B, Byrne C: A review of current approaches used to help children and parents cope with health care procedures, *Matern Child Nurs J* 13:145-165, 1984.

Programs that prepare children for hospitalization are designed to inform the child about what will happen and to familiarize the child with the hospital environment. Even though the reason that information is beneficial is unclear, benefits have been demonstrated. Information about health care procedures was provided through modeling, procedural and sensory information, and stress-point nursing. The research findings tended to oppose the notions that young children should not receive information, that all children benefit equally from the same type and timing of preparation, that a child who has had a previous experience requires less preparation, and that a one-time preadmission program provides adequate preparation. Techniques that assist the child in gaining a sense of control suggest that children can benefit from being helped to gain a sense of mastery over a stressful event. Progressive muscle relaxation and desensitization have been shown to reduce anxiety and discomfort during health care procedures.

Janz NK, Becker MH, Hartman PE: Contingency contracting to enhance patient compliance: a review, *Patient Educ Counsel* 5:165-178, 1983.

The contingency contract is a specific negotiated agreement that provides for the delivery of positive consequences or reinforcers contingent on desirable behavior. It has its theoretical roots in operant conditioning. The 15 studies reviewed demonstrated at least short-term positive effects from contingency contracting across a variety of medical conditions and health-related behaviors. Most of the studies were conducted with motivated volunteers rather than with random samples of some defined population.

Janz NK and others: Interventions to enhance breast self-examination: a review, *Public Health Rev* 17:89-169, 1989/90.

Intensive interventions result in better outcomes. The provisions of information seem sufficient to obtain breast self-examination (BSE) initiation but not necessarily adequate to maintain practice or to establish proficiency. The addition of skills training and corrective feedback leads to significantly improved proficiency in BSE. Prompts and reminder aids seem also to contribute to long-term frequency.

Jones LC: A meta-analytic study of the effects of childbirth education on the parent-infant relationship, *Health Care Women Int* 7:357-370, 1986.

Twenty-seven studies of the effect of childbirth education on knowledge, behavior, or attitude in the parent-infant relationship (completed from 1960 to 1981) were analyzed. Average effect size was 0.38 (equivalent to a correlation of 0.20) even though the major focus of these childbirth classes was on helping women cope with labor and delivery with few medications and minimum pain. Compared with parents who did not take childbirth education, parents participating in it were more attentive and responsive to their infants, were more satisfied with the behavior of the infants, reported fewer feeding problems, had more positive feelings and attitudes toward their infants, and spent more time playing with and cuddling their infants. Few negative effects of childbirth education were found. Larger effect sizes were obtained for middle-income parents (0.40) compared with parents of low income (0.16). Flaws in the research included the researchers' acknowledging allegiance to childbirth education, conducting the research while knowledgeable of the composition of the groups or while teaching the classes, or using instruments that could be easily controlled by the investigator.

Kirscht JP: Preventive health behavior: a review of research and issues, *Health Psychol* 2:277-301, 1983.

Preventive behavior is any behavior that people engage in spontaneously or can be induced to perform with the intention of alleviating the impact of potential risks and hazards in their environment. Sociocultural perspectives and cognitive and behavioral models were used to explain the behavior, with each point of view having its own intervention strategies.

Kottke TE and others: Attributes of successful smoking cessation interventions in medical practice: a meta-analysis of 39 controlled trials, *JAMA* 259:2883-2889, 1988.

Group and individual sessions combined were better than either alone. Success was the product of personalized smoking cessation advice and assistance repeated in different forms by several sources over the longest feasible period. It is reinforcement—the number of contacts and the number of people making them—that produces results. Withdrawing reinforcement contributes to relapse.

Levy SR, Iverson BK, Walberg HJ: Adolescent pregnancy programs and educational interventions: a research synthesis and review, *J Soc Health* 3:99-103, 1983.

Research from 1970 to 1980 contained in studies of educational programs designed for the adolescent parent in diverse settings such as schools, communities, hospitals, and clinics was synthesized. Examples of topics emphasized in these various settings include family life, parenting, birth defects, nutrition, and prenatal care. The mean overall effect size was 0.35 standard deviation unit. (An effect size contrasts the average performance of a treatment group with that of another treatment or control group.) The programs being evaluated were not being compared with true control groups, which receive no treatment. They were being compared with different groups of clients who receive some services similar to those of the target program; therefore the effect size can be considered both statistically significant and an advantageous result of educa-tional programs. Interestingly, the effect size for reducing or delaying repeat pregnancies was only 0.177.

Lindeman CA: Patient education, *Annu Rev Nurs Res* 6:29-60, 1988.

Patient-education influences learning, with the greatest impact on knowledge and skills. Most teaching strategies, such as booklet, programmed instruction, modeling, and lecture-discussion, are effective. Group teaching is as effective as individual teaching. The organizational structure of the hospital is less important than the value the staff and administration attaches to patient-teaching. The effectiveness of patient education as a nursing intervention is clearly established.

Linden W, Stossel C, Maurice J: Psychosocial interventions for patients with coronary artery disease; a meta-analysis, *Arch Intern Med* 156:745-752, 1996.

This is a meta-analysis of 23 randomized controlled trials that evaluated the additional impact of psychosocial treatment. Benefits of reduction in mortality and morbidity, psychological distress, and some biological risk factors were clearly evident.

Lipsey MW, Wilson DB: The efficacy of psychological, educational and behavioral treatment; confirmation from meta-analysis, *Am Psychol* 48:1181-1209, 1993.

This study examined large bodies of meta-analyses of treatment research, many focused on mental health but including some on patient education. It is most useful as a reference work.

Lorig K, Konkol L, Gonzalez V: Arthritis patient education: a review of the literature, *Patient Educ Counsel* 10:207-252, 1987.

Patient education can influence a variety of arthritis-related behaviors, such as exercise, relaxation, and joint protection. With patient education, 61% of health status measures of pain, disability, count of painful joints, depression, and quality of life demonstrated improvement. The effect of arthritis patient education is potentially similar to that of other standard arthritis treatment, such as nonsteroidal anti-inflammatory drugs.

Mazzuca SA: Does patient education in chronic disease have therapeutic value? *J Chron Dis* 35:521-529, 1982.

From a pool of 320 articles on patient education, 30 were found that documented controlled experiments in chronic disease. These experiments had dependent variables that included (1) compliance with a therapeutic regimen, (2) physiological progress of patients, or (3) long-range health outcomes. Diseases in the sample included hypertension (10), other heart disease (5), asthma and obesity (3 each), and others.

A summary of all experimental effects shows that patient education was most successful in altering compliance (average improvement = 0.67 standard deviation over control) but was also statistically significant in improving physiological progress (0.49 standard deviation) and health outcomes (0.20 standard deviation).

Studies were divided according to those in which (1) the emphasis was didactic, having a standard presentation to all subjects, with information transfer accomplished by numerous vehicles, or (2) the emphasis was behavioral, focusing on the patient's own regimen and daily routine as the content of instruction, with attempts made to affect the patient's home or work environment in ways that promoted effective self-management, use of social support, medication monitoring, and telephone follow-up.

Behaviorally oriented programs were found to be consistently more successful in improving the clinical course of chronic disease.

McCain NL, Lynn MR: Meta-analysis of a narrative review: studies evaluating patient teaching, *West J Nurs Res* 12:347-358, 1990.

This meta-analysis summarized studies previously summarized in narrative reviews and found a clear benefit of patient teaching. The score of the average individual in the experimental group exceeded that of 69% of the individuals in the control group.

Meyer TJ, Mark MM: Effects of psychosocial interventions with adult cancer patients: a meta-analysis of randomized experiments, *Health Psychol* 14:101-108, 1995.

This study summarizes results of 45 studies of psychosocial interventions intended to improve the quality of life of adult cancer patients. The analysis found an effect size of 0.24 for emotional adjustment, 0.19 for functional adjustment, and 0.26 for treatment and disease-related symptoms. These are moderate effect sizes.

Mullen PD: Health promotion and patient education benefits for employees, *Annu Rev Public Health* 9:305-332, 1988.

For reducing risk of disease and promoting well-being, group programs at the worksite or those contracted by the employer in the community can be moderately effective in changing behavior for some groups of employees. For increasing competence in self-care of minor complaints, several rigorous studies suggest that providing materials and support to guide and encourage self-care for common complaints can safely reduce outpatient visits. Education is an important component of programs to substitute home care for hospital and outpatient care. Currently, however, a patient cannot rely on usual providers of medical care to offer adequate education.

Mullen PD, Green LW, Persinger GS: Clinical trials of patient-education for chronic conditions: a comparative meta-analysis of intervention types, *Prev Med* 14:753-781, 1985.

The findings of 70 published evaluations of education programs for people with long-term health problems and regimens that include drugs were synthesized. The overall effect size was 0.37, indicating a substantially decreased number of drug errors. Effect size for decreased drug errors for one-to-one counseling was 0.43; for group education, 0.34; for written or other audiovisual materials except patient package inserts (PPIs), 0.43; for PPIs, 0.01 (almost no effect on increasing patients' knowledge); for counseling or group plus materials, 0.44; for labels, special containers, or memory aids, 0.42; for behavior modification and self-administration, 0.50. The higher the educational quality of an intervention in terms of relevance, individualization, feedback, reinforcement, and so on, the larger the effect size value for decreased drug errors.

Mullen PD, Mains DA, Velez R: A meta-analysis of controlled trials of cardiac education, *Patient Educ Counsel* 9:143-162, 1992.

Twenty-eight controlled studies of cardiac patient education programs showed an average effect size of 0.51 for blood pressure and 0.24 for mortality.

Mullen PD, Ramirez G, Groff JY: A meta-analysis of randomized trials of prenatal smoking cessation interventions, *Am J Obstet Gynecol* 171:1328-1334, 1994.

Most of the programs included individual counseling sessions of no more than 10 minutes; all used material specifically directed to pregnancy rather than to a general audience. More intensive interventions with multiple contacts, multiple formats, and some form of follow-up reaped a larger effect.

Mullen PD and others: Efficacy of psychoeducational interventions on pain, depression, and disability in people with arthritis: a meta-analysis, *J Rheumatol* 14(suppl 15):33-39, 1987.

This summary of 15 studies of the effects of psychoeducational interventions in individuals with arthritis showed moderate effect sizes of 0.2 for pain, 0.27 for depression, and 0.13 for disability.

Mullen PD and others: A meta-analysis of trials evaluating patient education and counseling for three groups of preventive health behaviors, *Patient Educ Counsel* 32:157-173, 1997.

The authors focused on primary prevention areas of contraceptive use, breast and testicular self-examination, exercise, injury prevention, nutrition, stress management, substance abuse, and weight control. They excluded studies of patients with diagnosed disease and those with extremely specialized learning needs. Use of essential principles of education and more than one patient contact were important predictors of treatment effect. The average member of the experimental group was 44% better off than was the average member of the control group. When the goal was subtracting an existing behavior (smoking/alcohol, nutrition/weight control) behavioral techniques, especially self monitoring, were important.

Mumford E, Schlesinger HJ, Glass GV: The effects of psychological intervention on recovery from surgery and heart attacks: an analysis of the literature, *Am J Public Health* 72:141-151, 1982.

Thirty-four controlled experimental studies were reviewed. On the average, surgical or coronary patients, who were provided information or emotional support to help them master the medical crisis, did better than patients who received only ordinary care. The effect size was 0.50 standard deviation, consistent across studies. A combination of both approaches seems clearly superior to either alone.

A review of 13 studies that used hospital days after surgery or after heart attack as outcome indicators showed that, on average, psychological intervention reduced hospitalization approximately 2 days below the control group's average of 9.92 days.

Most of the interventions were modest, and in most studies they were not matched in any way to the needs or coping styles of particular patients. Beyond the intrinsic value of offering humane and considerate care, the evidence shows that psychological care can be cost-effective.

Nunes EV, Frank KA, Kornfeld DS: Psychologic treatment for the type A behavior pattern and for coronary heart disease: a meta-analysis of the literature, *Psychosom Med* 48:159-173, 1987.

The type A behavior pattern (TABP) is a recognized risk factor for coronary heart disease; yet treatments aimed at its modification are not widely used. Eighteen controlled studies of the psychologic treatment of TABP found an effect size of 0.61. Treatment modalities include education about coronary heart disease, education about TABP, relaxation training, cognitive therapy, imaging, behavior modification, emotional support, and psychodynamic interpretation. A combination of treatment techniques is most effective.

O'Connor AM and others: Decision aids for patients facing health treatment or screening decisions: systematic review, *Br Med J* 319:731-734, 1999.

Seventeen studies met the inclusion criteria for decision aids for patients facing real (not hypothetical) treatment or screening decisions. Decision aids improve knowledge, reduce decisional conflict and stimulate patients to be more active in decision making without increasing their anxiety and do a better job than does usual care. They had a variable effect on decisions and virtually no effect on satisfaction.

Padgett D and others: Meta-analysis of the effects of educational and psychosocial interventions on management of diabetes mellitus, *J Clin Epidemiol* 41: 1007-1030, 1988.

Diet instruction showed an effect size of 0.68, and social learning and behavior modification interventions an effect size of 0.57. The weakest effect size was for relaxation training (0.30). Positive effects decreased but were retained at 6- and 12-month follow-up with the exception of weight loss.

Posavac EJ: Evaluation of patient-education programs: a meta-analysis, *Eval Health Prof* 3:47-62, 1980.

A literature search identified 23 evaluations of patient-education programs that used a randomly selected experimental or quasiexperimental design. The mean effect size was 0.74; for measures of compliance, it was 1.08, and for anxiety, 0.60.

Posavac EJ and others: Increasing compliance to medical treatment regimens: a meta-analysis of program evaluation, *Eval Health Prof* 8:7-22, 1985.

A total of 58 studies evaluating the effectiveness of programs to increase compliance with medical treatment regimens were quantitatively integrated to assess their impact on the behavior of clients. Mean effect size was 0.47. The advantage of the program groups dropped as the amount of life-style changes required by the treatment regimen increased. The most successful interventions involved improving the facility providing care and helping patients to incorporate the treatment regimen into their daily routine. One program using several interventions had the largest impact, and two based on the behavioral principle of rewarding successive approximations of outpatient compliant behavior were very strong as well.

Reading AE: The short-term effects of psychological preparation for surgery, *Soc Sci Med* 13A:641-654, 1979.

Accumulating evidence exists on the short-term effects of psychological preparation for surgery; however, the way in which these effects are produced is not clear. Worry, information, and coping models have been used. It seems likely that the effects of psychological preparation will vary according to the nature of the situation as well as the personality of the patient.

Roter DL and others: Effectiveness of interventions to improve patient compliance; a meta-analysis, *Med Care* 36:1138-1161, 1998.

This is a summary of the results of 153 studies published between 1977 and 1994 that evaluated the effectiveness of interventions to improve patient compliance with medical regimens. Patients with chronic diseases including those with diabetes and hypertension, persons with cancer, and those with mental health problems especially benefited from interventions. Comprehensive interventions combining cognitive, behavioral, and affective components were more effective than were single-focus interventions. No single intervention strategy appeared consistently stronger than any other—direct education, group processes, familial support, or behavioral modalities.

Suls J, Wan CK: Effects of sensory and procedural information on coping with stressful medical procedures and pain: a meta-analysis, *J Consult Clin Psychol* 57:372-379, 1989.

Combined sensory-procedural preparation yielded the strongest and most consistent benefits in terms of reducing negative affect, pain reports, and other-rated distress. Procedural details provide a map of specific events, whereas sensory information facilitates their interpretation as nonthreatening.

Superio-Cabuslay E, Word MM, Lorig KR: Patient education interventions in osteoarthritis and rheumatoid arthritis: a meta-analytic comparison with nonsteroidal anti-inflammatory drug treatment, *Arthritis Care Res* 9:292-301, 1996.

The purpose of this meta-analysis was to compare the effects of education interventions and nonsteroidal anti-inflammatory drug treatment on pain and functional disability. Nineteen patient education trials were included. The weighted average effect size for pain was 0.17 and for functional disability was 0.03; effects of education were much larger in rheumatoid arthritis studies than in osteoarthritis studies, with average effect sizes for tender joint at 0.34. Because patients in the educational trials were being treated with medications, the effect sizes of these trials represent the additional effects of patient education interventions beyond those achieved by medication.

Taal E, Rasker JJ, Wiegman O: Group education for rheumatoid arthritis patients, *Semin Arthritis Rheum* 26:805-816, 1997.

This is a narrative review of 31 studies of group education for patients with rheumatoid arthritis. Group education increased knowledge, which was maintained over long intervals. In 60% of studies, physical health status was improved but almost never maintained over long intervals and seldom led to improvement in psychosocial health status. Behavioral methods are necessary to improve health status.

Theis SL, Johnson JH: Strategies for teaching patients: a meta-analysis, *Clin Nurse Spec* 9:100-120, 1995.

This meta-analysis synthesized the body of research examining teaching strategies used in patient education—a total of 72 studies. The mean effect size was a moderate 0.41, indicating that 66% of subjects receiving planned teaching had better outcomes than did control group subjects receiving routine care. Structure yielded the highest effect size, with reinforcement, independent study, and use of multiple strategies also above the study mean.

Thompson RH: Where we stand: twenty years of research on pediatric hospitalization and health care, *Child Health Care* 14:200-210, 1986.

More than 300 research reports appearing since 1965 were summarized. This literature encompassed children's responses to hospitalization and health care, the effects of separation and parental rooming-in, parental responses to hospitalization, the hospital environment, play, and preparation for hospitalization.

Turley MA: A meta-analysis of informing mothers concerning the sensory and perceptual capabilities of their infants: the effects on maternal-infant interaction, *Matern Child Nurs J* 14:183-197, 1985.

Twenty research studies conducted between 1970 and 1981 were analyzed. These studies investigated the effects of providing information to mothers concerning the sensory and perceptual capabilities of their newborns and the effects this treatment had on maternal-infant interaction. The overall effect size in terms of maternal-infant interaction was significantly increased by the intervention. The fourth week after discharge was shown to be the most effective time to present the information.

Vallejo BC: Is structured presurgical education more effective than nonstructured education? *Patient Educ Counsel* 9:283-290, 1987.

None of the literature synthesis techniques showed that structured presurgical education was more effective than unstructured education in promoting compliance with the postsurgical therapeutic regimen.

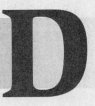

Patient Education: Rights, Standards, Guidelines, Accreditation, and Organizational Statements

A PATIENT'S BILL OF RIGHTS

Introduction

Effective health care requires collaboration between patients and physicians and other health care professionals. Open and honest communication, respect for personal and professional values, and sensitivity to differences are integral to optimal patient care. As the setting for the provision of health services, hospitals must provide a foundation for understanding and respecting the rights and responsibilities of patients, their families, physicians, and other caregivers. Hospitals must ensure a health care ethic that respects the role of patients in decision making about treatment choices and other aspects of their care. Hospitals must be sensitive to cultural, racial, linguistic, religious, age, gender, and other differences as well as the needs of persons with disabilities.

The American Hospital Association presents *A Patient's Bill of Rights* with the expectation that it will contribute to more effective patient care and be supported by the hospital on behalf of the institution, its medical staff, employees, and patients. The American Hospital Association encourages health care institutions to tailor this bill of rights to their patient community by translating and/or simplifying the language of this bill of rights as may be necessary to ensure that patients and their families understand their rights and responsibilities.

A Patient's Bill of Rights was first adopted by the American Hospital Association in 1973. This revision was approved by the AHA Board of Trustees on October 21, 1992. ©1992 by the American Hospital Association, 840 North Lake Shore Drive, Chicago, Illinois 60611. Printed in the U.S.A. All rights reserved. Catalog no. 157759.

Bill of Rights*

1. The patient has the right to considerate and respectful care.

2. The patient has the right to and is encouraged to obtain from physicians and other direct caregivers relevant, current, and understandable information concerning diagnosis, treatment, and prognosis. Except in emergencies when the patient lacks decision-making capacity and the need for treatment is urgent, the patient is entitled to the opportunity to discuss and request information related to the specific procedures and/or treatments, the risks involved, the possible length of recuperation, and the medically reasonable alternatives and their accompanying risks and benefits.

   Patients have the right to know the identity of physicians, nurses, and others involved in their care, as well as when those involved are students, residents, or other trainees. The patient also has the right to know the immediate and long-term financial implications of treatment choices, insofar as they are known.

3. The patient has the right to make decisions about the plan of care prior to and during the course of treatment and to refuse a recommended treatment or plan of care to the extent permitted by law and hospital policy and to be informed of the medical consequences of this action. In case of such refusal, the patient is entitled to other appropriate care and services that the hospital provides or transfer to another hospital. The hospital should notify patients of any policy that might affect patient choice within the institution.

4. The patient has the right to have an advance directive (such as a living will, health care proxy, or durable power of attorney for health care) concerning treatment or designating a surrogate decision maker with the expectation that the hospital will honor the intent of that directive to the extent permitted by law and hospital policy. Health care institutions must advise patients of their rights under state law and hospital policy to make informed medical choices, ask if the patient has an advance directive, and include that information in patient records. The patient has the right to timely information about hospital policy that may limit its ability to implement fully a legally valid advance directive.

5. The patient has the right to every consideration of privacy. Case discussion, consultation, examination, and treatment should be conducted so as to protect each patient's privacy.

6. The patient has the right to expect that all communications and records pertaining to his/her care will be treated as confidential by the hospital, except in cases such as suspected abuse and public health hazards when reporting is permitted or required by law. The patient has the right to expect that the hospital will emphasize the confidentiality of this information when it releases it to any other parties entitled to review information in these records.

7. The patient has the right to review the records pertaining to his/her medical care and to have the information explained or interpreted as necessary, except when restricted by law.

8. The patient has the right to expect that, within its capacity and policies, a hospital will make reasonable response to the request of a patient for appropriate and medically indicated care and services. The hospital must provide evaluation, service, and/or referral as

---

*These rights can be exercised on the patient's behalf by a designated surrogate or proxy decision maker if the patient lacks decision-making capacity, is legally incompetent, or is a minor.

indicated by the urgency of the case. When medically appropriate and legally permissible, or when a patient has so requested, a patient may be transferred to another facility. The institution to which the patient is to be transferred must first have accepted the patient for transfer. The patient must also have the benefit of complete information and explanation concerning the need for, risks, benefits, and alternatives to such a transfer.

9. The patient has the right to ask and be informed of the existence of business relationships among the hospital, educational institutions, other health care providers, or payers that may influence the patient's treatment and care.

10. The patient has the right to consent to or decline to participate in proposed research studies or human experimentation affecting care and treatment or requiring direct patient involvement, and to have those studies fully explained prior to consent. A patient who declines to participate in research or experimentation is entitled to the most effective care that the hospital can otherwise provide.

11. The patient has the right to expect reasonable continuity of care when appropriate and to be informed by physicians and other caregivers of available and realistic patient care options when hospital care is no longer appropriate.

12. The patient has the right to be informed of hospital policies and practices that relate to patient care, treatment, and responsibilities. The patient has the right to be informed of available resources for resolving disputes, grievances, and conflicts, such as ethics committees, patient representatives, or other mechanisms available in the institution. The patient has the right to be informed of the hospital's charges for services and available payment methods.

The collaborative nature of health care requires that patients, or their families/surrogates, participate in their care. The effectiveness of care and patient satisfaction with the course of treatment depend, in part, on the patient fulfilling certain responsibilities. Patients are responsible for providing information about past illnesses, hospitalizations, medications, and other matters related to health status. To participate effectively in decision making, patients must be encouraged to take responsibility for requesting additional information or clarification about their health status or treatment when they do not fully understand information and instructions. Patients are also responsible for ensuring that the health care institution has a copy of their written advance directive if they have one. Patients are responsible for informing their physicians and other caregivers if they anticipate problems in following prescribed treatment.

Patients should also be aware of the hospital's obligation to be reasonably efficient and equitable in providing care to other patients and the community. The hospital's rules and regulations are designed to help the hospital meet this obligation. Patients and their families are responsible for making reasonable accommodations to the needs of the hospital, other patients, medical staff, and hospital employees. Patients are responsible for providing necessary information for insurance claims and for working with the hospital to make payment arrangements, when necessary.

A person's health depends on much more than health care services. Patients are responsible for recognizing the impact of their life-style on their personal health.

Conclusion

Hospitals have many functions to perform, including the enhancement of health status, health promotion, and the prevention and treatment of injury and disease; the immediate and ongoing care and rehabilitation of patients; the education of health professionals, patients, and the community; and research. All these activities must be conducted with an overriding concern for the values and dignity of patients.

NATIONAL STANDARDS FOR DIABETES SELF-MANAGEMENT EDUCATION PROGRAMS AND AMERICAN DIABETES ASSOCIATION REVIEW CRITERIA*

In 1993, the National Diabetes Advisory Board charged the American Diabetes Association to coordinate a task force of representatives of diabetes and other organizations to review, and revise if indicated, the National Standards for Diabetes Patient Education Programs. The Task Force consisted of representatives from the following organizations: The American Association of Diabetes Educators, The American Diabetes Association, The American Dietetic Association, the Centers for Disease Control and Prevention, the Department of Defense, the Department of Veterans Affairs, the Diabetes Research and Training Centers, the Indian Health Service, and the Juvenile Diabetes Foundation. The task force decided to revise the standards to reflect recent research and current health care trends. Thus, the standards were revised and are now termed the National Standards for Diabetes Self-Management Education Programs. These revised standards have been endorsed by the organizations involved in their development.

National Standards for Diabetes Self-Management Education Programs and American Diabetes Association Review Criteria

Diabetes mellitus is a chronic metabolic disorder. Individuals affected by diabetes must learn self-management skills and make lifestyle changes to effectively manage diabetes and avoid or delay the complications associated with this disorder. For these reasons, self-management education is the cornerstone of treatment for all people with diabetes. These National Standards, which were developed in collaboration with diabetes organizations, will provide guidance for the establishment and maintenance of quality diabetes self-management education programs.

The process whereby people with chronic diseases, such as diabetes, learn to take care of these disorders has traditionally been termed "patient education." However, over time, this designation has changed and is currently termed "self-management training" and "self-management education," as well as patient education. This document will use the term self-management education to refer to the process whereby individuals learn to manage their diabetes.

These standards provide:

1. Diabetes educators with the means to:
   - develop quality self-management education programs
   - assess the quality of their education programs
   - identify areas in their programs where changes and improvements are needed
2. People with diabetes with the means to:
   - assess the quality of the diabetes-related services they receive
   - gain an understanding of the skills needed for self-management
3. Referral sources, insurers, employers, government agencies, and the general public with:
   - a description of quality self-management education services for people with diabetes
   - an awareness of the importance of comprehensive self-management education

---

*The recommendations in this paper are based on the evidence reviewed in the following publications: Diabetes self-management education (Technical Review). *Diabetes Care* 18:1204-1214, 1995; and National standards for diabetes self-management education programs (Technical Review). *Diabetes Care* 18:100-116, 1995. (From American Diabetes Association, National Standards for Diabetes Self-Management Education Programs and American Diabetes Association Review Criteria, *Diabetes Care* 22(Suppl 1) 111-114, 1999.

to enable people with diabetes to effectively manage this disorder

Quality diabetes self-management education programs can be measured in terms of structure, process, and outcomes. Each of these program components includes one or more elements with specific standards. The broad outline of the National Standards for Diabetes Self-Management Education Programs is as follows:

Structure

- Organization
- Needs assessment
- Program management
- Program staff
- Curriculum
- Participant access

Process

- Assessment
- Plan and implementation
- Follow-up

Outcomes

- Program outcome evaluation
- Participant outcome evaluation

Structure

The structure necessary to provide quality diabetes self-management education consists of the human and material resources and the management systems needed to achieve program and participant goals. Such structure includes the support and commitment of the organization that is sponsoring the program, the program administration and management systems, the qualifications and diversity of the personnel involved in the program, the curriculum and instructional methods and materials, and the accessibility of the program.

Organization

The sponsoring organization must provide the support and structure within which the program functions. Organizational commitment to self-management education including operational support and adequate space, personnel, budget, and materials must be clearly evident. Since multiple health care professionals from a variety of disciplines are involved in diabetes care, clear lines of authority and efficient communication systems should be established.

Standard 1. The sponsoring organization shall have a written policy that affirms education as an integral component of diabetes care.
Review Criterion
1-1. There is a written statement from the sponsoring organization to reflect that self-management education is an integral component of diabetes care.

Standard 2. The sponsoring organization shall identify and provide the educational resources required to achieve its educational objectives in terms of its target population. These resources include adequate space, personnel, budget, and instructional materials.
Review Criterion
2-1. For both individual and group instruction, resources (including space, staff, budget, and educational materials) are adequate to support the programs offered and the participants served.

Standard 3. The organizational relationships, lines of authority, staffing, job descriptions, and operational policies shall be clearly defined and documented.
Review Criteria
3-1. The relationships among the sponsoring organization and the diabetes program coordinator, staff, and advisory committee are clearly defined.
3-2. There is a description of the following for the coordinator and each instructional staff member:

- Role in the program
- Teaching responsibilities
- Other program responsibilities
- Amount of time spent in the program

3-3. There are written policies approved by the advisory committee concerning the operation of the program.

Needs Assessment

A successful program is based on the needs of the population that the program is intended to serve. Because diabetes populations vary, each organization should assess its service area and match resources to the needs of the defined target population. Needs assessments should guide program planning and management. Periodic reassessment should be done to allow the program to adapt to changing needs.

Standard 4. The service area shall be assessed in order to define the target population and determine appropriate allocation of personnel and resources to serve the educational needs of the target population.

Review Criterion

4-1. The target population is defined (specifically the potential number to be served, types of diabetes, age range, language, ethnicity, unique characteristics, and special educational needs).

Program Management

Effective management is essential to implement and maintain a successful program and to ensure that resources are adequate for the defined tasks. To ensure that management policies and program design reflect broad perspectives relevant to diabetes, the organization should designate a standing advisory committee that includes health care professionals and people with diabetes to assist staff with program planning and review. Involvement and support from the medical community are also necessary. At times resources outside the sponsoring institution may be required to enable individuals affected by diabetes to maximize their health outcomes.

Standard 5. A standing advisory committee consisting of a physician, a nurse educator, a dietitian, an individual with behavioral science expertise, a consumer, and a community representative, at a minimum, shall be established to oversee the program.

Review Criteria

5-1. The advisory committee members specified above attend at least two meetings a year.

5-2. The health professional members include at least one physician, one nurse educator, and one registered dietitian, each with expertise in diabetes.

5-3. The individual with behavioral science expertise is any professional with academic preparation in the behavioral sciences: e.g., counseling, health behavior, psychology, social work, sociology.

5-4. The consumer is any individual with diabetes or the caretaker thereof.

5-5. The community representative is any individual not employed by the institution.

5-6. There is a written policy concerning the membership and responsibilities of the advisory committee.

5-7. There is documentation that the advisory committee is fulfilling its responsibilities to approve the program plan, recommend and approve policy, and review the program annually.

Standard 6. The advisory committee shall participate in the annual planning process, including determination of target audience, program objectives, participant access mechanisms, instructional methods, resource requirements (including space, personnel, budget, and materials), participant follow-up mechanisms, and program evaluation.

Review Criterion

6-1. There is documentation that the advisory committee approves a written program plan each year that includes the items specified above.

Standard 7. Professional program staff shall have sufficient time and resources for lesson planning, instruction, documentation, evaluation, and follow-up.

Review Criterion

7-1. The instructors' available hours and resources are adequate to meet the needs of the program and the participants.

Standard 8. Community resources shall be assessed periodically.

Review Criterion

8-1. There is a list (including name, address, and telephone number) of community resources within the service area that serve the target population and their families. This list is reviewed and updated yearly by the advisory committee.

Program Staff

Qualified personnel are essential to the success of a diabetes self-management education program. The sponsoring organization should identify the program personnel, which must include a program coordinator who has overall responsibility for the program. Because diabetes is a chronic disorder requiring lifestyle changes, instructors need to be skilled and experienced health care professionals with recent education in diabetes, educational principles, and behavior change strategies.

Standard 9. A coordinator shall be designated who is responsible for program planning, implementation, and evaluation.

Review Criteria

9-1. The job description for the program coordinator includes his/her responsibility for the following:

- Acting as a liaison between the program staff, the advisory committee, and the administration of the institution
- Providing and/or coordinating the orientation and continuing education for the professional program staff
- Participating in the planning and review of the program each year
- Participating in the preparation of the program budget
- Evaluating progam effectiveness
- Serving as the chair or a member of the advisory committee
- Overseeing the program with on-site supervision

9-2. The program coordinator is a Certified Diabetes Educator (CDE) or has completed at least 24 h of approved continuing education that includes a combination of diabetes, educational principles, and behavioral strategies.

Standard 10. Health care professionals with recent didactic and experiential preparation in diabetes clinical and educational issues shall serve as the program instructors. Certification as a diabetes educator by the National Certification Board for Diabetes Educators (NCBDE) is recommended. Multidisciplinary instructional staff who are collectively qualified to teach the required content areas shall include at least *1)* a registered dietitian and *2)* either a registered nurse or other health professional who is a CDE.

Review Criteria

10-1. Program instructors are professional staff who routinely teach in the diabetes self-management education program and include at least *1)* a registered dietitian and *2)* either a registered nurse or other health professional who is a CDE.

10-2. Program instructors are health care professionals with a valid license, registration, or certification and who are CDEs or have completed at least 16 h of approved continuing education that includes a combination of diabetes, educational principles, and behavioral strategies.

Standard 11. Professional program staff shall obtain education about diabetes, educational principles, and behavioral change strategies on a continuing basis.

Review Criterion

11-1. The program coordinator and all instructors complete at least 6 h per year of approved continuing education that includes a combination of diabetes, educational principles, and behavioral strategies.

Curriculum

A quality diabetes self-management education program should provide comprehensive instruction in the content areas relevant to the target population and to the participants being served. The curriculum, instructional methods, and materials should be appropriate for the specified target population, considering type and duration of diabetes, age, cultural influences, and individual learning abilities.

Standard 12. Based on the needs of the target population, the program shall be capable of offering instruction in the following content areas:

a. Diabetes overview
b. Stress and psychosocial adjustment
c. Family involvement and social support
d. Nutrition
e. Exercise and activity
f. Medications
g. Monitoring and use of results
h. Relationships among nutrition, exercise, medication, and blood glucose levels

i. Prevention, detection, and treatment of acute complications

j. Prevention, detection, and treatment of chronic complications

k. Foot, skin, and dental care

l. Behavior change strategies, goal setting, risk factor reduction, and problem solving

m. Benefits, risks, and management options for improving glucose control

n. Preconception care, pregnancy, and gestational diabetes

o. Use of health care systems and community resources.

Review Criteria

12-1. There is a written curriculum that includes educational objectives, content outline, instructional methods and materials, and the means for evaluating achievement of the objectives for each content area or session of the program.

12-2. The curriculum is current and includes all 15 content areas as appropriate for the identified target population.

Standard 13.   The program shall use instructional methods and materials that are appropriate for the target population and the participants being served.

Review Criterion

13-1. Instructional methods and materials are appropriate for the target population and participants in terms of cultural relevance, age, language, reading level, and special educational needs.

Participant Access

Quality programs must be readily accessible to those in need of education. The sponsoring organization should facilitate access to self-management education for the target population identified in the needs assessment. Access is promoted by a commitment to routinely inform referral sources and the target population of the availability and benefits of the program.

Standard 14.   A system shall be in place to inform the target population and potential referral sources of the availability and benefits of the program.

Review Criterion

14-1. The program reviews marketing strategies for the target population and potential referral sources annually.

Standard 15.   The program shall be conveniently and regularly available.

Review Criterion

15-1. Program utilization, program completion rate, and waiting periods are assessed yearly.

Standard 16.   The program shall be responsive to requests for information and referrals from consumers, health care professionals, and health care agencies.

Review Criterion

16-1. There is a procedure for responding to requests for information and referrals.

Process

Process refers to the methods or means by which resources are used to attain stated goals. The process of providing diabetes self-management education involves the integration of an individual assessment, goal setting, education plan development, implementation, evaluation, and follow-up. Each component requires documentation that can be evaluated.

Assessment

Because individuals are unique, their educational needs will vary with age, disease processes, culture, and lifestyles. Effective instruction can only be accomplished by a collaborative effort between educators and participants to identify individualized educational needs.

Standard 17.   An individualized assessment shall be developed and updated in collaboration with each participant. The assessment shall include relevant medical history, present health status, health service or resource utilization, risk factors, diabetes knowledge and skills, cultural influences, health beliefs and attitudes, health behaviors and goals, support systems, barriers to learning, and socioeconomic factors.

Review Criterion

17-1. An initial assessment of the items specified above is documented in the education record and updated as needed.

Plan and Implementation

For the educational experience to meet the participant's needs, an individual assessment should be used to develop the education plan. All information about the educational experience should be documented in the participant's permanent medical or education record. Since different health care professionals may be involved in the provision of the educational experience, effective communication and coordination is essential.

Standard 18. An individualized education plan, based on the assessment, shall be developed in collaboration with each participant.

Review Criterion

18-1. The participant's pre-program knowledge and skill level in relation to the fifteen content areas of the National Standards is assessed. Educational needs are identified with the participant and documented in the education record.

Standard 19. The participant's educational experience, including assessment, intervention, evaluation, and follow-up, shall be documented in a permanent medical or education record. There shall be documentation of collaboration and coordination among program staff and other providers.

Review Criteria

19-1. The participant's progress through the program is documented in the education record and includes the following:

- The initial assessment and education plan as specified above
- An indication of the content taught, dates of instruction, and the instructors
- Post-program assessment of the participant's knowledge and skill level of each of the appropriate content areas of the National Standards
- Behavioral goals
- A plan for follow-up
- Communication of participant's progress and any follow-up recommendations to the primary care provider
- Follow-up assessment and any resulting interventions

19-2. Each program instructor documents his/her own interventions with the participants.

19-3. Communication and collaboration among program staff are facilitated by and documented in the education record.

Follow-Up

Because diabetes is a chronic disorder requiring a lifetime of self-management, follow-up services will be needed. Participants' lifestyles, knowledge, skills, attitudes, and disease characteristics change over time, so that ongoing education is necessary and appropriate. Programs should be able to offer periodic reassessment and education as part of comprehensive services.

Standard 20. The program shall offer appropriate and timely educational interventions based on periodic reassessments of health status, knowledge, skills, attitudes, goals, and self-care behaviors.

Review Criteria

20-1. At least one follow-up assessment of the items specified above and any interventions are documented in the education record.

20-2. Participant achievement of behavioral goals is assessed and documented 1-3 months after goal setting.

Outcomes

Outcomes are the desired results for the program and participants. For programs, the desired results include achievement of stated objectives, reaching the defined target population, and helping participants improve their health outcomes. For participants, outcomes include the knowledge and skills necessary for self-management, desired self-management behaviors, and improved health outcomes. Assessing outcomes and using the assessments in regular program evaluation and subsequent planning are essential to maintain quality programs.

Program Outcome Evaluation

The advisory committee should periodically review the program to ascertain that the program continues to meet the National Standards for Diabetes Self-Management Education Programs.

The results of this review should be documented and used in subsequent program planning and modification.

Standard 21. The advisory committee shall review program performance annually, including all components of the annual program plan and curriculum, and use the information in subsequent planning and program modification.

Review Criteria

21-1. The advisory committee conducts and documents the results of an annual review of the program including the following:

- Program objectives
- The curriculum, instructional methods, educational materials, and community resource list
- Actual audience compared to the target population
- Participant access and follow-up mechanisms
- Program resources (space, personnel, and budget)
- Program effectiveness/participant outcomes
- Marketing strategies to the target population and any potential referral sources.

21-2. The results of the annual review are reflected in the next annual program plan.

Participant Outcome Evaluation

Participant outcomes, such as success in incorporating self-management into their lifestyles, should be periodically reviewed. The specific outcomes evaluated will vary with the program, but the program's effectiveness in helping participants improve their health outcomes should be documented and used for future program planning and modification.

Standard 22. The advisory committee shall annually review and evaluate predetermined outcomes for program participants.

Review Criteria

22-1. Participants' outcomes are measured and evaluated, specifically, the degree to which the participants achieve their behavioral goals and **one** other outcome measure (e.g., monitoring for

complications, lost work or school days, metabolic control, or others).

22-2. The program's effectiveness at improving outcomes among participants is evaluated by the advisory committee and the results of this evaluation are reflected in the next annual program plan.

Bibliography

1. Clement S: Diabetes self-management education (Technical Review). *Diabetes Care* 18:1204-1214, 1995.
2. Funnell MM, Haas LB: National standards for diabetes self-management education programs (Technical Review). *Diabetes Care* 18:100-116, 1995.

SCOPE OF PRACTICE FOR DIABETES EDUCATORS*

Purpose

The American Association of Diabetes Educators developed the Scope of Practice to delineate: (1) selected beliefs and definitions related to the practice of diabetes education, and (2) the dimensions of this practice in relation to other components of care for persons with diabetes, their families, and appropriate support systems. This Scope of Practice describes the present practice of diabetes education by multidisciplinary health care professionals.

Beliefs and Definitions

Living well with diabetes requires a positive psychosocial adaptation to achieve self-care management of the disease. To achieve effective self-management of diabetes mellitus, a patient must learn the body of knowledge, attitudes, and self-management skills related to the control of this chronic disease. *Diabetes education* is defined as an interactive, collaborative, ongoing process involving the person with diabetes and the educa-

---

*From American Association of Diabetes Educators: The 1999 scope of practice for diabetes educators and the standards of practice for diabetes educators, *Diabetes Educ* 26:519-525, 2000.

tor. This process includes: 1) assessment of the individual's specific education needs; 2) identification of the individual's specific diabetes self-management goals; 3) educational and behavioral intervention directed toward helping the individual achieve identified self-management goals; 4) evaluation of the individual's attainment of identified self-management goals. This planned educational experience is most effectively provided by qualified diabetes educators. Diabetes education is considered a therapeutic modality and is integral to the care of people with diabetes and their families, support systems, and caregivers.

A *diabetes educator* is defined as a health care professional who has mastered the core of knowledge and skills in the biological and social sciences, communication, counseling, and education, and who has experience in the care of people with diabetes. The role of the diabetes educator can be assumed by various health care professionals, including, but not limited to: registered nurses, registered dietitians, pharmacists, physicians, mental health professionals, podiatrists, and exercise physiologists. A goal for all diabetes educators should be to meet the academic, professional, and experiential requirements to become a Certified Diabetes Educator (CDE).

Dimensions of Practice

The role of the diabetes educator is multidimensional, with boundaries for accountability that interface with other members of the health care team. This role involves the education of people with diabetes, their families, and appropriate support systems, as well as other health care professionals who do not specialize in diabetes management, such as policy makers and the public. A multidisciplinary team approach is the preferred delivery system for diabetes education. This specialty practice can occur successfully in a wide variety of settings and formats.

The primary area of responsibility for diabetes educators is the education of people with diabetes, their families, and appropriate support systems about diabetes self-care management and related issues. The content of this educational experience should include, but not be limited to, the following topics:

- Describing the diabetes disease process and treatment options
- Incorporating appropriate nutritional management
- Incorporating physical activity into lifestyle
- Using medications (if applicable) for therapeutic effectiveness
- Monitoring blood glucose and urine ketones (when appropriate), and using results to improve control
- Preventing, detecting, and treating acute complications
- Preventing (through risk reduction behavior), detecting, and treating chronic complications
- Goal setting to promote health and problem solving for daily living
- Integrating psychosocial adjustment into daily life
- Promoting preconception care, management during pregnancy, and gestational diabetes management (if applicable)

The diabetes educator should present the necessary information using established principles of teaching/learning theory and life-style counseling. The instruction is individualized for persons of all ages, incorporating their cultural preferences, health beliefs, and preferred learning styles. The goal is to assist the person with diabetes discover how to manage their diabetes. The diabetes educator should perform the following:

- Assessment of educational needs
- Planning of the teaching/learning and behavioral change process
- Implementation of the educational plan
- Documentation of the process including follow-up with the primary care provider
- Evaluation based on outcome criteria

The scope of practice of a diabetes educator intersects with the practice of other members of the health care team. The diabetes educator should appreciate the impact of acute or chronic problems on a person's health behaviors, life-style, and on the teaching/learning process. Such appreciation is essential for the development of a comprehensive plan for continuing education and cost-effective, self-care management.

Members of the various health care professions who practice diabetes education bring their particular focus to the educational process. This phenomenon widens or narrows the scope of practice for individual educators, as is appropriate within the boundaries of each health profession, which may be regulated by national or state agencies or accrediting bodies. Other roles for the diabetes educator may involve program management, case management, clinical management, healthcare consultancy with other providers, organizations and industry, public and professional education, public health and wellness promotion, and research in diabetes management and education.

Diabetes education occurs in a variety of settings depending on the needs of the patient, the practice of the educator, and the local environment. Acute and ambulatory settings, home and pharmacy settings, as well as electronic professional diabetes education can be used effectively for both individual and group education. Diabetes education should be a planned, individualized, and evaluated activity wherever it occurs.

Summary

This Scope of Practice incorporates definitions of diabetes educator and diabetes education, while providing statements of beliefs regarding the educational process inherent in this practice. The general scope of practice of a diabetes educator has changing dimensions because of the multidisciplinary nature of the health care professionals who provide it and the changing health care system. The primary role of a diabetes educator is to provide an accessible therapeutic experience for people with diabetes, their families, and appropriate support systems that enhance effective self-care management and improve health outcomes and quality of life. Thus, the Scope of Practice delineates the multifaceted role and responsibilities of the health care professional who

engages in this teaching-learning process. This Scope of Practice does not constitute an exhaustive description of diabetes education as a specialty practice because there are local, regional, and national variations in the functions of the diabetes educator within a health care team.

STANDARDS OF PRACTICE FOR DIABETES EDUCATORS*

Purpose

This document has been developed by the American Association of Diabetes Educators to: (1) provide standards for a nationally acceptable level of practice for diabetes educators and (2) assure quality in the professional practice of diabetes education. The individual diabetes educator is responsible for adhering to these Standards.

The Standards of Practice will provide:

1. Diabetes educators with
   - direction to assess and improve the quality of their practice
   - a framework within which to practice
2. Patients with
   - a means of assessing the quality of diabetes education services provided
   - a basis for forming expectations of the diabetes education experience
3. Health care professionals who do not specialize in diabetes management with a means of
   - understanding the role of the diabetes educator
   - assessing the quality of diabetes education services provided
   - understanding diabetes education as an integral component of diabetes patient care

*From American Association of Diabetes Educators: The 1999 scope of practice for diabetes educators and the standards of practice for diabetes educators, *Diabetes Educ* 26:519-525, 2000.

4. Insurers, policy makers, purchasers, employers, government agencies, industry, and the general public with
   - a description of the specialized educational services provided by a diabetes educator
   - information about the benefits of diabetes education in developing self-care management skills
   - an awareness of the importance of diabetes education in improving the quality of life and health care for people with diabetes

Standards of Education

Standard I. Assessment The diabetes educator should conduct a thorough, individualized needs assessment with the participation of the patient, family, or support systems, when appropriate, prior to the development of the education plan and intervention. Integral to this assessment is an ongoing analysis and interpretation of the data and consultation with the referring primary care provider.

The needs assessment should include the following information from the patient:

1. Health history
2. Medical history
3. Previous use of medication
4. Nutritional history
5. Current mental health status
6. Family and social supports
7. Previous diabetes education, actual knowledge, and skills
8. Current self-care management practices
9. Use of healthcare delivery systems
10. Lifestyle practices such as occupation, vocation, education level, financial status, and social, cultural, and religious practices
11. Physical and psychosocial factors including age, mobility, visual acuity, hearing, manual dexterity, alertness, attention span, and ability to concentrate
12. Factors that influence learning such as education and literacy levels, perceived learning needs, motivation to learn, and health beliefs

Standard II. Use of Resources The diabetes educator should strive to create an educational setting conducive to learning, with adequate resources to facilitate the learning process. The diabetes educator must provide accessible services or make reasonable accommodations to make services accessible.

Appropriate resources for effective teaching should include:

1. A teaching environment that provides
   - privacy, safety, and accessibility
   - ample and appropriate teaching and storage space, furniture, lighting, and ventilation
2. Teaching materials and audiovisual teaching aids to meet the individual patient's needs
3. Adequately trained staff for the needs of the patient population
4. Adequate number of staff

Standard III. Planning The written educational plan should be developed from information obtained from the client-centered needs assessment and based on the components of the educational process: assessment, planning, implementation, and evaluation. The educational plan reflects an integration of current diabetes care practices, teaching/learning principles, a flexible approach to teaching, and respect for lifestyle and health beliefs. The plan is coordinated among diabetes health team members, and the person with diabetes, the family, and their support system.

The written educational plan should include the following:

1. Collaboratively defined goals of the educational intervention
2. Measurable, behaviorally stated objectives established by the patient based on a clear explanation of options and choices
3. A content outline

4. Instructional methods and processes accessible and appropriate to the culture of the individual and the community, including discussion, demonstration, role playing, and simulations

5. Learner outcomes based on the evaluation process

Standard IV. Implementation As a member of the healthcare team and in collaboration with other resources and services, the diabetes educator must provide accessible services and should provide individualized education based on a progression from basic survival skills to advanced information for daily self-care management, and improved outcomes.

Considerations in developing the individualized education plan should include:

1. The need for diabetes education to be lifelong because of the chronicity of the condition

2. The need for a dynamic education plan that will reflect the inevitable changes in life-style

3. Survival skills that include safe practices of medication administration, meal planning, self-monitoring for glycemic control, and recognition of when to access professional assistance for emergencies

4. Advanced information for daily self-care management practices that may include prevention and management of chronic complications, problem-solving skills, exercise, psychosocial adjustment, medication adjustment, stress management, travel situations, and pattern management

5. Oportunity for peer support

6. Follow-up and continuity of education

Standard V. Documentation The diabetes educator should completely and accurately document the educational experience. Accurate documentation

1. Establishes a record to document the delivery of education and behavioral strategies and patient goals

2. Contributes information for retrospective, concurrent, and prospective reviews

3. Provides data for scientific and economic analysis

4. Serves as a resource for continuity of care

5. Participates in planning subsequent diabetes education

6. Tracks clinical, behavior, and economic outcomes

7. Addresses short-, intermediate-, and long-term outcomes

8. Reports to the referring primary care provider the progress and outcomes from the education experience

Standard VI. Evaluation and Outcome The diabetes educator should participate in at least an annual review of the quality and outcome of the education process.

Evaluation of the diabetes education process should

1. Occur periodically and as part of a comprehensive, outcome-driven, quality improvement program

2. Be consistent with the National Standards for Diabetes Self-Management Education as originally established by the National Diabetes Advisory Board

3. Determine the impact of education on patients, institutions, and the community

4. Use outcome measures such as
   - Cost-effectiveness
   - Changes in use of healthcare delivery systems (e.g., emergency room visits, acute care visits, hospital length of stay, regular prevention-based providers visits and complication monitoring)
   - Changes in knowledge, attitudes, skills, and behaviors (e.g., smoking cessation, self-managing blood glucose, foot care)
   - Changes in physiological measures (e.g., HbA_{1c} values, weight or body mass index, lipid profile, microalbuminuria, blood pressure)
   - Changes in healthcare beliefs

Standards of Professional Practice

Standard VII. Multidisciplinary Collaboration The diabetes educator should collaborate with a multidisciplinary team of health care professionals and integrate their knowledge and skills to provide comprehensive health care interventions.

The multidisciplinary education team should

1. Include, but not be limited to, the registered nurse, registered dietitian, physician, pharmacist, social worker, psychologist, exercise physiologist, and podiatrist
2. Observe professional practice boundaries in light of each member's discipline
3. Have a responsibility to:
   - integrate the patient education plan into the plan of care of the referring primary care provider
   - share with other team members information from individual patient assessments
   - prioritize learning needs
   - make education relevant to medical management
   - promote delivery of consistent information from various team members to patients
   - conduct patient management conferences in collaboration with other team members and the patient on a regular basis
   - provide referrals for appropriate follow-up

Standard VIII. Professional Development The diabetes educator should assume responsibility for professional development and pursue continuing education to acquire current knowledge and skills.

The diabetes educator should

1. Incorporate into practice the generally accepted new techniques and knowledge acquired through continuing education
2. Deliver education based on a continuous process of review and evaluation of scientific theory, clinical and educational research, and study of behavioral changes strategies and positive health care outcomes
3. Pursue professional education based on progression from basic through advanced curriculum
4. Strive to meet the academic, professional, and experiential requirements to become a Certified Diabetes Educator (CDE)

Standard IX. Professional Accountability The diabetes educator should accept responsibility for self-assessment of performance and peer review to assure the delivery of high quality diabetes education.

The diabetes educator should

1. Participate in an annual systematic review and evaluation of practice
2. Incorporate into practice the appropriate changes based on the results of self-evaluation, peer and primary care provider reviews, and patients' evaluations

Standard X. Ethics The diabetes educator should respect and uphold the basic human rights of all persons.

The diabetes educator should

1. Maintain confidentiality of appropriate information
2. Encourage freedom of expression, decision making, and action
3. Demonstrate concern for personal dignity, culture, and health beliefs
4. Recognize that people with diabetes balance many daily tasks for self-care management that may require a gradual incorporation into their lifestyles
5. Appreciate the impact of diabetes management on daily living so that reasonable expectations are established with patients
6. Display nonjudgmental honesty, warmth, and openness to reinforce positive behavior change

Developed under the aegis of a multidisciplinary task force of the American Association of Diabetes Educators.

Bibliography

American Diabetes Association. Standards of medical care for patients with diabetes mellitus. *Diabetes Care* 2000;23(suppl 1):532-542.

American Dietetic Association. Scope of practice for qualified professionals in diabetes care and education. J Am Diet Assoc. 1995;95:607-608.

American Dietetic Association. Nutrition Practice Guidelines for Type 1 and Type 2 Diabetes Mellitus. Chicago: American Dietetic Association; 1996.

American Nurses' Association and American Association of Diabetes Educators. Standards of diabetes nursing; 1998.

Bartlett E. At last a definition of patient education [Editorial]. *Patient Educ Couns* 1985;7: 323-24.

Brookfield SD. *Understanding and facilitating adult learning.* San Francisco: Jossey-Bass, 1986.

Dunst C, Trivette C, Deal A. *Enabling and empowering families: principles and guidelines for practice.* Cambridge, Mass: Brookline Books, 1988.

Franz MJ, Splett PL, Monk A, et al. Cost-effectiveness of medical nutrition therapy provided by dietitians for persons with non-insulin-dependent diabetes mellitus. *J Am Diet Assoc.* 1995;95:1018-1024.

Funnell MA, ed. *A core curriculum for diabetes education.* 3rd ed. Chicago: American Association of Diabetes Educators; 1998.

Green LW, Kreuter MW. *Health promotion planning: an educational and environmental approach.* 2d ed. Mountain View, Calif: Mayfield Publishing Co, 1991.

Kulkami K, Castle G, Gregory R, et al. Nutrition practice guidelines for type 1 diabetes mellitus positively affect dietitian practices and patient outcomes. *J Am Diet Assoc.* 1998;98:62-70.

National standards for diabetes self-management education programs and American Diabetes Association review criteria. *Diabetes Care.* 1999;22(suppl 1): S111-S114.

Peeples M, Mulcahy K. Diabetes education outcomes and measurements. *AADE News.* 1999;6:4-5.

Redman BK. *The process of patient education.* 6th ed. St. Louis: CV Mosby, 1988.

Report of the ADA Task Force on the clarification of the roles and responsibilities in providing diabetes self-management education. *Diabetes Spectrum.* 1997; 10:155-158.

Report of the Task Force on the delivery of self-management education and medical nutrition therapy. *Diabetes Spectrum.* 1999;12(1):44-47.

Van Hoozer HL. *The teaching process: theory and practice in nursing.* East Norwalk, Conn: Appleton and Lange, 1987.

ARTHRITIS AND MUSCULOSKELETAL PATIENT EDUCATION STANDARDS*

I. Introduction

Background. Patient education is a powerful strategy intervention that can improve the lives of persons with rheumatic disease. Most forms of arthritis are chronic in nature and extend over many years. Therefore, along with the routine, ongoing education given by caregivers during individual clinical contacts, the patient needs a formal body of knowledge and skills in order to manage the disease on a day-to-day basis. Effective, efficient management of chronic disease is possible only when patients are knowledgeable participants in decisions about their care and are able to follow through on these decisions.

Patient education is considered an integral part of the treatment of the more than 100 forms of rheumatic disease. More than 75 education programs, reported in the literature, have shown beneficial effects on various aspects of health status, such as functional ability, psychological state, and pain. Furthermore, considerable effort has been made to develop and/or test instruments to evaluate important health outcomes of rheumatic disease care.

This document addresses suggested standards for formal rheumatic disease patient education programs. The purposes of the standards are to: (1) assure the quality of patient education programs, (2) promote the easy access to education for the patient with rheumatic disease, and (3) secure documentation of outcomes of patient education that can be used to improve care.

Definitions. The following terms are defined for use in this document.

1. **Patient Education.** Patient education is planned, organized learning experiences designed to facilitate voluntary adop-

---

*From Burckhardt CS and others: Arthritis and musculo-skeletal patient education standards, *Arthritis Care Res* 7:1-4, 1994.

tion of behaviors or beliefs conducive to health. It is a set of planned educational activities that are separate from clinical patient care. The activities of a patient education program must be designed to attain goals the patient has participated in formulating. The primary focus of these activities includes acquisition of information, skills, beliefs and attitudes which impact on health status, quality of life, and possibly health care utilization.

2. **Program.** A program consists of three parts:
   a. Specific objectives oriented to each individual or group
   b. Content tailored to meet these objectives
   c. Education processes which deliver the content in a manner which enables the patient to achieve the objectives
   A program can be delivered in a variety of ways and in different settings dependent upon the needs of patients and the availability of resources.
3. **Standards.** Standards are written statements that describe the expectations of the quality of a given education program.
4. **Review Criteria.** Review criteria are measurable methods of determining whether the standards have been met.
5. **Provider.** The provider may be an individual practitioner, an organization or an institution. In all cases the provider is responsible for upholding the standards.
6. **Approved Program.** An approved program is one that has been found to meet the rheumatic disease patient education standards as determined by the designated authority.

II. Needs Assessment Standards

Standard. The numbers and needs of persons with rheumatic disease vary. Therefore, patient education programs must begin with an assessment of the needs of the target population. This includes the patient and his/her family members and significant care providers.

The provider of the patient education program will conduct an educational needs assessment of the target patient population. This assessment will include, but not be limited to, problems cased by the rheumatic disease, skills needed to manage the disease, and current level of knowledge and skills. Preferred language of instruction and reading level will also be assessed, if applicable. Additional need assessments, as appropriate, may be conducted with health care providers, administrators, or family members and significant others.

Review Criterion

1. The provider will document how the needs assessment was conducted and the findings of the needs assessment.

III. Planning/Management Standards

Standard. Planning is a comprehensive process that should involve health professionals and educators as well as persons with rheumatic diseases and members of their families.

In addition, it entails good communication and clearly delineated responsibilities and functions. Communication must occur among program personnel, health care givers, community health agencies, patients, and their family members. A program coordinator with ultimate responsibility and authority for the quality and operation of the program should be designated. The program should be readily accessible to all patients for whom it has been designed.

Review Criteria

1. Provider will document the participation of a rheumatologist, one or more other health professionals and patients in the selection or planning of a program.
2. Each provider will designate one person as coordinator. At a minimum, this person will be responsible for coordinating and documenting patient education activities and is responsible for the quality and operation of the program.
3. Information about patient participation in educational programs shall be documented.

4. Information about each patient's participation shall be retained in a patient's record or similar file for at least 5 years. This record will be available for the patient's personal or other consented use.

IV. Curriculum Standards

Standard. The program curriculum organizes the content and documents the educational process. It is also expected that the educational program will be reasonably supported by professional consensus and the research literature on arthritis patient education.

The provider periodically assesses the availability of community resources for their potential contribution to rheumatic disease education. In addition, programs should be updated in a timely manner.

Review Criteria

1. The program shall have written patient outcome objectives which reflect the findings of the needs assessment(s) and the patients' goals.
2. The program shall offer information and skills in the content areas determined by the needs assessment and patients' goals. These will be documented by a written curriculum plan which includes content outlines, instructional methods, and instructional materials.
3. Documentation is available to show that curriculum and instructional materials are appropriate for the specified target audience.
4. The curriculum is reviewed and updated as necessary or at least every 5 years.
5. The provider shows evidence of an initial assessment of community resources and repeats the assessment at least every 2 years. The assessment includes the name, address, telephone number and a brief statement of what the particular resource offers.

V. Instructor Standards

Qualified personnel are essential to the success of a rheumatic disease education program. Instruc-

tors should have recent training and experience in both rheumatic disease and educational principles, including teaching approaches specific to the target audience (e.g., children, adults, geriatric, culturally diverse population).

Review Criteria (instructor-led patient education)

1. Instructors are health professionals or lay persons with special education and/or training and experience appropriate to the instructional needs of the program.
2. Documentation of rheumatic disease related training and/or experience is provided.
3. Personnel are expected to participate in continuing education in their areas of expertise on a regular basis.
4. Evidence is provided of regular meetings between instructors and program coordinator.

Review Criteria (mediated patient education)

1. Some educational programs such as those utilizing interactive computers, interactive video, or packages utilizing written, audio tape, and/or video components do not require an instructor. When such programs are used, a person knowledgeable in program content and rheumatology care must be readily available to answer questions or assist with problems. Access may be in person or by telephone. Resource persons for mediated programs must meet the same criteria as outlined in section V, 1-4.

VI. Evaluation Standards

Standard. In order for a program to meet the standards of this document, it must demonstrate is effectiveness in maintaining or improving health status (i.e., pain, functional ability, psychological state, social functioning, and/or quality of life). For example, decreased pain, depression, disability, fatigue, and improvement of quality of life can be determined by assessing the patient with a standardized measurement tool. Maintenance and/or improvement may be shown in terms of group or individual change (e.g., a third of a standard deviation) or other definitions that can be justified by the provider. In addition, satisfaction data from patients and family members must be collected and reviewed annually.

Review Criteria. For new, not previously approved, programs.

1. Effectiveness is documented by scores on standard validated instruments.
2. Providers do not need to present new evaluation data when using already approved programs.
3. Any provider who chooses to use an approved program which has been demonstrated to meet the criteria in section VI, 1 for patients who differ in some major way from the patient groups for which the program was designed, must show evidence that the program is effective for this new patient group.

VII. Documentation Standards

Standard. Documented program planning and evaluation serves as the basis for future program development and modification. All aspects of the program shall be recorded by the program coordinator or other designated person.

Review Criteria

1. Documentation shall include:
   a. How needs assessment(s) were conducted
   b. Results of needs assessment
   c. Curriculum
   d. Instructors/resource persons—qualifications, training, retraining, supervision, evaluation by participants
   e. Program outcome evaluation for new program
   f. Number of participants entering the program

g. Number of participants completing the program
   h. Satisfaction data from patients and family members
   i. Any other documentation required by this document
2. The provider shall conduct and record a yearly internal review of the program documentation.

NATIONAL GUIDELINES FOR ENTEROSTOMAL PATIENT EDUCATION*

Prepared by the Standards Development Committee of the United Ostomy Association with the Assistance of Prospect Associates (See acknowledgements for complete list of contributors and affiliations.)

Background on the National Guidelines for Enterostomal Patient Education

In October 1988, the National Digestive Diseases Advisory Board (NDDAB) sponsored a conference where patients and health care professionals developed recommendations to improve enterostomal patient education. These recommendations may be used as a model for improving patient education on other digestive diseases. Following the conference, a task group, which included an enterostomal nurse, a gastroenterologist, and a patient, met to develop an action plan and identify the lead organizations responsible for implementing the conference recommendations. One recommendation was to develop national standards for enterostomal patient education as a tool for planning, implementing, and evaluating quality of care. The task group identified the United Ostomy Association (UOA) as the appropriate lead organization for coordinating the development of these standards. The UOA invited other relevant professional and

---

*From Standards Development Committee of the United Ostomy Association: National guidelines for enterostomal patient education. *Dis Colon Rectum* 37:559-563, 1994.

voluntary organizations to participate. This document is a result of their efforts. A list of the individuals and organizations that contributed to this document is provided. At its May 1993 meeting, the Board reviewed and endorsed the original document with the provision that they be called "guidelines," not standards, consistent with current terminology used by the medical community (e.g., practice care guidelines).

Introduction

The following guidelines for enterostomal patient education have been formulated to assist the educator in providing the self-care skills and psychosocial support needed by patients to successfully manage their stomas. Studies have suggested that ostomy patient education reduces the patient's hospital length of stay, postoperative complications, need for additional surgery, and hospital readmissions. Additionally, teaching self-management techniques may improve the patient's compliance with treatment and reduce excessive use of medications and supplies.

The term "educator," as used in this document, includes various members of the multidisciplinary health care team who play important roles in caring for the ostomy patient. The educator may be a surgeon (e.g., general, colorectal, urologic, pediatric), a gastroenterologist, a nurse, a psychosocial health care professional, a registered dietitian, or a trained volunteer from a lay organization (e.g., UOA, ACS, CCFA). Each area of information should be administered by the appropriate educator (i.e., a surgeon should discuss surgical procedures, a registered dietitian should provide diet counseling, etc.). Many resources are available to assist the educator in meeting these guidelines and achieving optimal patient outcomes. A list of individuals and organizations that may serve as important resources is provided.

The term "patient," as used in this document, is defined as the enterostomal patient (temporary or permanent) as well as spouse, parent, guardian, or other home care provider. The patient encompasses all age groups from neonates to the elderly. Age, stage of developmental maturation, or disability of the patient may influence expected outcomes. Therefore, the educator will need to adapt his or her approach to accommodate such differences. Also in this context, the term "self-care," as used in this document, may refer when applicable to care or assisted care by a home care provider.

These guidelines are designed to ensure continuing patient education from diagnosis through rehabilitation. The guidelines are divided into three segments: preoperative, postoperative, and long-term rehabilitation. Guidelines, rationale, outcome criteria, and interventions have been identified for each segment. Ideally, the enterostomal patient's education begins in the preoperative period and continues throughout the hospital stay and after discharge. However, in emergency situations, the patient may be unable to receive information before an operation. In these cases, it is appropriate that the education process begin after the operation for the patient, and before the operation for the person giving permission for surgery.

The long-term outcome of an ostomy operation is highly dependent on patient education. Educators provide patient education to potentially reduce the length of hospital stay for the patient, to avoid stoma-related postoperative complications, and to reduce fears, depression, and negative feelings associated with having an ostomy. The UOA Ostomate Bill of Rights states that the ostomy patient has the right to have access to and obtain systematic teaching from knowledgeable individuals.

These guidelines are directed to educators responsible for delivering enterostomal patient education and may improve patient awareness and knowledge concerning life with an ostomy.

National Guidelines for Enterostomal Patient Education

Preoperative Period

Guidelines

Patient education begins during the preoperative period. At this stage, the educator(s) will:

Review changes in anatomy and physiology as it relates to the planned surgery.

Define the structure, care, and function of an ostomy, including related equipment and supplies.

Explain the anticipated surgical procedure, indications, alternative procedures, reason for stoma site selection, anticipated postoperative course, expectations for self-care, potential complications, and follow-up care.

Describe the relationship between the planned procedure and the disease process, including the potential effects on prognosis and future interventions.

Explain the physiological and psychological changes that may be associated with the ostomy, including potential effects on body image, self-esteem, sexuality, social function, nutrition, employment or schooling, and growth and development where applicable.

Inform the patient of the existence of community resources and support systems.

Rationale

Providing the patient with adequate and accurate information during the preoperative period should facilitate self-care in the rehabilitative process and should reduce postoperative apprehension and complications related to ostomy care and function.

Outcome criteria

The patient will:

Describe the stoma and its function including related equipment and supplies.

List community resources for equipment, supplies, and emotional support.

Describe the anticipated surgical procedure, changes in anatomy and physiology, indications, alternative procedures, reason for stoma site selection, anticipated postoperative course, expectations for self-care, potential complications, and follow-up care.

Describe the disease process, including prognosis, potential future therapies, and expected outcomes.

Discuss the potential impact of the stoma on body image, self-esteem, sexuality, social function, and employment or schooling as applicable.

Describe dietary modifications to prevent/ manage diarrhea, constipation, bloating, stoma obstruction, food blockage, malnutrition, flatulence, dehydration, urinary tract infection, and urinary calculus formation.

Explain potential effects of the stoma on growth and development, as appropriate.

Interventions

Suggested interventions include:

Provision of educational materials (see resource section).

Nutrition counseling.

Enterostomal consultation.

Educator/patient conferences including lay visitor.

Social services consultation.

Postoperative Period

Guidelines

To facilitate the patient's recovery and return to self-care, the educator will:

Provide strategies for attaining an appropriate level of self-care.

Clarify the patient's understanding of the changes in anatomy and physiology, structure, care, and function of the ostomy, including related equipment and supplies.

Reinforce the patient's knowledge of the surgical procedure and its implications.

Clarify the relationship between the surgical procedure and the disease process, including the prognosis.

Discuss the impact of the stoma on body image, self-esteem, sexuality, employment, and social function.

Provide strategies for the prevention and management of stoma-related complications.

Instruct the patient regarding the continued need for adequate nutritional and fluid intake, including individual requirements and those related to the specific surgery.

Inform the patient of the existence of community resources and support systems.

Instruct the patient regarding sources of obtaining and receiving reimbursement for equipment.

Rationale

Providing postoperative education and psychosocial support should lead to improved patient function and facilitate recovery.

Outcome criteria

The patient will:

Demonstrate an appropriate level of self-care.

Describe the prevention and management of potential complications resulting from ostomy surgery.

Demonstrate an understanding of types of equipment needed in ostomy management and reasons for use.

Explain ostomy management within activities of daily living, work, play, and sexual life.

Communicate concerns and potential problems related to altered body image and function.

Describe dietary means to prevent/manage diarrhea, constipation, bloating, stoma obstruction, food blockage, malnutrition, flatulence, dehydration, urinary tract infection, and urinary calculus formation.

Identify sources of equipment and resources for reimbursement.

Demonstrate an appropriate understanding of stoma-related complications.

List community resources for mutual aid and support, rehabilitation, and education.

Interventions

Suggested interventions include:

Provision of educational materials (see resource section).

Educator/patient conferences, including lay visitor.

Nutrition counseling.

Enterostomal consultation.

Social services consultation.

Long-Term Rehabilitation Period

Guidelines

To prepare the patient for the long-term rehabilitation period, the educator will:

Explain long-term nutritional, social, pharmacologic, and other therapeutic needs.

Assist the patient in achieving optimal physiologic and psychosocial status and level of activity.

Define long-term follow-up approaches including monitoring for potential complications and ongoing education to facilitate self-care.

Explain the difference between the effects of the disease process and the effects of the ostomy on long-term rehabilitation.

Rationale

Optimal understanding, acceptance, and management of the ostomy and possible ongoing disease process should minimize complications and maximize the patient's quality of life. Educational activities should prepare the patient for the long-term rehabilitation period. The patient must be prepared for possible adjustments in areas of medication, equipment, diet, fluid intake, routines of daily living, and self-care expectations.

Outcome criteria

The patient will:

Manage care of the stoma and appropriately select and utilize equipment and supplies.

Identify and describe prevention, detection, and management strategies related to potential complications, adaptive and environmental changes, and the disease process, within the limits of the patient's level of education and understanding.

Use professional, community, family, and personal resources to maximize level of functioning and, when applicable, to optimize growth and development.

Interventions

Suggested interventions include:

Referral to appropriate support group(s).

Provision of educational materials (see resource section).

Nutrition counseling.
Enterostomal consultation
Educator/patient conferences, including lay
   visitor.
Social services consultation.
An appropriate, individualized follow-up
   protocol.

Resources

Numerous professional and voluntary organizations provide relevant materials and information on ostomy patient education that assist educators in implementing these standards. Health care professionals located within local communities are also excellent resources. These include: surgeons (e.g., general, colorectal, urologic, pediatric), gastroenterologists, enterostomal therapy nurses, registered dietitians, pharmacists, gastrointestinal nurses and associates, social workers, trained lay visitors, and psychotherapists. In addition, manufacturers and suppliers of ostomy equipment and pharmaceuticals produce patient education materials.

The following organizations provide a variety of useful information related to ostomy patient education and may have local chapters, support services, or representatives in the educator's community.

American Cancer Society, Ostomy Rehabilitation Program, 1599 Clifton Road, N.E., Atlanta, Georgia 30329. 1-800-227-2345.

American Dietetic Association, 216 West Jackson Boulevard, Suite 800, Chicago, Illinois 60606-6995. (312) 899-0040.

American Society of Colon and Rectal Surgeons, 800 East N.W. Highway, Suite 1080, Palatine, Illinois 60067. (708) 359-9184.

American Urological Association Allied, Inc., 11512 Allecingie Parkway, Richmond, Virginia 23235. (804) 379-1306.

Association of Rehabilitation Nurses, 5700 Old Orchard Road, First Floor, Skokie, Illinois 60077. (708) 966-3433.

Crohn's & Colitis Foundation of America, Inc. (formerly National Foundation for Ileitis and Colitis), 444 Park Avenue, S., 11th

floor, New York, New York 10016-7374. 1-800-343-3637.

International Association for Enterostomal Therapy, 27241 LaPaz Road, Laguna Niguel, California 92656. (714) 476-0268.

National Digestive Diseases Information Clearinghouse, Box NDDIC, 9000 Rockville Pike, Bethesda, Maryland 20892. (301) 468-6344.

Society of Gastroenterology Nurses and Associates, 1070 Sibley Tower, Rochester, New York 14604. (716) 546-7241. 1-800-245-SGNA.

United Ostomy Association, Inc., 36 Executive Park, Suite 120, Irvine, California, 92714-6744. (714) 660-8624. 1-800-826-0826.

Acknowledgments

Coordinated for the United Ostomy Association (UOA) by Marilyn A. Mau, Past President

STANDARDS DEVELOPMENT STEERING
   COMMITTEE
CHAIR: James Fleshman, M.D.
Washington University School of Medicine,
   St. Louis, MO
Chair, UOA Medical Advisory Committee
INVITED TO PARTICIPATE
American Cancer Society (ACS)
American College of Physicians (ACP)
American Dietetic Association (ADA)
American Gastroenterological Association
   (AGA)
American Nephrology Nurses Association
   (ANNA)
American Nurses' Association (ANA)
American Society of Colon and Rectal
   Surgeons (ASCRS)
American Society of Gastroenterology
   Endoscopy (ASGE)
American Urological Association Allied, Inc.
   (AUAA)
Association of Rehabilitation Nurses (ARN)
Crohn's and Colitis Foundation of America
   (CCFA)

Digestive Disease National Coalition (DDNC)

National Digestive Diseases Information Clearinghouse (NDDIC)

North American Society for Pediatric Gastro-enterology (NASPG)

Society of Gastroenterology Nurses and Associates (SGNA)

Wound, Ostomy and Continence Nurses Society (WOCN)

CONTRIBUTORS TO THE STANDARDS

Linda K. Aukett,* UOA

Rebecca Bonsaint, ASGE

Cheryl Corbin, M.S., R.D., ADA

Frederick Daum, M.D., NASPG

Judy Ebbert, ACP

Linda Farah, ANNA

John Farrar, M.D., DDNC

Jim Fleshman,* M.D., UOA and ASCRS

Linda Gabrielson,* M.S., R.D., ADA

Michael Gray, Ph.D., AUAA

Cecilia Grindel,* Ph.D, R.N., ANA

TennieBee Hall,* UOA, CCFA, past member of the NDDAB

Marsha Hardick, R.N., CGC and SGNA

John Latimer,* M.D., NASPG

Malcolm Malooh, M.S., R.N., R.N.C.

Marilyn A. Mau,* Past President, UOA

Kenneth Mirkin,* M.D., AGA

Nancy J. Reilly, R.N., M.S.N., C.U.R.N., AUAA

Dale Singer,† Prospect Associates

Beth Stevenson, M.P.H., ACS

Kristy Wright, R.N., B.S.N., C.E.T.N., WOCN

References

Bartlett EE. How can patient education contribute to improved health care under prospective pricing? *Health Policy* 1986;6:283-94.

Karam JA, Sundre SM, Smith GA. Cost/benefit analysis of patient education. *Hosp Health Serv Adm* 1986;31: 82-90.

Kreps GL, Ruben BD, Baker MW, Rosenthal SR. Survey of public health knowledge about digestive health and diseases: implications for health education. *Public Health Rep* 1987;102:270-7.

Ostomate bill of rights. United Ostomy Association. Irvine, California, 1977.

IAET Standards Committee. Outcome standards for the ostomy client. *J Enterostomal Ther* 1983;10:128-31.

Stanton M. Patient education-implications for nursing. *Todays OR Nurse* 1987;9:16-20.

Wainwright P. Information and the surgical patient. *Nurs Times* 1982;78:1480-2.

Williams D. Preoperative patient education: in the home or in the hospital? *Orthop Nurs* 1986;5:37-41.

Ziemer MM. Effects of information on postsurgical patient coping. *Nurs Res* 1983;32:282-7.

SELECTIONS FROM JCAHO 1999 HOSPITAL ACCREDITATION STANDARDS

Education*

Overview

The goal of patient and family† education function‡ is to improve patient health outcomes by promoting healthy behavior and involving the patient in care and care decisions.

Education promotes healthy behaviors, supports recovery and a speedy return to function, and enables patients to be involved in decisions about their own care. The goals of patient and family education are met when a hospital performs the following processes well:

- Assessing organization-wide patient education programs and activities
- Formulating patient education program goals
- Allocating resources for patient education
- Determining and prioritizing specific patient educational needs

---

*Represents members of the Steering Committee.

†This document was prepared with the assistance of Prospect Associates under a contract with the United Ostomy Association.

---

*From Joint Commission for the Accreditation of Health Care Organizations, *Hospital Accreditation Standards*, Oakbrook Terrace, IL, 1999, The Association.

†**family** The person(s) who plays a significant role in the individual's life. This may include a person(s) not legally related to the individual. This person(s) is often referred to as a surrogate decision maker if authorized to make care decisions for an individual should the individual lose decision-making capacity.

‡**function** A goal-directed, interrelated series of processes, such as continuum of care or management of information.

- Providing education to meet identified patient needs

The standards in this chapter address activities involved in these processes, including the following:

- Promoting interactive communication between patients and providers
- Improving patients' understanding of their health status, options for treatment, and the anticipated risks and benefits of treatment
- Encouraging patient participation in decision making about care
- Increasing the likelihood that patients will follow their therapeutic plans of care
- Maximizing patient self-care skills
- Increasing the patient's ability to cope with his or her health status
- Enhancing patient participation in continuing care
- Promoting healthy life-styles
- Informing patients about their financial responsibilities for treatment when known

Psychosocial, spiritual, and cultural values also affect patients' responses to care and their willingness to participate actively in care and education.* Recognizing the impact these values have, a hospital supports its patients' involvement in their care and the educational process. The hospital makes sure its education process supports ongoing interaction between patients and staff.

Note: *While the standards in this chapter recommend a systematic approach to education, they do not require any specific structure, such as an education department, a patient education committee, or the employment of an educator. More important is a philosophy that views the educational function as an interactive one in which both parties are learners. These standards help the hospital focus on how education is consistent with the patient's plan of care, level of care, the educational setting, and continuity of care.*

Standards

The following is a list of all standards for this function.

PF.1
The patient's learning needs, abilities, preferences, and readiness to learn are assessed.

PF.1.1 The assessment considers cultural and religious practices, emotional barriers, desire and motivation to learn, physical and cognitive limitations, language barriers, and the financial implications of care choices.

PF.1.2 When called for by the age of the patient and the length of stay, the hospital assesses and provides for patients' academic education needs.

PF.1.3 Patients are educated about the safe and effective use of medication, according to law and their needs

PF.1.4 Patients are educated about the safe and effective use of medical equipment.

PF.1.5 Patients are educated about potential drug-food interactions, and provided counseling on nutrition and modified diets.

PF.1.6 Patients are educated about rehabilitation techniques to help them adapt or function more independently in their environment.

PF.1.7 Patients are informed about access to additional resources in the community.

PF.1.8 Patients are informed about when and how to obtain any further treatment the patient may need.

PF.1.9 The hospital makes clear to patients and families what their responsibilities are regarding the patient's ongoing health care needs, and gives them the knowledge and skills they need to carry out their responsibilities.

PF.1.10 With due regard for privacy, the hospital teaches and helps patients maintain good standards for personal hygiene and grooming, including bathing, brushing teeth, caring for hair and nails, and using the toilet.

PF.2
Patient education is interactive.

---

*This aspect of patient education relates to standard R1.1.2 in the "Patient Rights and Organization Ethics" chapter of this book.

PF.3

When the hospital gives discharge instructions to the patient or family, it also provides these instructions to the organization or individual responsible for the patient's continuing care.

PF.4

The hospital plans, supports, and coordinates activities and resources for patient and family education.

PF.4.1 The hospital identifies and provides the educational resources required to achieve educational objectives.

PF.4.2 The patient and family educational process is collaborative and interdisciplinary, appropriate to the plan of care.

Standards and Intent Statements for Patient and Family Education and Responsibilities

Standards

PF.1

The patient's learning needs, abilities, preferences, and readiness to learn are assessed.

PF.1.1 The assessment considers cultural and religious practices, emotional barriers, desire and motivation to learn, physical and cognitive limitations, language barriers, and the financial implications of care choices.

PF.1.2 When called for by the age of the patient and the length of stay, the hospital assesses and provides for patients' academic education needs.

PF.1.3 Patients are educated about the safe and effective use of medication, according to law and their needs.

PF.1.4 Patients are educated about the safe and effective use of medical equipment.

PF.1.5 Patients are educated about potential drug-food interactions, and provided counseling on nutrition and modified diets.

PF.1.6 Patients are educated about rehabilitation techniques to help them adapt or function more independently in their environment.

PF.1.7 Patients are informed about access to additional resources in the community.

PF.1.8 Patients are informed about when and how to obtain any further treatment the patient may need.

Intent of PF.1 Through PF.1.8

Hospitals offer education to patients and families to give them the specific knowledge and skills they need to meet the patient's ongoing health care needs. Clearly, such instruction needs to be presented in ways that are understandable to those receiving them.

Openness and flexibility are important elements in patient education, and can make a critical difference in whether the patient follows instructions. In assessing a patient's needs, abilities, and readiness for education, staff members take into account such variables as the following:

- The patient's and family's beliefs and values
- Their literacy, educational level, and language
- Emotional barriers and motivations
- Physical and cognitive limitations
- The financial implications of care choices

When school-age children or adolescent patients are hospitalized for long periods of time, state or local laws may specify the requirements for meeting the child's schooling needs. Although the hospital may not provide school teachers directly, it is responsible for providing access to schooling, according to state education law.

In addition, the hospital uses guidelines in educating patients on the following topics:

- Safe and effective use of medication
- Safe and effective use of medical equipment
- Diet and nutrition
- Rehabilitation
- Educational resources in the community
- Follow-up care

The appropriate disciplines are involved in developing these guidelines.

Standard

PF.1.9

The hospital makes clear to patients and families what their responsibilities are regarding the patient's ongoing health care needs, and gives them the knowledge and skills they need to carry out their responsibilities.

Intent of PF.1.9

Hospitals are entitled to reasonable and responsible behavior on the part of patients and their families—always keeping in mind, of course, the nature of the illness and the constraints it imposes. To facilitate such behavior, hospital staff members clearly identify for patients and families what their responsibilities are, and educate them accordingly. Hospital policies and procedures make clear how and by whom this is done.

Patient responsibilities generally include at least the following:

- **Providing information.** The patients and family are responsible for providing, to the best of their knowledge, accurate and complete information about present complaints, past illnesses, hospitalizations, medications, and other matters relating to the patient's health. They are responsible for reporting unexpected changes in the patient's condition to the responsible practitioner.
- **Asking questions.** The patient and family are responsible for asking questions when they do not understand what they have been told about the patient's care or what they are expected to do.
- **Following with instructions.** The patient and family are responsible for following the treatment plan developed with the practitioner. They should express any concerns they have about their ability to follow the proposed course of treatment; the hospital, in turn, makes every effort to adapt the treatment plan to the patient's specific needs and limitations. Where such adaptations are not recommended, the patient and family should understand the consequences of failing to follow the recommended course of treatment, or of using other treatments.
- **Accepting the consequences of not following instructions.** If the patient or family refuses treatment or fails to follow the practitioner's instructions, they are responsible for the outcomes.
- **Following hospital rules and regulations.** The patient and family are responsible for following the hospital's rules and regulations concerning patient care and conduct.
- **Acting with consideration and respect.** Patients and families are expected to be considerate of other patients and hospital personnel by not making unnecessary noise, smoking, or causing distractions. Patients and families are responsible for respecting the property of other persons and that of the hospital.

Standard

PF.1.10

With due regard for privacy, the hospital teaches and helps patients maintain good standards for personal hygiene and grooming, including bathing, brushing teeth, caring for hair and nails, and using the toilet.

Intent of PF.1.10

Personal hygiene and grooming is maintained or even improved during a hospital stay. The patient has a primary responsibility for these activities; however, the hospital supports, encourages, and provides education when necessary to help the patient.

Standard

PF.2
Patient education is interactive.

Intent of PF.2

Interactive patient education is an integral part of patient care. An "interactive" education process is one in which hospital staff, while imparting information to patients and families, continuously elicits feedback to ensure that the information is understood, and that it is appropriate, useful, and usable in practical terms. There are several crucial steps in this process:

- Identifying the patient's learning needs. This depends on many factors, including not only the patient's medical diagnosis but also the anticipated length of stay, tasks the patient can or cannot accomplish, resources available to the patient in the community, and the patient's own preferences regarding education. It also depends on the ability of the patient and family to understand and implement the education provided.
- Setting priorities on individual learning needs. Staff should understand that not all patients need education concerning their plan of care, and that particular elements of education should be given when the patient is ready to receive them.
- Implementing the education plan, including feedback to make sure it is understood and effective.

Standard

PF.3
When the hospital gives discharge instructions to the patient or family, it also provides these instructions to the organization or individual responsible for the patient's continuing care.

Intent of PF.3
The purpose of discharge planning is to help develop a workable plan for care following the patient's release from the hospital. Education as well as continuity of care are integral to effective discharge planning. Education in preparation for the patient's discharge includes several elements:

- Helping the patient and family understand the patient's treatment and the need for continuing care

- Teaching the patient and family what they need to know about care after discharge
- Making life-style changes
- Managing continuing care, whether it is carried out at home (with or without home health care services) or at another facility

Instructions for care after discharge are given not only to the patient and family, but to anyone responsible for the patient's health care needs so that ongoing education can be provided as necessary. For example, the hospital forwards a copy of the discharge summary and instructions to the patient's primary care provider.

Standard

PF.4
The hospital plans, supports, and coordinates activities and resources for patient and family education.

Intent of PF.4
Within the context of its mission and scope of services, the hospital plans for and provides patient education. In this planning, the hospital considers two major factors:

- The types of patients who will need education, including their illnesses, ages, and sociocultural backgrounds, and the community resources that will be available to them to support life-style changes
- The settings in which patients will be educated, including outpatient and inpatient settings

While the primary goal of patient education is to promote and maintain patients' health, it may also contribute to other hospital activities and patient outcomes, such as risk management, obtaining informed consent, and patient satisfaction.

Planning can be an informal process; it does not require a written plan. However, a well-planned patient education strategy will encompass these steps:

- Establish an environment that encourages patients and families to ask questions, learn, and participate in decision making and care.
- Provide for the competency of staff members who provide patient and family education.
- Establish processes and procedures to identify and respond to individual learning needs, requests, abilities, and resources. (This includes the identification of community resources.)
- Help staff members think about and understand the environment in which the patient will apply the education they provide.
- Provide for appropriate, available, effective, and efficacious educational resources.
- Provide for the delivery of education in a continuous, safe, timely, efficient, caring, and respectful manner.
- Ensure that explanations and instructions are understandable to the patient and family, and that they take into consideration the patient and family's culture, religion, language, age, abilities, resources, and physical disabilities.
- Assess and improve educational systems and outcomes as part of the hospital's performance improvement process.

Standard
PF.4.1
The hospital identifies and provides the educational resources required to achieve its educational objectives.

Intent of PF.4.1
As part of its commitment to patient and family education, the hospital selects and makes available a variety of educational resources, based on the learning needs of its patient population. These resources may include the following:

- Direct teaching by appropriate members of the health care team
- Educational materals such as pamphlets and videotapes
- Materials and resources that accommodate persons with disabilities (for example, braille, audio tape, or large print for the sight impaired)
- Community resources for education
- Referrals to programs that can meet special needs

Standard
PF.4.2
The patient and family educational process is collaborative and interdisciplinary, as appropriate to the plan of care.

Intent of PF.4.2
When health care professionals understand one another's contributions to patient education, they can collaborate more effectively. Collaboration, in turn, ensures that the information patients and families receive is comprehensive, consistent, and as effective as possible.

Collaboration is not always necessary or appropriate. Sometimes patient education is best provided by a single discipline—for example, the physician or the nurse—in the hospital or a private office. However, when patient education is *multidisciplinary*—involving, for example, the physician, nurse, and physical therapist—it should be *interdisciplinary,* that is, coordinated among the various disciplines involved.

Box 1	*Oncology Nursing Society's Standards*

Patient/Family Education
Standard 1
Oncology nurse
The oncology nurse at both the generalist and advanced practice levels is responsible for patient/family education related to cancer.

Standard II
Resources
Adequate resources to achieve the objectives of patient/family education related to cancer care are available and appropriate.

Standard III
Curriculum
Knowledge, skills, and attitudes related to the management of human responses to cancer are reflected in the educational activity for the patient/family experiencing cancer.

Standard IV
Teaching-learning process
Teaching-learning theories are applied to the development, implementation, and evaluation of learning experiences related to cancer care.

Standard V
Learner: the patient family
The patient/family apply knowledge, skills, and attitudes to management of actual or potential human responses to the cancer experience.

Public Education
Standard 1
Oncology nurse
The oncology nurse provides formal and informal cancer-related public education commensurate with personal education and experience.

Standard II
Resources
Adequate resources for public education related to cancer prevention, detection, treatment, and care are current and appropriate to achieve education objectives.

Standard III
Curriculum
Knowledge, skills, and attitudes related to the physical and psychosocial aspects of cancer prevention, early detection, treatment, and care are included in public education activities.

Standard IV
Teaching-learning process
Teaching-learning theories are applied to the development, implementation, and evaluation of learning experiences related to cancer education for the public.

Standard V
Learner: the public
Personal behaviors and public policy related to cancer prevention, detection, treatment, rehabilitation, and supportive care are influenced by formal and informal cancer public education.

From Oncology Nursing Society: *Standards of oncology education: patient/family and public nursing,* Pittsburgh, 1995, The Society.

Examples of Exemplary Patient Education

Blanchard MA and others: Using a focus group to design a diabetes education program for an African American population, *Diabetes Educ* 25:917-924, 1999.

Among African Americans the incidence of diabetes is 1.6 times that for white Americans, and 25% of all African-American women older than age 55 have diabetes. Focus groups showed that there were significant differences between what was being offered for diabetes education in the facility and what the focus group desired. They did not want a classroom setting but rather wanted a support group with an ongoing informal educational component; peer leadership with more than common knowledge about the facts of diabetes and availability of clinicians as experts; a balance of focused and spontaneous discussion; aggressively pursued publicity using ethnically sensitive brochures, fliers, and contacts; and education that was ongoing, frequent, easily accessible, and free. A successful program should focus on how to incorporate diabetes self-care into real life and give patients a sense of control over diabetes.

The lesson to be learned is that learning styles are culturally related and that program organiz-ers need to ask persons in the target population what they want.

Karl DJ: The interactive newborn bath, *MCN Am J Matern Child Nurs* 24:280-286, 1999.

Teaching parents about bathing their newborn has always been a cornerstone of postpartum nursing practice. An interactive bath adds interpretation of infant behavior, models ways to respond to this behavior including calming and orienting newborns and eliciting reflexes, and supports parental strategies for doing so. Newborns usually demonstrate a range of behaviors in the course of the bath as they experience a progression of different stimuli, including undressing, temperature changes, the touch of the washcloth and water, drying, dressing, and wrapping. Most infants cry at some time during the bath and may calm themselves or require calming intervention. Many have quiet, alert periods during which they are able to respond to sights and sounds around them. Some close their eyes to protect themselves from overstimulation. This behavioral range offers an opportunity to help parents observe and interpret behavior. Ideal timing is half-way between feedings when the baby is neither hungry nor just fed.

The article describes the continuum of newborn states, how to point out these states during the interactive bath, and calming interventions.

Meng A: An asthma day camp, *MCN Am J Matern Child Nurs* 22:135-141, 1997.

Asthma specialty camps have improved attitudes toward asthma, promoted participation in sports activities, improved self-management skills and reduced school absences and hospital visits. The camp better represents a child's world than the hospital does, and self-management concepts become more meaningful when they are integrated into a child's usual daily activities.

A local children's theater company provided 5 hours of musical theater, taught diaphragmatic breathing, and directed the children's show on the last day of camp. A local fitness instructor known for his motivational teaching style taught aerobics to demonstrate that with proper planning any child with asthma can participate in some level of physical activity. Rhythmic breathing was integrated into swimming. Children learned trigger-control concepts via horseback riding as they changed into long pants, medicated as needed, and learned to avoid touching their faces after petting the horses.

The article describes content of classes and other instructional approaches, including learning diaries kept by campers.

Index

Page numbers in *italics* indicate boxes and illustrations; page numbers followed by *t* indicate tables.